Relational Perspectives in Psychoanalysis

edited by

Neil J. Skolnick
Susan C. Warshaw

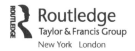

Routledge
Taylor & Francis Group
New York   London

First published 1992 by The Analytic Press

This edition published 2013 by Routledge
711 Third Avenue, New York, NY 10017
27 Church Road, Hove, East Sussex BN3 2FA, UK

First issued in paperback 2015

Routledge is an imprint of the Taylor & Francis Group, an informa business

Library of Congress Cataloging-in-Publication Data

Relational perspectives in psychoanalysis / edited by Neil J.
  Skolnick, Susan C. Warshaw.
    p.   cm.
  Includes bibliographical references and index.
  ISBN 0-88163-107-8
  1. Psychoanalysis.   2. Object relations (Psychoanalysis)
  3. Interpersonal relations.   4. Self psychology.   5. Child analysis.
  6. Psychotherapy.   I. Skolnick, Neil J.   II. Warshaw, Susan C.
  [DNLM: 1. Object Attachment.   2. Psychoanalytic Theory.
  3. Psychoanalytic Therapy.   4. Self Concept.   WM 460.5.E3 R382]
  BF175.5.O24R45   1992
  150.19′5 – dc20
  DNLM/DLC
  for Library of Congress   92-49413
                                                                CIP

ISBN 13: 978-1-138-87231-8 (pbk)
ISBN 13: 978-0-8816-3107-4 (hbk)

Dedicated to the New York University Postdoctoral Program in Psychotherapy and Psychoanalysis. The sustained commitment of members of this community to the academic values of scholarship and open discourse have furthered immeasurably the study and practice of psychoanalysis.

Acknowledgments

We would like to thank several people who have given consistent support and encouragement to our efforts on this project. We are grateful to Paul Stepansky, our editor, for his recognition of the significance of evolving relational perspectives in psychoanalytic theory and his generous advice throughout. We would also like to thank Stephen Mitchell, John Kerr, Doris Silverman, Lewis Aron, and Judith Alpert.

We are in no small way indebted to Eleanor Starke Kobrin, managing editor of The Analytic Press, for her good humor and her indefatigably patient assistance throughout.

We are thankful to Pauline Gooden, Rose Etelson, and Agnes Conte, who helped in the preparation of parts of the manuscript.

We are also appreciative of the cooperation of the publishers of *Contemporary Psychoanalysis* and *Psychoanalytic Psychology*.

Acknowledgments

Contents

Contributors

Neil Altman, Ph.D. — Supervisor, New York University Postdoctoral Program in Psychotherapy and Psychoanalysis; Faculty and Supervisor, National Institute for the Psychotherapies.

Lewis Aron, Ph.D. — Faculty and Supervisor, New York University Postdoctoral Program in Psychotherapy and Psychoanalysis; Clinical Associate Professor and Supervisor, Adelphi University Postdoctoral Program in Psychoanalysis and Psychotherapy.

Beatrice Beebe, Ph.D. — Faculty, New York University Postdoctoral Program in Psychotherapy and Psychoanalysis; Visiting Associate Professor of Psychology, New York State Psychiatric Institute, Columbia University.

Jessica Benjamin, Ph.D. — Faculty, New York University Postdoctoral Program in Psychotherapy and Psychoanalysis; Faculty, Program in Psychoanalytic Studies, New School for Social Research.

Philip M. Bromberg, Ph.D. — Fellow and Training and Supervising Analyst, William Alanson White Institute of Psychiatry, Psychoanalysis, and Psychology, New York; Faculty, New York University Postdoctoral Program in Psychotherapy and Psychoanalysis.

Jody Messler Davies, Ph.D. — Adjunct Associate Professor of Psychology, Derner Institute, Adelphi University; Supervisor, Center for the Study and Treatment of Abuse and Incest, Manhattan Institute for Psychoanalysis.

James L. Fosshage, Ph.D. — Cofounder and Board Director, National Institute for the Psychotherapies; Faculty and Supervisor, New York University Postdoctoral Program in Psychotherapy and Psychoanalysis.

Adrienne Harris, Ph.D. – Associate Professor of Psychology, Rutgers University; Faculty, New York University Postdoctoral Program in Psychotherapy and Psychoanalysis.

Irwin Hirsch, Ph.D. – Former Director, Manhattan Institute for Psychoanalysis; Professor of Psychology and Supervisor, Adelphi University Postdoctoral Program in Psychoanalysis and Psychotherapy.

Joseph Jaffe, M.D. – Professor of Clinical Psychiatry, Department of Clinical Psychiatry (in Neurological Surgery), Columbia University; Chief, Department of Communication Sciences, New York State Psychiatric Institute.

Frank M. Lachmann, Ph.D. – Senior Supervisor and Training Analyst, Postgraduate Center for Mental Health, New York; Core Faculty, Institute for the Psychoanalytic Study of Subjectivity, New York.

Stephen A. Mitchell, Ph.D. – Training and Supervising Analyst, William Alanson White Institute for Psychiatry, Psychoanalysis, and Psychology, New York; Faculty and Supervisor, New York University Postdoctoral Program in Psychotherapy and Psychoanalysis.

Steven Reisner, Ph.D. – Director of Psychology, Regent Hospital, New York; Adjunct Assistant Professor of Psychology and Education, Teachers College, Columbia University.

Doris K. Silverman, Ph.D. – Faculty and Supervisor, New York University Postdoctoral Program in Psychotherapy and Psychoanalysis; Teaching and Supervising Analyst, and Fellow, IPTAR.

Neil J. Skolnick, Ph.D. (editor) – Associate Professor, Ferkauf Graduate School of Psychology, Yeshiva University; Faculty and Supervisor, New York University Postdoctoral Program in Psychotherapy and Psychoanalysis; Codirector, Faculty, and Supervisor, National Institute for the Psychotherapies, Regional Psychoanalytic Training Program at Kansas City.

Susan C. Warshaw, Ed.D. (editor) – Associate Professor, Ferkauf Graduate School of Psychology, Yeshiva University; Supervisor, New York University Postdoctoral Program in Psychotherapy and Psychoanalysis; Supervisor, Institute for Child, Adolescent, and Family Studies.

Benjamin Wolstein, Ph.D. – Faculty, New York University Postdoctoral Program in Psychotherapy and Psychoanalysis; Faculty, Training and Supervising Analyst, William Alanson White Institute of Psychiatry, Psychoanalysis, and Psychology, New York.

Foreword

EMMANUEL GHENT

The title of this book, *Relational Perspectives in Psychoanalysis*, sets a rather complex stage before us; it situates the reader within a theater in the round, inviting him or her to move around freely so as to experience the play from a variety of angles. The drama presents a panorama of issues, clinical and theoretical, that populate the world of psychoanalysis; we are asked to view them from a variety of vantage points, all of which have at least one thing in common, namely that the adjective *relational* is apposite.

The critical term, then, is *relational*. Rather than trying to define it, I believe it would be more fruitful to do in microcosm what the book attempts in the hands of its numerous contributors. Seldom do we learn new words by finding them in the dictionary. Much more naturalistically we come to know them by encountering them in their contexts and usage. An appropriate point of departure would be how the term *object relations* came to be used in psychoanalysis. The term *object* owes its origin to the very beginnings of Freud's drive theory, where it was defined as the largely human target or influencer of an instinctual impulse, or drive. Most usually, it meant *person*.[1] Melanie Klein's (1925, p. 121) first use of the term *object relations* dates to 1925, where its meaning again was relations with people. By 1932 Klein had begun to develop the notions of internal objects and relations among

Emmanuel Ghent, M.D. is Training and Supervising Analyst and faculty member, New York University Postdoctoral Program in Psychotherapy and Psychoanalysis. He is also Clinical Professor of Psychology, New York University.

[1]Ferenczi (1921), for example, observed that, in "hysteria . . . the repressed pathogenic material belongs to the memory-traces in the unconscious for things that belong to the libido objects (persons)" (p. 172).

them, as well as phantasy as the repository of phylogenetically based images of good and bad internal objects. In 1935, in connection with introducing the conception of the depressive position, and with it the newly developed capacity of the infant of five or six months to internalize whole rather than part objects, Klein (1935) began a subtle shift in theory in which object relations played an increasingly important role (Greenberg and Mitchell, 1983). Beginning in 1940, Fairbairn (1952) began formulating his object relations theory of personality as a radical departure from drive theory. For many years he wrote not of object relations but rather of *object relationships*. Endopsychic structure, as he referred to the internal world, was no longer based on built-in phantasy, but instead was seen as deriving entirely from relations of the infant and child with significant people. Clinging to terms that belong to drive theory while totally trans-forming their meaning, Fairbairn reconceptualized libido as, at root, object seeking rather than pleasure seeking. What came to be called the object relations school of psychoanalysis stemmed largely from the work of Fairbairn, Winnicott, and Balint in particular, notwith-standing the significant differences among them; since the 1950s it has generally been known as the Independent Group in the British Psycho-Analytical Society (Hinshelwood, 1991).

Meanwhile, across the ocean in America, Harry Stack Sullivan had, in the early 1930s, begun developing what he referred to as the interpersonal theory of psychiatry. As early as 1931, in what may be the first reference to "interpersonal relations," he wrote, "psychiatry . . . is not an impossible study of an *individual* suffering mental disorder; it is a study of disordered interpersonal relations nucleating more or less clearly in a particular person" (p. 978), and, a little further on, "the mental or psychobiological . . . has a meaningful existence only in interpersonal complexes, real or *fancied*" (p. 979). "Fancied" was to become Sullivan's quasi-operational code word for what we would today call "internalized." By 1938, Sullivan had started publication of a new journal, *Psychiatry, a Journal of the Biology and the Pathology of Interpersonal Relations.* Not long after, in the early 1940s, the William Alanson White Institute of Psychiatry, Psychoanal-ysis and Psychology was founded and became the training ground for several generations of interpersonal psychoanalysts.

It will not easily escape notice that what is common to the two phrases—British object relations theory, and the American theory of interpersonal relations—is the word *relation*. Only slightly less ap-parent is the overlap in meaning of the terms object and person.

About 20 years later, in 1961, Bernard Kalinkowitz, then Director of the Doctoral Program in Clinical Psychology at New York University and a graduate of the White Institute, brought to realization a vision he had long cherished of providing a center for psychoanalytic studies in a university setting. The inauguration of the Postdoctoral Program in Psychotherapy and Psychoanalysis set in motion a long chain of events that, among many other gratifying sequelae, has resulted in the publication of the present book. The Program answered several pressing needs. It opened the door to clinical psychologists to be trained as full-fledged psychoanalysts without having to take the onerous oath that they would not practice as psychoanalysts, as was the case with those few psychologists who were admitted on a research basis to the principal medical institutes of the time. As a university-based center for training in psychoanalysis, it provided for the first time an alternative to the ubiquitous institute model of psychoanalytic training. Fundamental to the formation of a psychoanalytic program for psychologists were the academic values of scholarship, diversity of thinking, efforts at integration and synthesis, and, above all, open discourse, research, and debate. All the existing institutes in the past, including those which accepted a few psychologists on a restrictive basis, were committed to a single theoretical approach. It was Freud *or* Sullivan; never Freud *and* Sullivan, let alone Klein, Winnicott, Mahler, and Kohut. The unique intent of the NYU Postdoctoral Program was to offer in-depth study and training in the major theoretical orientations in a tradition of comparative study. The goal has been to examine basic assumptions and epistemological premises underlying the differing psychoanalytic points of view. In striking contrast to what obtains in psychoanalytic institutes, the very design of the Program was to facilitate and encourage open debate and high-level discourse.

Early in the history of the Program, it was decided to form two tracks or orientations, one classical Freudian, the other Interpersonal; matriculants were encouraged to partake of courses offered by both. Much more recently, a new outlook, one that was not represented in the existing track system, began to make itself felt.

Here is where we return to pick up the thread of the evolution of the term *relational*. A small group of faculty members (Bernard Friedland, Emmanuel Ghent, and Stephen Mitchell) technically affiliated with the interpersonal track had been teaching for some time about exciting developments in the field of psychoanalysis that seemed to extend and enhance the conceptions of interpersonal relations theory, particularly the work of the British object relations theorists, the self psychologists, and some ego psychologists, most notably Loewald, who, in one or other way, were marking out a new paradigm in psychoanalytic theory and practice. What was most striking, indeed exhilarating, was that despite substantial differences in theoretical baggage and in language, one element seemed to be held in common—the notion that human *relations* played the central role both in human development and in psychopathology. Another major element was that all rejected, in one way or another, the classical metapsychology that was rooted in the notion that two biologically given instincts or drives, sex and aggression, were the root determinants of all human motivation.

The year 1983 marked the publication of two very significant works, one a paper by Merton Gill (1983) and the other a book by Greenberg and Mitchell (1983). In Gill's thinking, the fundamental question facing the field, the question from which all others flow, was the dichotomy between an energy discharge model of mind and a "person" model. Gill recognized that to label his point of view "interpersonal" carried too heavily the political and theoretical weight of Sullivanian thinking. To label his point of view a "self" point of view implied, in the current terminological atmosphere, a global embracing of Kohut's thinking. To label it an "object relations" point of view slanted it incorrectly, in that the term failed to distinguish with sufficient clarity between the work of Klein, where energy discharge remained superordinate to object relations, and that of Fairbairn, where the reverse obtained. He proposed a new term, a "person point of view," to define an inclusive position, one that is opposed to classical metapsychology and its energy discharge point of view and that is currently in the foreground in the evolution of psychoanalytic thinking. Gill noted that although Winnicott approached a person point of view, he did not attempt a systematic and consistent formulation in terms of points of view.[2]

Gill forthrightly opted for abandoning the energy discharge model. He noted, however, that this did not mean abandoning some notion of drive; in fact, along with Bowlby, he proposed that the need for interpersonal attachment is an innately organized drive, with vast and far-reaching consequences for human ontogeny. One might add here that, but for his eschewal of the term, the drive for interpersonal attachment is a cornerstone of Sullivan's theory. Gill's goal clearly was to combine the best strands of these three schools with the best

---

[2]Gill sees Loewald also as being on the edge: "Loewald describes drive as developing in the matrix of object relations rather than as the matrix within which object relations develop, but his concept of drive remains ambiguous between the person and energy discharge points of view, and he does not propose the major reorientation which his formulation requires" (p. 494).

of Freudian clinical theory and experience while avoiding the political-theoretical implications of singularly endorsing any one of them.

Meanwhile, in the same year, Greenberg and Mitchell (1983) published their landmark book, in which, by careful analysis of the structure and underlying assumptions of current psychoanalytic theoretical systems, they were able to demarcate two mutually exclusive models of mind, a drive/structure model and a relational/structure model. Although a variety of hybrid theories have been propounded in an effort to bridge these models, none has been able to surmount the incompatibility of the almost axiomatic assumption that underpins each. As Greenberg and Mitchell put it,

> [t]here have been two major strategies for dealing with the problem of object relations. The first, employed originally by Freud, has been essentially preservative and consists of stretching and adapting his original model based on drive to accommodate their clinical emphases on object relations. . . . [T]o solve the problem of object relations while preserving drive theory intact requires the derivation of relations with others (and the individuals' inner representation of those relations) as vicissitudes of the drives themselves. Freud and subsequent theorists employing this first strategy understand the role of objects largely in relation to the discharge of drive: they may inhibit discharge, facilitate it, or serve as its target. The second, more radical strategy for dealing with object relations has been to replace the drive theory model with a fundamentally different conceptual framework in which relations with others constitute the fundamental building blocks of mental life. The creation, or re-creation, of specific modes of relatedness with others replaces drive discharge as the force motivating human behavior [p. 3].

At the Postdoctoral Program, the mid-1980s were marked by intense ferment in the area of psychoanalytic theorizing and practice. Finally, in early 1988, owing in no small measure to the efforts of the matriculant body, a new track, or "orientation," came into being. Although we referred to it as the relational perspective, it could with equal advantage be thought of, following Gill, as representing "the person point of view." While the term "person point of view" retained a reasonably euphonious ring, a "person track" would have been rather jarring. We chose, therefore, the name *relational orientation* or *relational track*. The choice, however, was not made without misgivings. Placing the emphasis strongly, if not solely, on human relations tends to minimize both the role of the self and the role of the biologically given in theory building. In addition, its origins in the context of specifically human relations tend to constrict the meaning of the term "relation," which otherwise could signify relations of all sorts and at many levels of meaning.

The last four years have witnessed remarkable changes both at the Postdoctoral Program and in the field at large. Starting with a faculty of five (Philip Bromberg, Bernard Friedland, James Fosshage, Emmanuel Ghent, and Stephen Mitchell), the Relational Track faculty has burgeoned into a very substantial force of over 30 members, many of whom have participated in the creation of this volume. Peace, mutual respect, a spirit of collaboration, and an atmosphere of healthy discourse have come to prevail at the Program. Several books published by Relational Track faculty (for example, Eagle, 1984; Benjamin, 1988; Mitchell, 1988; Eigen, 1991; Greenberg, 1991) have achieved national and international prominence in recent years, and others are currently in press. A new journal, *Psychoanalytic Dialogues: A Journal of Relational Perspectives* (The Analytic Press), has achieved, within the brief space of a year, remarkable salience in the field.

One might ask, "How does one recognize a relational psychoanalyst?" There is no such thing as a relational analyst; there are only analysts whose backgrounds may vary considerably, but who share a broad outlook in which human relations—specific, unique human relations—play a superordinate role in the genesis of character and of psychopathology, as well as in the practice of psychoanalytic therapeutics.

Relational theorists have in common an interest in the intrapsychic as well as the interpersonal, but the intrapsychic is seen as constituted largely by the internalization of interpersonal experience mediated by the constraints imposed by biologically organized templates and delimiters. Relational theorists tend also to share a view in which both reality and fantasy, both outer world and inner world, both the interpersonal and the intrapsychic, play immensely important and interactive roles in human life. Relational theorists do not substitute a naive environmentalism for drive theory. Due weight is given to what the individual brings to the interaction: temperament, bodily events, physiological responsivity, distinctive patterns of regulation, and sensitivity. Unlike earlier critics of drive theory, relational theorists do not minimize the importance of the body or of sexuality in human development. Relational theorists continue to be interested in the importance of conflict, although conflict most usually is seen as taking place between opposing relational configurations rather than between drive and defense. Relational theory is essentially a psychological, rather than a biological or quasi-biological, theory; its primary concern is with issues of motivation and meaning and their vicissitudes in human development, psychopathology and treatment.

Human experience, from the prenatal period onward, is what writes the software, the programming, and in the earliest stages probably even modulates the very hard wiring that provides the capacities and limitations for the integration of experience. What ensues ultimately is an enormously complex perceptual, cognitive, affective, and motivational system in which prior experience, by now patterned into templates that are unique for each individual, in turn molds and patterns experience. And yet experience, in turn, influences and modifies the template; what hope would there be for psychotherapy or psychoanalysis were this not true?

The word *intrapsychic* is the buzzword that for many interpersonalists is experienced as virtually hyphenated to drive theory, with its associated conception of the primacy of fantasy over reality. For me the intrapsychic is not in opposition to the interpersonal but is complementary to, and in constant flux, with it. Substitute the word *template*, qualify it by adding that templates are in large measure created out of human experience and in turn play a major role in contributing to and controlling human experience; include the notion that the psychological expression of these dynamic templates is what we call *fantasy* and the activities of an inner world; then we have no further need for the term intrapsychic—except that it is a convenient way of referring to internal psychic patterning (or "structure") as against the interpersonal.

The reader will note here that I have used the word *interpersonal* in the sense that it has customarily been used even by interpersonalists. By contrast, when Sullivan first introduced the term, his meaning was grand (see Schecter, 1972). His heuristic conception was that all of psychopathology—indeed, even the structure of personality, or at least all of it that was relevant to the therapeutic situation—was rooted in early human interactions and that these interactions continued to reverberate outside of awareness in such a way as to control a person's entire way of being. Sullivan developed conceptions of good-me, bad-me and not-me, and of the self system; they all represent what might be called the intrapsychic.

The grand vision that Sullivan offered was that the intrapsychic *is* interpersonal. Although his penchant for operationalism kept him from using terms like inner world, it did not stop him from speaking and thinking in those terms as, for example, when he would refer to the eight or more people who were in the room at any one time even though to all external appearances there were only two physical presences.

Years later, when Loewald (1978, p. 494), eschewing the notion of built-in structure with more or less built-in contents, redefined id, ego and superego in terms of interpersonal experience, it was clear that he was not only drastically revising classical metapsychology, but also formulating the intrapsychic as interpersonal. It should be noted that this inclusive meaning of the term interpersonal is quite different from its current, more constricted and superficial usage; in the current vernacular it is used almost exclusively to refer to the "what's going on in the here and now" between people. It is exactly because the term interpersonal has lost its more profound meaning that we continue to need a term like intrapsychic while at the same time taking pains to divest it of its drive theory penumbra.

Parenthetically, it is worth noting that the term relational is beginning to suffer the same fate that has already befallen the term interpersonal, that of being banalized by constricting its meaning to here-and-now interactions. To my mind, the more profound significance of the term relational is that it stresses relation not only between and among external people and things, but also between and among internal personifications and representations. It stresses process—as against reified entities—and the relations among processes all the way along the continuum from the physical and physiological, through the neurobiological, ultimately the psychological, and, for some, even the spiritual. Everything is context dependent; nothing has meaning without relation to other processes. I believe "relational analysis" represents a step in the direction of moving beyond the idiosyncratic languages and conceptions that parented it—an effort to push past the political polemics that separated the speakers of these dialects from one another and an effort to explore the commonalities and divergencies in the theoretical gropings that came, respectively, to be called interpersonal theory, British object relations theory, self psychology, and what I would refer to as advanced ego psychology.

Earlier I noted that the choice of name *the Relational Track* as representing this new orientation at the Postdoctoral Program was not made without some misgiving; a number of issues remain unaddressed by the overcondensed title. By placing the emphasis firmly on human interrelation or what might be considered a two-person psychology, the result is an implicit defocusing of the one-person aspects of psychological theory (Ghent, 1989).

From the perspective of the evolution of psychoanalytic thinking, Sullivan's radical interpersonalism was heuristically invaluable. It provided the means to probe the extent to which all human motivation could be understood solely in terms of interhuman experience; that purpose has been well served, and the gains from it have by no means been exhausted. At the same time, I believe that we are now at a point in theory building that invites exploration of the balance between the contributions of the software and hardware, and the ways in which they influence each other. The self as a center of activity and agency has somehow been neglected by placing the emphasis so firmly on a two-person psychology. As elusive as the self is, so, too, is it tangible, even if illusory; certainly the mainte-nance of security and self-coherence are needs central to human life and their lack spells psychopathology. Somewhat more controversial, but of great interest, are such needs as the quest for growth in the sense of the expansion of one's capacities. Is it exactly here that the lines between hardware and software, between a one-person and a two-person psychology, become blurred. Is it that the growth ten-dency is simply built into the human organism, or does it require facilitating and structuralizing experience at the hands of others for it to come into being?

In my view, a further proposition underlies a global view of the relational perspective. In its most general form, it can be stated that there are two basic opposing motivational thrusts in all living beings. They could be called expansive versus conservative, centrifugal versus centripetal, growth-oriented versus status-quo oriented, and so on. While we look upon the self-perpetuating motivational thrust as "resistance," we recognize the expansive tendency as the indis-pensable ally in our therapeutic efforts; in fact, in many ways we, as analysts, are midwives to this thrust. Recently, Greenberg (1991) has advanced persuasive arguments for a model of the mind that eschews the dual-instinct theory of sex and aggression while retaining the duality of two newly defined basic drives, the "safety drive" and the "effectance drive." Although very different in structure, Greenberg's model has a certain family resemblance to the dual-thrust model of Angyal (1965), who proposed two basic trends, one toward auton-omy, the other toward homonomy. One can trace the resemblance even as far back as Buber (1947, pp. 85–88), who interestingly referred to somewhat similar dual trends, the "originator instinct"–the human need to make things–and "the instinct for communion"–the need to enter into mutuality and to share in a common undertaking. It is not difficult to see how the vistas offered by Angyal or Buber, although foreign to the language of psychoanalysis, nonetheless can be located in the two broad categories of motivation (see Ghent, 1989). Also related is the distinction made by Schachtel (1959, ch. 2) between activity affects and embeddedness affects. Implicit in Sul-livan are the twin givens, the need for satisfaction and the need for security. In all these systems, the "drives" are in some ways and under certain circumstances adversarial and at other times quite complementary.

Clearly, relational thinking has had a long and rich history, although the designation "relational" is a relative newcomer on the psychoanalytic scene. The present volume is a testament to its continuing evolution and clarification; the varied contributions point to the areas of commonality and, as well, draw attention to the unresolved conflicts, both explicit and implicit, in points of view. As I see it, this opportunity to air and discuss such differences is the very essence of what is needed to nurture the development of psychoanalysis both as a theory and as a therapeutic procedure.

REFERENCES

Angyal, A. (1965), *Neurosis and Treatment: A Holistic Theory*. New York: Wiley; reprinted. New York: Da Capo Press, 1982.

Benjamin, J. (1988), *The Bonds of Love*. New York: Pantheon.

Buber, M. (1947), *Between Man and Man*. London: Routledge & Kegan Paul.

Eagle, M. (1984), *Recent Developments in Psychoanalysis*. New York: McGraw-Hill.

Eigen, M. (1991), *Coming Through the Whirlwind*. Wilmette, IL: Chiron.

Fairbairn, W. R. D. (1952), *Psychoanalytic Studies of the Personality*. London: Tavistock.

Ferenczi, S. (1921), Psycho-analytical observations on tic. In: *Further Contributions to the Theory and Technique of Psycho-Analysis*. London: Hogarth Press, 1950.

Ghent, E. (1989), Credo: The dialectics of one-person and two-person psychologies. *Contemp. Psychoanal.*, 25:169–211.

Gill, M. M. (1983), The point of view in psychoanalysis: Energy discharge or person? *Psychoanal. Contemp. Thought*, 6:523–552.

Greenberg, J. (1991), *Oedipus and Beyond*. Cambridge, MA: Harvard University Press.

——— & Mitchell, S. A. (1983), *Object Relations in Psychoanalytic Theory*. Cambridge, MA: Harvard University Press.

Hinshelwood, R. D. (1991), *A Dictionary of Kleinian Thought*. London: Free Association Books.

Klein, M. (1925), A contribution to the psychogenesis of tics. In: *Love, Guilt and Reparation*. London: Hogarth Press.

——— (1935), A contribution to the psychogenesis of manic-depressive states. In: *Love, Guilt and Reparation*. London: Hogarth Press.

Loewald, H. (1978), Instinct theory, object relations and psychic structure formation. *J. Amer. Psychoanal. Assn.*, 26:493–506.

Mitchell, S. A. (1988), *Relational Concepts in Psychoanalysis*. Cambridge, MA: Harvard University Press.

Schachtel, E. (1959), *Metamorphosis*. New York: Basic Books.

Schechter, D. E. (1972), Two of Sullivan's conceptions. *Contemp. Psychoanal.*, 8:71–75.

Sullivan, H. S. (1931), Socio-psychiatric research: Its implications for the schizophrenia problem and for mental hygiene. *Amer. J. Psychiat.*, 10:979–991.

Introduction

NEIL J. SKOLNICK
SUSAN C. WARSHAW

As psychoanalysis prepares to enter its second century, a number of prominent scholars have noted the fundamental conceptual shifts that have occurred within the discipline, shifts that many believe present major challenges to the classical metapsychology (see, e.g., Gedo, 1979; Eagle, 1984; Greenberg and Mitchell, 1983; Mitchell, 1988). There is increasing focus on, and acceptance of, the primacy of relationships with others in the development of the personality, with major ramifications for conceptions of psychic structure, theories of motivation and pathogenesis, and clinical technique.

Since the very beginnings of psychoanalysis there have been attacks on Freud's instinctual drive theory, attacks that have led to the development of alternative models of mind based on different motivational and developmental premises. Writing almost a decade ago, Greenberg and Mitchell (1983) suggested that

> the most significant tension in the history of psychoanalytic ideas has been the dialectic between the original Freudian model . . . and an alternative comprehensive model initiated in the works of Fairbairn and Sullivan, which evolves structure solely from the individual's relations with other people [p. 20].

They designated models belonging to the alternative perspective as "relational/structure" models, with Fairbairn and Sullivan representing its purest forms. Currently many theorists are attempting to integrate relational concepts into their work. There is no single relational model or theory. Rather, some who identify with this perspective are interpersonalists; others, British object relations theorists; still others, self psychologists. Some may not completely align themselves with a purely relational model and differ in the extent to which they dissociate themselves from drive theory. All have a common concern with the centrality of relationship in the development and structure of personality.

The past decade has seen major attempts to increase communication among psychoanalytic theorists and practitioners from diverse orientations. Greenberg and Mitchell (1983) expressed the hope that a careful and respectful comparison of theories would increase clarity, mitigate confusion generated by diverse schools of thought, and highlight commonalities as well as differences among metapsychological approaches. The contributors to the present volume, each of whom identifies with a relational perspective, have their roots in different psychoanalytic traditions, including British object relations, interpersonal, self psychology, as well as Freudian psychoanalysis. All the contributors have been involved with describing and elucidating aspects of their theoretical and clinical approaches in order to promote an openness of inquiry and a comparison of diverse metapsychologies. Some have undertaken comprehensive explorations of the possibilities for integration and synthesis of ideas from different models. The unifying focus of all the authors has been the primary significance of relational configurations as both the building blocks of mind and the central concern of the psychoanalytic situation. Contemporary developmental research focusing on early mother–infant interaction as well as on attachment theory has provided empirical support for the evolution of relational points of view.

The chapters in this book represent a sampling of issues being addressed by contemporary psychoanalytic clinicians and theoreticians writing from a relational point of view. Some authors concern themselves with reconceptualizing aspects of metapsychology; others believe that relational thinking has in fact permeated psychoanalytic theory from its earliest days. Others take as their focus revision of developmental theory. Still others are concerned with clinical applications. The issues addressed here by no means represent all those with which current relational thinkers are wrestling.

Historically, a central focus of relational theorists has been with the definition and description of the concept of self, particularly in regard to its roles in development, psychopathology, and the analytic process. The first three chapters discuss problematic issues that surface when one attempts to consider the concept of self from a relational point of view. Stephen Mitchell notes that locating the core of the self presents a particular difficulty for relational theorists. Whereas Freud located the core, or center, of the self in the biologically based id, most relational theorists have difficulty locating such a core, or center, in a model that takes as its basic assumption an inherently interactive definition of self. Mitchell suggests that previous attempts to conceptualize the locus of individuality, or the true self, as rooted in a spatial metaphor, are misleading. Offering as an alternative a temporal definition of self, he defines the self as the subjective organization of meanings a person creates as he or she moves through time, experiencing ideas and feelings, including self-reflective ideas and feelings. Mitchell offers authenticity as a substitute for the concept of true self or core self. Defining authenticity, however, is problematic since its illusiveness is rooted in distinguishing internal from external considerations.

James Fosshage argues that the concept of self can and should be considered from the vantage point of a synthesis of one- *and* two-person psychologies. He discusses the emergent theoretical synthesis in regard to its usefulness for understanding and explaining issues in development, pathogenesis, transference, and therapeutic action.

Jessica Benjamin discusses the significance of our relationships with "the other" in the development of our experience of our self. The concept of the other as object has its historical roots in intrapsychic theory, essentially a one-person psychology. Acknowledging the significance of the object in the development of the self, Benjamin argues that object relations theories and self psychology theory provide us with only a partial understanding of the significance of the relationship to the other in our development. Drawing on the theory of intersubjectivity (originally brought into psychoanalysis from philosophy), Benjamin notes that there is another relationship that we have to the other which is of equal significance to our development of self, and that is our relationship to the other as a separate "subject" with a separate and equivalent center of self. Benjamin proposes that the two dimensions of experience with the object/other (the intrapsychic and the intersubjective) are complementary even though they sometimes stand in an oppositional relationship.

Advancements in developmental research with mothers and young children have provided support for an evolving relational model of mind. The next two chapters present recent and innovative research on the interaction of mothers and children at different developmental stages. Beatrice Beebe, Joseph Jaffe, and Frank Lachmann review the contributions of infant research literature to illustrate a "Dyadic Systems View of Communication." They believe that the elucidation of the nature of interpersonal process and interactive regulation in the dyad has implications for the conceptualization of psychic structure and its development. It is their contention that early interaction structures, represented in presymbolic form in the first year of life, provide the basis for emerging symbolic forms of self- and object representations. Interaction structures are characteristic patterns of mutual regulation between infant and caregiver, patterns that the infant comes to remember and expect. They believe that the elucidation of the nature of interpersonal process and interactive regulation in the dyad has implications for the conceptualization of psychic structure and its development.

Adrienne Harris explores the manner in which the process of language development is interwoven with the evolution of the self and subjectivity. She reviews many important concepts emerging out of, developmental psycholinguistics. She perceives a relationship between certain key psycholinguistic concepts and certain ideas emanating from British object relations theory, particularly Winnicott's "transitional space." By using vignettes derived from her mother–toddler research, Harris illustrates the multiple ways in which parent–child dialogues become sites for the construction of the experience both of self and of social consciousness.

The six clinically oriented chapters represent a sampling of the possibilities for conceptualizing treatment issues and phenomena and formulating intervention approaches once a shift to a relational perspective is taken. Two chapters focus specifically on the implications of a relational perspective for doing clinical work with children.

Susan Warshaw reviews the contributions to child psychoanalysis of several key child clinicians whose work has in one way or another been contributory to an evolving relational perspective. Explicating aspects of the work of Melanie Klein, Anna Freud, D. W. Winnicott, and Margaret Mahler, she notes that these primary contributors to the child psychoanalytic treatment literature were practitioners whose work was rooted in instinct theory. Warshaw discusses the place of relational thinking within each of their treatment perspectives and the conceptions of each with respect to mutative factors in child treatment. She then discusses the implications of attempting to develop a child-treatment approach using a non-drive-relational model of mind.

Neil Altman focuses specifically on the concept of transference in child treatment and attempts to develop a relational perspective that is useful for child work. He begins with a comparison of the concept of transference in the works of Anna Freud and Melanie Klein, and he further develops an object-relational perspective that is rooted in the works of Bion. Presenting two clinical vignettes, he attempts to clarify the ways in which his relational perspective assists in understanding and working with the transference.

The following four authors all present arguments, substantiated and illustrated by clinical observations, for the viability and utility of applying a relational emphasis to some aspect of adult clinical work. All make respectful comparisons with other models, with the expressed or implicit purpose of highlighting the change in clinical approach that is shaped and informed by a relational perspective. Doris Silverman provides us with a comprehensive overview of research related to attachment theory. She draws from three sources of intersecting data to demonstrate the establishment and internalization of attachment patterns, which she believes may become relatively unconscious and exert motivational force. She suggests a way that motivations rooted in attachment patterns can exist alongside, as well as become integrated with, motivations originating in bodily experience. The case material she presents illustrates the interdependency of sensual/sexual and aggressive strivings and thwarted early attachment relationships.

Neil Skolnick and Jody Messler Davies consider the issues of secrets and secrecy as they manifest in normal development, psychopathology, and the clinical situation. After a historical overview of psychoanalytic conceptualizations of secrets, they present a developmental and clinical understanding of secrecy that has its foundation in relational concerns. They consider the process of forming and maintaining secrets to be supraordinate to the actual content of a secret. Making this shift to a focus on process, they argue, allows us to regard the meaning and importance of secrets as residing in relational requisites of the self. These requisites include establishing intimacy; defining secure, flexible boundaries between internal and external experience; mitigating primitive omnipotence; and aiding in the discovery and development of an intersubjective sense of self and others.

At another level of discourse, Lewis Aron and Irwin Hirsch approach a long-neglected topic, routinely ignored by theoreticians and clinicians alike. With an admirable degree of candor, they consider the various aspects of the issue of money as it emerges in the transference/countertransference matrix. Invoking an interpersonal understanding of the nature of the analytic situation, they focus on the patient's awareness of the analyst's subjectivity, a focus rooted in Gill's (1982) theory of transference. The authors provide a clinical example to illustrate how the patient's perspective of the external reality and the analyst's attitudes toward money are worked within the clinical setting.

In the final chapter, Philip Bromberg describes the schizoid personality and its development from an interpersonal perspective. While acknowledging the insights derived from a drive perspective, he expands the conceptualization of the schizoid character structure by postulating its genesis as rooted in a tightly regulated balance between relatedness and detachment. Arguing that an interpersonally rooted approach provides a more comprehensive perspective than one based on libidinal concerns, he explains the appearance of the Isakower phenomenon during the middle phases of treatment as a reemergence of a developmentally earlier unsuccessful struggle to deal creatively and adaptively with potentially catastrophic interpersonal experience.

We conclude with two chapters that take as their exclusive focus the historical underpinnings of relational perspectives in psychoanalytic theory. Steven Reisner returns to Freud's text and argues that throughout Freud's writings a relational component can be discerned that exists in a dialectic tension with his drive-discharge model. Reisner claims, as a point of departure, that Eros, which Freud posited in his final dual-drive theory as one of the two irreducible primal human motivations, was intended to represent an incontrovertably relational concept. To truly appreciate the meaning of Eros, he argues, is to understand it as representing an unyielding motivation for relationship. He places it squarely in the realm of an object-seeking rather than a pleasure-seeking motive. He then focuses on what have been considered major turning points in classical drive theory: the abandonment of the seduction hypothesis of 1897, the articulation of the infantile sexual drive in "The Three Essays on the Theory of Sexuality" (Freud, 1905) and the elaboration of the metapsychology in "Instincts and Their Vicissitudes" (Freud, 1915). Throughout, he proposes that Freud continually counterposed his emphasis on bodily and genetic tensions with a decided concern for interactional experiences and their subjective meanings.

Benjamin Wolstein approaches the history of relational theorizing from another perspective. He differentiates between psychoanalytic psychology and metapsychology and traces the evolution of each. By psychoanalytic psychology, he is referring to the process of therapeutic inquiry that all psychoanalysts are involved in, such as making observations and inferences about transference, countertransference, resistance and counterresistance, anxiety and counteranxiety, and the self. Interpretively, analysts differ in their appeal to diverse myths and metaphors about the conjectured and reconstructable meanings of those observations and inferences. These diverse myths and metaphors are reflective of differing metapsychologies. Wolstein argues that Freud's metapsychology was only one of many possible explanatory systems that could be utilized to organize and provide meaning to the data gathered from his method of psychoanalytic inquiry. Despite Freud's use of a biological model of mind, Wolstein continues, from its inception as a method of therapeutic inquiry, psychoanalytic psychology has gathered its data from a primarily relational field of experience created and shared by two coparticipants, the analyst and the patient. This was always the case even when a metapsychology was invoked that did not focus on the relational underpinnings of the psychoanalytic explanatory system.

The range and depth of issues addressed by the contributors to this volume, while by no means comprehensive in scope, are representative of the extent to which clinicians and theoreticians writing from a relational point of view are presenting a serious challenge to more traditional metapsychologies. Although such challenges are far from new, it is our contention that a shift to a broad-based focus on relational concerns is emblematic of a momentous shift in the center of gravity in psychoanalytic theory and practice. Given the diverse traditions and backgrounds of those writing from relational perspectives, it is inevitable that differences among relational theorists will continue to be elucidated and debated. All, however, share a conviction of the centrality of relationships in human development and personality structure.

REFERENCES

Eagle, M. (1984), *Recent Developments in Psychoanalysis*. New York: McGraw-Hill.

Freud, S. (1905), Three essays on the theory of sexuality. *Standard Edition*, 7:125–245. London: Hogarth Press, 1953.

———— (1915), Instincts and their vicissitudes. *Standard Edition*, 14:117–140. London: Hogarth Press, 1957.

Gedo, J. (1979), *Beyond Interpretation*. New York: International Universities Press.

Gill, M. M. (1982), *Analysis of Transference*, Vol. 1. New York: International Universities Press.

Greenberg, J. & Mitchell, S. A. (1983), *Object Relations in Psychoanalytic Theory*. Cambridge, MA: Harvard University Press.

Mitchell, S. (1988), *Relational Concepts in Psychoanalysis*. Cambridge, MA: Harvard University Press.

True Selves, False Selves, and the Ambiguity of Authenticity

STEPHEN A. MITCHELL

The major influences on Freud's thought include not only the rationality of the 18th-century Enlightenment, which laid the philosophical foundation for the modern scientific world view, but also the powerful romantic vision of 19th-century poets and painters. Central to the vision of the latter was a call for the shedding of the trappings of civilization and a return to the power and immediacy of the "natural" world. For Freud, the embodiment of the "natural" world in man is the "id," where he locates the instincts, at the core of the self; they represent "the true purpose of the individual organism's life. This consists of the satisfaction of its innate needs" (Freud, 1940, p. 148); the ego and the superego are secondary formations, social adaptations, formed on the surface of the id. For Freud, it is an understanding of the body-based instincts that makes psychoanalysis a "depth" psychology, grounded in the most central, most "primitive" wellsprings of the individual.

The commitment of many contemporary analysts to Freud's drive theory is based on the belief that only in an appreciation of drives is the deepest understanding of the individual found, underneath the more superficial, cultural, adaptive overlays. Just as society requires us to wear clothing to cover our physical nakedness, social necessities create layers of regulatory and defensive adaptations to cover our true

I would like to express my gratitude to Emmanuel Ghent and Neil Altman, both of whom carefully read and challenged the ideas in earlier drafts of this essay in a way that helped develop my own thinking about these problems.

animal motives and nature. Waelder's (1960) homage to what he called the "imperative, majestic, power of *Trieb*" (p. 98) is emblematic of the elemental and elevated primacy attributed to the drives.

From this viewpoint, various relational theories including self psychology, interpersonal psychoanalysis, and some versions of object relations theories, by abandoning the theory of drives have lost the basis for an understanding of the individual in any depth. They have given up the tools for exploring true, passionate, authentic individuality, in contrast to the more superficial, shallow, interpersonal and social overlays. In fact, many European analysts see the movement away from an exclusive focus on drives in contemporary American Freudian theory, exemplified by ego psychology, as an abandonment of the individual, personal depths of human psychology. The call for a "return to Freud" and much of the contemporary loyalty to classical theory derive from the concern that the increasing emphasis on relational factors throughout recent psychoanalytic theorizing threatens to eliminate the personal, the uniquely individual, which Freud located in the body-based, sexual and aggressive impulses of the presocial id.

Where is the core of the self within a relational perspective? This is a real problem. In most relational theorizing, consistent with most contemporary infancy research as well as with contemporary linguistics, it is assumed that the self cannot exist in isolation. "There is no such thing as a baby," Winnicott's startling epigram reminds us, "only the mother–infant couple." The very capacity to have experiences necessarily develops in and requires an interpersonal matrix, and the organization, the patterning of all experiences is an extremely complex product of the interactions between the baby (with its temperamental sensitivities and thresholds) and the semiotic and interactive styles of the caregivers. There is no experience that is not interpersonally mediated. The meanings generated by the self are all interactive products.

But where is the center, the heart, the core of the individual in such a perspective? How can we find a place in the self where the individual *qua* individual might be thought to begin or reside? With the relational emphasis on attachment, interpersonal relations, identifications, and so on, how can psychoanalysis fail to become a form of sociology or social learning theory, in which the individual is viewed as a product of the social environment? If there are no body-based drives to represent "nature" at the intrapsychic core of the individual, how does psychoanalysis retain its most important and precious legacy as an instrument for inquiry into the depths of personal experience? The distinction between the true self and false, between the superficial and the more deeply felt, between conformistic adaptations and the more truly personal, between the authentic and the inauthentic: these distinctions are crucial to the analytic enterprise, and these distinctions seem to require that we locate the core or center of the self for use as a reference point.

There have been various attempts to deal with this problem as alternatives to retaining Freud's outmoded concept of drives as preexperiential, prelinguistic, archaic, phylogenetic residues.

One strategy has been to grant primary importance to the body, its parts and processes, and particularly to infantile bodily experiences, yet without Freud's notion of "drives." Why would the body be important if not for drives? There might be lots of reasons. Schafer (whose identity as a Freudian despite his disavowal of drive theory is based largely on the importance he places on infantile sexuality and aggression) believes that infantile body parts and experiences are the cognitive paradigms for organizing all experience. Our early life is dominated by powerful and absorbing physical events—eating, urinating, defecating, arousal, quiescence—and these events and processes become the basic categories, the underlying metaphors through which all subsequent experience is patterned.

This extremely valuable approach makes possible a reinterpretation of Freudian and Kleinian concepts of instincts from energic into cognitive and linguistic terms, and characterizes some of the most important contemporary contributions to psychoanalytic theorizing (see Ogden, 1986, 1989). Yet it does not help solve our problem of locating the core of the self. Freud thought that body parts and processes are represented directly and invariably in experience; that the ego is first and foremost a body ego, and that "anatomy is destiny." This makes sense within the context of drive theory, because the bodily tensions drive the mental apparatus, because instinctual experiences are the sole motivational energy for the mind, and because the self as a whole is derivative of and superimposed upon the vicissitudes of body-based drives. But if we eliminate drive theory as a motivational substructure, how do we understand the *meaning* that body parts and experiences take on for the individual? They must derive to a significant degree from the mutually regulatory, interpersonal, linguistic, and cultural matrix into which the individual is born. In most relational approaches, in contrast to drive theory metapsychology, it makes no sense to talk about *raw* bodily experience, which is subsequently controlled or regulated through cultural processes. As Lakoff and Johnson (1980), who have made important recent contributions to our understanding of the metaphorical structure of language, argue:

What we call "direct physical experience" is never merely a matter of having a body of a certain sort; rather, *every* experience takes place within a vast background of cultural presuppositions. It can be misleading, therefore, to speak of direct physical experience as though there were some core of immediate experience which we then "interpret" in terms of our conceptual system. Cultural assumptions, values, and attitudes are not a conceptual overlay which we may or may not place upon experience as we choose. It would be more correct to say that all experience is cultural through and through, that we experience our "world" in such a way that our culture is already present in the very experience itself [p. 57].

It is also true that the individual experiences culture *through* their own body. In that sense, all experience is also bodily "through and through." The cultural input can sometimes be factored out, because it appears across individuals and its transmission is often visible and apparent (as in a particular cultural value system). Bodily experience only becomes known in necessarily social experience with others, and the very terms and categories through which it becomes known are shaped by linguistic and social experience.

The physical structure of the body probably provides constraints on body-based elaborations of meaning. The penis probably lends itself to a somewhat different, although overlapping, array of possible meanings and metaphors than either the clitoris or the vagina, although this is impossible to ever really determine. Within the framework of drive theory it made sense to think one could separate out the universal from the socially elaborated in bodily experience and to assign the core of the individual to the former, as if the body were directly represented in experience in some sort of pure form. Without the presumption of primary drives as the underlying motivational push, it makes no sense to think about the distillation of a pure, "natural" dimension of experience.

Another way to relocate the importance of the body within a relational framework is to argue that intense bodily happenings—like sexual arousal, orgasm, eating, defecating, perhaps rage—have a preemptive physical claim and explosive power to them that inevitably places them at the core of personal experience. This seems to be what Winnicott for example, meant by "instinctual" experience, which has very little to with Freud's drive theory. This is a very useful approach, but once again, it does not help us with the problem of locating a core self.

Consider Winnicott's perspective, for example, where the self is derived from interactions between the baby and the mother. Instinctual experiences *can* facilitate and vitalize the development of the self, but they also can operate totally outside it. Winnicott (1963, p. 181) warns that the baby can be "fobbed off" by a good feed. What does that mean? The self does not develop out of instinctual experiences like feeding, but rather out of the subtle dialectic of maternal responsiveness. If feeding occurs in the context of good-enough mothering, it becomes a vehicle for growth of the self. If the mothering is inadequate, the power of the feeding experience actually detracts from self-development. The meaning of the bodily event depends on its position vis-à-vis the self.

There are people who experience sexual desire, or hunger for food, as a welcome sign of vitality. Others experience desire as a toxic impingement. Still others have no idea at all when they might be desirous of sex or of food, but decide by the clock. Finally, others never seem to experience desire or hunger at all. The location of experiences of anger or rage in relation to the self is similarly crucial; anger can vitalize, intrude upon, or deplete the self. The *meaning* of these bodily events, the psychological significance they contain regarding self, derives not from their inherent properties, but from the way early relational patterns have structured them vis-à-vis the self. Such physical experiences can not represent the core of the self, since they operate rather as vehicles to self-experience, in either authentic or inauthentic ways.

Another aspect of constitutional, bodily factors—temperament—has been similarly appropriated as a route to finding the core of the self. The history of psychoanalytic ideas is a history of overcorrections. In their eagerness to jettison the concept of innate drives, early relational theorists often wrote as if all babies were the same and the course of development derived purely from environmental input. Critics now correctly argue that babies are quite different from each other and that these temperamental differences have major implications for development. Those differences has been amply demonstrated empirically over the past several decades, and recent models of infant–mother interactions stress the "fit" or lack of fit between particular mothers and particular babies. Bollas (1989) has explored and extended this factor in stressing the importance of constitutionally based temperamental differences leading to particular personality style or personal "idiom" and to a sense of "destiny."

Differences in temperament, although extremely important, are nevertheless a problematic place to locate the core of the self. Temperament is not in any obvious sense motivational, and it is not represented directly in experience. The experience and meaning of temperamental differences is interpreted, often through identifications and counteridentifications. What is "high energy" in one family is hyperactivity in another. What is "sensitivity" in one family is weakness and inadequacy in another. Temperamental factors, like bodily configurations and processes, can be used by the self to fill out and represent various self-expressions and self-definitions. But they do not in themselves lead to particular forms of self-formation outside of complex social interaction.

There have been other attempts to search for a new locus of individuality, apart from the body per se, but located in very early experience. In the place previously occupied by Freud's id Kohut (1977) puts a preprogrammed "destiny"; Guntrip (1969) places a regressed, schizoid baby; Winnicott designates a creative omnipotence, and so on. Each theorist wants to divide the content of the self, to cut up the pie into socially negotiated segments and something else, which exists prior to social interaction and which can be considered the core of the self.

The latter approach is closely connected with a linear perspective on development and developmental arrests. The infant is presumed to begin life with a whole, or integral, self at least in potentiality, and that self is either facilitated by the human environment or blocked and thwarted in some fashion. If the self is blocked, the potential for authentic experience is frozen at that developmental point, and a reanimation of the true self is only possible through a regeneration of those developmental needs. One artifact of this strategy for locating the core of the self outside of and prior to the relational field is that it leads to a regressive cast in theorizing. Earlier is presumed to be somehow more primary, more personal, more "primitive," as if the core of the individual existed preverbally, even preexperientially *before* the infant encountered others.

One way in which this sort of developmental approach is framed is to speak of the self of the child-to-be as existing in potentiality in the infant and intuited and reflected by the mother (Loewald, 1960; Kohut, 1977). I have no problem with this notion if it is understood that the child has many potentialities with respect to self-development and that the one intuited by the mother is regarded as also partially a reflection of the mother's own subjectivity. The father, after all, may very likely intuit a quite different child in potential. In fact, it is precisely because the mother's child is somewhat different from the father's child that conflict between different organizations of self is so universally generated. So, to speak of the core of the self as existing in potentiality is to beg the question. Either it exists in already organized fashion and unfolds in a receptive environment, a notion that I find implausible; or unorganized temperamental differences exist, organized and selected through interaction with care-givers.

This brings us straight back to the problem of locating the core of the self.

An interesting variant of this strategy has been developed recently by Slavin and Kriegman (1990), who have proposed a new paradigm for psychoanalysis derived from evolutionary biology and broad considerations concerning genetics and adaptation. They argue that the basic conflict in human experience is intergenerational—the clash in self-interest between parent and child. Because the offspring represent the survival of the parents' gene pool, the parents sacrifice individual self-interest to care for the child. Because the child exists in a prolonged period of dependence on the parent, the need to continually connect with the parents' goals and values is paramount; his own self-interested motives are rendered secondary and repressed, only to return later in life (that is, in adolescence), when primary attachments are less functionally necessary. Slavin and Kriegman suggest that Freud's concept of endogenous instinctual drives, representing peremptory, aggressively self-interested, asocial, exclusively personal needs, can be thought to refer to that aspect of the personality which shapes and maintains the self as individual versus the self as embedded in a relational matrix. "In the drives we have a mechanism that guarantees access to some types of motivation that *arise from non-relational sources* and are, in a sense, *totally dedicated toward the promotion of our individual interests*" (p. 37).

The evolutionary perspective of Slavin and Kriegman provides interesting angles on many traditional psychoanalytic issues. However, their attempt to use the classical concept of "drives" as the core of the individually-configured self does not really work in the way they claim. A close reading suggests that they alter Freud's notion of "drives" in order to make it work within their larger scheme.

> Drives, and the structural model of drive-defense conflict, assumes a *subsidiary* role within a larger, relationally designed and configured psyche. But, to the extent that the classical agenda is read as a "narrative of conflict," it captures certain major, significant features of the relational world and the inherently "divided" way we are adapted to it [p. 47].

In my view, "drives" relocated and reset into a relationally configured psyche are no longer Freud's "drives," prewired, endogenous pressures whose meaning is represented within the mind unmediated by the semiotic, metaphoric meaning systems of the relational world. Once again, the effort to portray a part of the psyche as separate from, prior to, and sheltered from the interactive, mutually regulatory structures of the relational matrix proves problematic.

There has been considerable interest in contemporary philosophy and linguistics in the way metaphor shapes understanding and experience. Concepts as vague and insubstantial as "psyche," "mind," or "self" are impossible to grasp in precise, denotative terms. We understand and come to experience them in terms of other, generally more concrete kinds of experiences and activities (see Lakoff and Johnson, 1980). Schafer (1976) has demonstrated that in most psychoanalytic theorizing in general and especially in psycho-analytic formulations about self, the self is thought about, either explicitly or implicitly, in concretely spatial terms. This way of thinking comes directly from Freud.[1] In both the topographical and the structural models, Freud grounds his theorizing in a clearly defined spatial metaphor: "the hypothesis we have adopted for a psychical apparatus extended into space" (1940, p. 196).

If we think about mind in terms of spatial metaphors, as if it existed in space, with structures, within a topography, then it makes sense to approach it as one would an onion, to try to locate its "core" or "heart," to delineate its layers, to differentiate its authentic pieces from its false, protective covering, and so on. Some of the more careful psychoanalytic theorists like Rapaport and Loewald have taken pains to point out that the concept of psychic structure refers not to something substantive but to recurring patterns of experience and behavior over time. Thus, Rapaport (1957) defines structure as a "relatively stable (having a slow rate of change), characteristic con-figuration that we can abstract from the behavior observed" (p. 701).

Yet in common usage, deriving from Freud's talking about the psyche as occupying spaces with structural properties, the spatial metaphor has become reified. All the strategies for theorizing about the "true" or "core" self that we have considered accept, explicitly or implicitly, this spatial metaphor and try to locate the elemental from the unessential features of the self, to distinguish its essential from its insignificant features, to locate its center or foundation. We want to get underneath the adaptations that the self has made in its negoti-ations with others, to get at its beginnings, its true, presocial essence. This search for a core is what continues to make Freud's id and its romanticization of a pure, animal nature so compelling.

Perhaps to think of the self as existing in space is misleading. Clearly, the brain exists in space, and the phenomenological *experience* of the self as layered and cloistered in space is common, perhaps

---

[1]Freud did not invent spatial metaphors for thinking about mind; they have a long history in western philosophy. (See Ryle, 1949, for an extended critique of this way of talking about mind.)

universal. But it seems more accurate and, I believe, more useful, to regard the self as a temporal rather than a spatial phenomenon. The self *is* nowhere; the self refers to the subjective organization of meanings a person creates as he or she moves through time, doing things, like having ideas and feelings, including some self-reflective ideas and feelings about oneself.

If the self moves in time rather than exists in space, it has no core; but it has many different ways of operating. Some of the ways in which I operate and express myself I consider more "authentic," more important to or representative of "me" than others. These are often difficult discriminations, but I think we are all involved in making them a good deal of the time. There are times when I feel more "myself" than others, when I feel I have presented my thoughts and feelings accurately and succinctly, when I have been comfortable enough to allow myself to reveal more of my spontaneous repertoire. At other times I feel less "myself," jumbled, unable or unwilling to make myself clear, too awkward or constrained to reveal myself in anything but a stereotyped or constricted fashion. We all operate in this range of possibilities. The extreme form of inauthenticity is deliberate lying. When I am lying, I am misrepresenting my feelings or events and am being less authentic than when I am trying to represent myself and events more accurately.

By using the terms "authentic" and "inauthentic," are we not measuring our experience against some implicit standard, some preconceived idea of what is "me"? Do these terms also imply a "core" or "true" or "real" me that exists somewhere (smuggling back the spatial metaphor)? No. One has a sense of one's experience over time. One can measure a new experience in terms of continuity or discontinuity with the past and present; a new experience can represent and express one's history and current state or deny and betray one's history and current state. Speaking of authenticity versus inauthenticity or true versus false *experience* frees us from the spatial metaphor in a way that speaking of a true or false *self* or a "core" or "real" *self* does not.

In speaking about authenticity and inauthenticity, the crucial difference lies not in the specific *content* of what I feel or do, but in the relationship between what I feel and do and the spontaneous configuration and flow of my experience at that point in *time*. A particular act of self-expression, a piece of self-revelation, for example, or a sexual overture, may feel extremely authentic at one point and extremely inauthentic at another. In the first case, it feels "right," suits both the external, interpersonal context and the internal emotional context. In the second case, it feels "off," forced, contrived, out of "sync" interpersonally, internally, or both. The degree to which an act or feeling represents or misrepresents the personal self depends not on its content (not on what is *in* it), but on its place in the context and configuration of experience as it is continually organized, disorganized, and reorganized in time.

Consider Winnicott's (1960, 1963) depiction of the earliest feeding experiences, which he establishes as the basis for the split between true and false selves. In pathological feeding, he suggests, the infant takes its cues from impingements from the outside. The baby's own impulses and needs are not met by the mother, and the baby learns to want what the mother gives, to become the mother's idea of who the baby is. Authentic feeding experience, on the other hand, derives from the baby's spontaneously arising gestures, which the good-enough mother meets and actualizes, creating what Winnicott terms the "moment of illusion."

What is the content of these spontaneous gestures? Even in the earliest feedings, Winnicott suggests, the baby's "readiness" to imagine a breast leads immediately to experiences in the real world out of which develops the baby's idea of the breast, which is further matched by the mother's responsiveness. It cannot be the content that differentiates authentic from inauthentic experience; the image of the breast in the two experiences is virtually the same. What is crucial is the point of origin of the idea at any given time, and that makes all the difference. At one moment a movement toward the breast occurs spontaneously in the baby; at another moment, it is a response to the mother's idea of what the baby wants, a compliance with external impingement. Does the idea of the breast at a particular moment come from the baby or the mother? Does it arise spontaneously in the baby, or is it suggested or even coerced from the outside? This is the crucial issue for Winnicott, and it is a very useful starting point for thinking about the problem of authentic individuality in general.

The individual discovers himself within an interpersonal field of interactions in which he has participated long before the dawn of his own self-reflective consciousness of himself. The mind of which he becomes self-aware is constituted by a stream of impulses, fantasies, bodily sensations, which have been patterned through interaction and mutual regulation with caregivers. The experience and meaning of all these have been established and continue to be established, through the physical and mental handling and holding of significant others (Stern, 1985). In Bollas's (1983) earlier work, he argues that there is no purely generic "holding environment"; the particularities of the individual mother's handling of the baby become the existential medium of the baby's world and are structured into the developing child's personal idiom. With the gradual dawning of self-awareness, that mental content becomes more fully one's own and can be used in various ways—it can be spontaneously expressed; it can be collaboratively coordinated in interactions with others; it can be deceptively packaged, disingenuously presented; it can be compromised; it can be betrayed.

In classical psychoanalysis, the central and most important question to be asked of the individual is: what are the patterns of gratification, frustration, and sublimation that shape this person's life? In contemporary psychoanalysis, in the work of its most visionary contributors (Winnicott, Bion, Schafer, Kohut, Lacan), the most important question to be asked has shifted to: how meaningful and authentic is a person's experience and expression of himself? Richness in living or psychopathology are the product not of instinctual vicissitudes, but of truth or falsity with respect to one's own experience. Why is the self so easily and commonly falsified, so routinely betrayed?

The self operates in the intricate and subtle dialectic between spontaneous vitality and self-expression on the one hand and the requirement, crucial for survival, to preserve secure and familiar connections with others, on the other. (Sullivan's, 1953, basic motivational distinction between the need for interpersonal security and needs for satisfaction reflect this duality.) Spontaneous self-expression serves as the ground for an array of authentic experience; the need for security leads to a concern with the impact of one's self-presentations on others. If I spontaneously express my feeling or thought or state of mind, do I make the other on whom I am greatly dependent anxious, angry, likely to withdraw? Do I have to conceal my spontaneous experience? disguise it? package it in a particular way, perhaps differently for different significant others? It is the necessity for mindfulness and some degree of control of one's impact on others that makes inevitable for all people at one time or another a whole array of inauthentic experiences. It is not differences in content that distinguish the authentic from the inauthentic; it is the way the content is organized, particularly in terms of the balance between internality and externality and the purpose to which the content is being put at any given moment.

Deciding what is true and what is false when it comes to self is a tricky business. Although Winnicott's idea of the "true self" is often used in a concrete and reified fashion, he himself suggests that "there is little point in formulating a True Self idea except for the purpose of trying to understanding the False Self, because it does no more than collect together the details of the experience of aliveness" (Winnicott,

1960, p. 148). Khan (1963), who wrote of the "privacy" of the self with such eloquence and subtlety, suggests that the "true self" is a conceptual ideal, known concretely mostly by its absence (p. 303).

We are often quietly aware of when we are being false or betraying ourselves, but authenticity does not often announce itself in such a stark and unambiguous way. In fact, a lack of *self*-consciousness, posturing, self-arranging, self-presenting, narcissistic pulse checking is often the hallmark of a truer form of experience, in which the self is taken for granted, unheralded and without banners. The patient who struggles to reveal his "true" feelings or to disclose what he is "really like" may reveal a conflict- or shame-ridden aspect of experience, but this is hardly the whole story. (Farber, 1976, chapter 12, provides a wonderful account of the deceptiveness of revelatory models of insight.) Khan (1963) thus alerts us to the elusiveness of the "true" self and chides Guntrip for having fallen prey to the seductive "danger of romantization of a pure self system" (p. 304).

Bollas (1983, p. 218) speaks of patients who seek him out looking for a "Winnicottian" analysis, envisioned as a totally regressive return to total dependency, a letting go of what they feel are their inauthentic yet perhaps highly effective ways of functioning in the world. The quest of these patients is clearly consistent with one aspect of Winnicott's contribution; Little (1985) notes that Winnicott "spoke of patients having to 'queue up' sometimes to go into such a state," to wait for their turn at "full regression" (p. 23). Yet Bollas points up the importance of *not* assuming that the functional self and the person's resources are any less "true" than the image of the regressed and wholly dependent infant the patient longs to be. The original reasons for someone to become resourceful and effective might well have been "inauthentic" and some distance from where the person genuinely was at the time. Nevertheless, what is crucial now is the use of misuse to which those capacities are put. The idea that one's "core" or "true" self is located in developmentally earlier states is both overly simplistic and also very compelling, as evidenced by the mileage given to "the child within" in much mass-market popular psychology. The claim to be helpless and the disclaiming of one's actual resources, although very understandable (it often operates as a testament to hope and an avoidance of coming to terms with irreversibly lost opportunities and experiences), nevertheless serves current purposes that are no longer *simply* authentic.

Consider the enormously delicate clinical problem involved in the psychoanalysis of victims of childhood abuse, sexual or otherwise. There are moments when to speak of anything else is false, inauthentic, a denial of what has taken place. Yet there are other moments when the account of the victimization is serving the purpose not of making oneself finally known, but of creating an impact, making a claim, often turning the tables via an identification with the original abuser (Davies and Frawley, 1992). In such moments, which Ferenczi (1988), in his tragic struggle with these issues, termed the "terrorism of suffering," the content is true, but the intent is laced with falseness. Any statement about the self and one's past can serve, and inevitably does begin to serve, other purposes in the present. This is what Sartre (1953) meant by his argument that we are all continually struggling to emerge from "bad faith." Yesterday's insight becomes today's resistance; yesterday's hard-fought self-understanding becomes today's familiar and comfortable refuge.

Part of the trickiness of distinguishing "true" from "false" experience is that both the distinction between internality and externality and the distinction between self and other become more complex the more closely one considers them. Winnicott's use of these distinctions for the infant vis-à-vis the breast provides an important starting point, but this is too simplified a situation when we consider adult experience. All personal motives have a long relational history. If the self is always embedded in relational contexts, either actual or internal, than all important motives have appeared and taken on life and form in the presence and through the reactions of significant others.

Let us say a little girl decides she will become a physician through a mixture of motives that we could divide into two groups. Group A includes genuine interest in the workings of nature in general and bodies in particular, sexual curiosity, a concern with helping others, and counterdependent defenses against being sick herself. Group B includes a strong desire to please her parents' thwarted longings to be educated as professionals, identification with their social-class aspirations, their anxieties about their daughter's future security, and so on. Let us assume that the little girl sensed the importance of this career path to her parents from the moment they gave her her first Fisher-Price doctor set. How do we evaluate the authenticity versus inauthenticity of this choice and life course? Since the motives in group A reflect internal concerns and those in group B reflect external concerns, the obvious starting point would be to assume that the balance between truth and falseness in this choice is determined by the balance between A motives and B motives. But a closer look suggests a greater complexity.

Group B motives *began* as external considerations. The girl likes to make her parents excited and happy by parading around with her toy stethoscope. But by the time she is applying to medical school, she has long since left home – her parents may even be dead. Externality now means something different. She certainly may still make the choice in order to please her parents; yet her parents are not actual people at this point but internal parents, internal objects. In making the choice to go to medical school, she feels a deep and pervasive connection with her parents, and her feelings of closeness with them perpetuate them as emotional presences in her experiences. So, these formerly external objects now operate internally.

Conversely, although group A motives seem to be purely self-generated, they cannot be wholly so. Allowing for the importance of constitutional, temperamental factors in terms of activity level, intellectual gifts, and sensibilities, we would have to assume that qualities like interest in nature, bodies, sexual curiosity, helping others, counterdependent defenses, and so on could not emerge in an interpersonal vacuum or flower in a simply mirroring, facilitating environment. They must have identificatory meanings embedded in interactions with important others, complex reverberations and resonances within various relational configurations. Group A motives, like group B motives, are complex blends of both internal and external factors.

It is not so easy therefore, to parse self from other, to neatly divide internal from external considerations. In fact, the extreme stickiness of this problem may be the reason why theories claiming to have located a center of the individual outside the relational field are so compelling.

We all have probably had the very private experience of connecting with oneself in solitude in a way that is not possible in the presence of others, the "incognito" subjective core of Winnicott (1963). And there is the experience of refinding what one really feels or wants to do through a sudden realization that one has been too concerned with the opinions and reactions of others. These considerations suggest that the core or foundation of the individual self is self-centered and perhaps omnipotent and egoistic.

Yet there are also experiences of losing oneself in private ruminations, self-alienation in solitude, and a sense of refinding oneself through engagement with another. There is a difference for most people between the relative hollowness of masturbation and the fullness of sex with another that probably has something to do with the perpetuation of the species. In sex with another, externality, compromise, and compliance are clearly features. If there is too much concern with externality, there is no spontaneous desire, and the experience lacks depth and passion. (Winnicott, 1968, depicts the importance of the capacity to "use" the other as a precondition for fully passionate experience.) On the other hand, if there is no sense of externality, there is no awareness of the other except as a masturbatory vehicle.

The richness of experience is generated in the subtle dialectics between internality and externality, desire and concern, destruction and reparation, self and other. Human beings use each other not just for safety, protection, control, and self-regulation; we also come alive, develop capacities, and expand personal consciousness through interaction in a way that is not possible in isolation. The simple distinction between internality and externality, although a very useful starting point, is not sufficient to distinguish true from false experience. What is crucial is the extent to which internal and external considerations, self and other, have been balanced and reconciled.

Loewald addresses himself to this process more than any other major psychoanalytic theorist. In the context of generational conflict and fratricide Loewald (1978) defines the self as "an atonement structure" and repeatedly depicts the richest form of experience as one which overcomes the compulsive separation between self and other, inside and outside, on different levels of organization. Bromberg (1991) has similarly noted the fluidity of the relationship between internality and externality in health and their forced separation in serious forms of psychopathology:

> Most people take their own subjective states of interiority for granted, and can routinely accept the fact that there is "more to them than meets the eye" as something that joins them to the rest of mankind without intrinsic emotional isolation. They can be both in the world and separate from it as a unitary experience that blends selfhood and relatedness. Others, more developmentally fragmented, protect their subjective interiors as a livelong task of emotional survival, while paying the price of never-ending efforts at self-validation, or desperate aloneness [p. 400].

From the perspective developed here, what is central to the analytic process is precisely an overcoming of the sense that one has to choose between being oneself in the "use" of others or betraying oneself in adaptation to others. Psychoanalysis becomes a struggle to find and be oneself in the process of atonement and reconciliation in relation to others, both actual others and others as internal presences.

Let us return to our would-be medical student. Most clinicians, regardless of ideological persuasion, would be concerned with the following considerations when thinking about her career deliberations: Is this choice consistent with enough dimensions of her personality to represent and work for her in a meaningful way? Will she use enough of herself, or does it draw her away from too much that is important to her? Is she anticipating pleasure in this work or primarily a fantasied security or fantastic solution to infantile anxieties? One could translate these considerations into different theoretical terms: Have the original motives attained sufficient secondary autonomy? Is she motivated by satisfactions or security? Are the identifications primarily superego identifications or ego identifications? Are her superego and ego reconciled or at odds? Are her internal objects happy? All these questions are concerned, in one way or another, with the *way* in which what was formerly external has become internal, the extent to which externality and internality have become reconciled or are pulling against each other in different directions, and the degree to which past interpersonal negotiations have been metabolized into nutriment for further growth and development.

Consider other kinds of experiences that provide for some people a deep sense of authenticity: athletic activities or artistic creation. If I am just learning to play tennis, the effort will feel unnatural, inauthentic, modeling or posturing, not representative of me. "Grip the racket just so; position your feet perpendicular to the net; keep your eye on the ball; keep your weight moving toward the net; swing through the ball." In learning the game I am learning a complex discipline created through a long history by a community of others. Some people are "naturals" with respect to sheer athletic ability, but no one can play tennis naturally, at least not very well. The techniques are essential if you are to get where you want to go.

Yet if I have played tennis for a long time, I may feel truly and deeply myself when I play. When I play well I am likely not only to feel free of any attention to technique or discipline, but also to free of self-consciousness altogether, playing "in the groove" or "out of my mind." The same techniques so painfully and awkwardly practiced over many years are now a part of me and make possible kinds of experiences not attainable in any other way. Tennis is a set of complex social conventions that make possible an individual, deeply subjective experience of potentially profound personal significance. Authenticity derives from the use of what has been socially negotiated to represent and express myself; inauthenticity derives from the use of what has been socially negotiated to create and manage impressions of me in others.

The use of an embedded spatial metaphor is prevalent not just in psychoanalytic literature but also in the way most people *experience* the self, at least part of the time. Certain areas of experience, different ones for different people, are difficult or impossible to risk exposing to others. It is as though they exist in secret, hidden recesses of being and constitute a core or center of the self. Other ways of being feel stereotyped, facile, and easily conjured; these ways of being seem to provide a protective buffer, a shell under which or within which more vulnerable, more hidden, and more authentic forms of experience can be concealed. For some people, sexual responses are impossible to express and integrate in interactions with others and have a "true" or pure quality to them, precisely because their sexuality has rarely been modulated through social interaction. For others, dissociated rage has a pure, deep quality about it, in contrast to the chronic characterological submission that may govern all other interactions (necessitating the dissociation of the rage in the first place). For others, a pure joy or spontaneous laughter remains hidden and unexpressed behind a dour demeanor or a hyperresponsible version of adulthood. For still others, certain kinds of preverbal experiences have been preserved as a refuge for the self, while language in general has been coopted by deception and self-betrayal. These experiences are sometimes organized into a sense that the thwarted spontaneity of the self as baby, is hidden behind the empty, conformistic adaptations of adulthood.

Clinical psychoanalysis, unless it becomes a sterile exercise in "rationality," operates within the phenomenology of the self. Analyst and patient enter spaces, explore recesses, traverse topographies. Previously inaccessible experiences, running the gamut from totally dissociated to concealed to conflict ridden, often make themselves known through personalized metaphors: animals, babies, explosions, elemental forces, closets, demons. These experiences can come alive in the analytic situation only on their own terms. The experience of self as a preverbal baby cannot be talked about, because it is the very corruption of language in the dynamics of particular families that initially makes it impossible for the patient to feel alive through words. The experience of the self as explosively rageful or demonically sexual cannot be translated into polite conversation, because it was precisely the disembodied and mannered forms of familial discourse that created the sense of rage and sexuality as dangerous and primitive. The metaphors around which versions of self are organized generally come in complementary pairs: the metaphor of the needy baby/the metaphor of pale and joyless adulthood; the metaphor of the beast/the metaphor of the civilized citizen; and so on. Versions of the self are states of mind accessible only on their own terms, and the collaborative struggle to discover and create these terms is a crucial dimension of the analytic process. Ironically, it is only as the analytic process enables the patient to live in what are felt to be secret, hidden, core spaces within the self that he begins to experience these states as versions of himself, among many other versions of himself, that emerge and are shaped over time.

Thinking about self in temporal as opposed to spatial terms forces a reconsideration of the relationship between body and experience of self. I have argued elsewhere (Mitchell, 1988) that it makes more sense to think about body-based experiences like sexual desire or rage not as continual, primitive, endogenous pressures located in a place within the psyche (like the "id"), but as *reactions* to stimuli, internal and external, always in particular relational contexts. From this perspective it makes no sense to say that desire and aggression are any more "primitive," basic, or fundamental than laughing or painting. It is not the content that is important, because no content is more central or primary than any other content. It is the function of the content in the larger context of experience. Does the desire, rage, laughter, or painting derive from and express spontaneous reactions to both internal and external stimuli, or is the desire, rage, laughter, or painting contrived to manage self-states and others?

From this perspective, body-based experiences of self are no more primary than verbal experiences of self; rather, different ways of organizing experience are seen as coterminous and in dialectical relationship with each other. Thus, Stern (1985) suggests that what he calls different "senses" of self—emergent, core, intersubjective and verbal—are not passed through sequentially in stages, but coexist together in adult experience. Ogden (1989) similarly argues that what he terms the "autistic-contiguous" mode of experience, involving a basic kinesthetic sense of sensory continuity and embodiment, operates in a continual interplay with paranoid-schizoid and depressive modes of organizing experience. Again, it is a mistake to think of one form of experience as more basic or deeper, because they are not layered in space; rather, they shift back and forth as forms of self-organization over time.

An interesting additional facet of the relationship between the body and the experience of self concerns the issue of gender. If one assumes, as did Freud, that "anatomy is destiny" and that the drives constitute the core of the psyche, one would think of the self and of experience in general as gendered. (Of course, Freud felt that the array of component drives makes us all bisexual, so that both genders are represented in each psyche.) In contrast, if one assumes that the self is organized in different ways at different points in time, some of those organizations may be gendered (monosexual or bisexual), while others may not. It may be developmentally necessary for a little boy or a little girl to feel very much like a little boy or a little girl, but very unnecessary and enormously constricting for any adult man or woman to need to experience themselves continually in a gendered way (Harris, 1991; Dimen, 1991). Gender identity, or a gendered identity, is, for most people, extremely important to establish. In fact, the most important function of sexual activity for many people is not the pleasure or release per se, but the establishment of the sense of oneself as a woman or as a man (see Person, 1980; Simon and Gagnon, 1973). Yet it may not be that a gendered sense of self always underlies experience. In fact, the capacity to organize experience in many ungendered (not bisexual) ways, without a compulsive need to evoke a gendered identity, might be considered a feature of mental health.

According to Lao-tsu, setting out to find the Tao (roughly speaking, Enlightenment) is like setting out in pursuit of a thief hiding in the forest by banging loudly on a drum. Setting out to find one's true self or trying to hold onto one's true self entails similar problems. The rushing fluidity of human experience through time makes authenticity essentially and necessarily ambiguous. It is the fascination with and pursuit of that ambiguity that lies at the heart of the analytic process. It is this fascination which is held in common by clinicians who love doing analytic work. It is in this sense that I do not agree with Schafer (1983) that doing analysis entails a "subordination" of the analyst's personality. Certainly there is a kind of discipline involved, but, like the discipline and technique in sports or artistic expression, the form makes possible a liberating kind of experience that is hard to come by in any other way. Doing analysis, either as a patient or as an analyst, involves a struggle to reach a fully authentic experience of a particular kind that, when fully engaged, makes possible a kind of freedom and authenticity which is both rare and precious.

What makes psychoanalysis a highly personal process is not deriving the individual mind from outside the social field, but its focus on the subjective meaning of any piece of mental life. Psycho-analytic theorizing will have more to contribute to our understanding of personal individuality if we can get away from a search for presocial or extrasocial roots of the core or true self and focus on what it means at any particular moment to be experiencing and using oneself more or less authentically.

REFERENCES

Bollas, C. (1983), *The Shadow of the Object*. New York: Columbia University Press.
_____ (1989), *Forces of Destiny*. London: Free Association Books.
Bromberg, P. (1991), On knowing one's patient inside out. *Psychoanal. Dial.*, 1:399–422.

Davies, J. & Frawley, M. (1992), Dissociation processes and transference-countertrans-ference paradigms in the psychoanalytically oriented treatment of adult survivors of childhood sexual abuse. *Psychoanal. Dial.*, 2:77–96.

Dimen, M. (1991), Deconstructing differences: Gender, splitting and transitional space. *Psychoanal. Dial.*, 1:335–352.

Farber, L. (1976), *Lying, Despair, Jealousy, Envy, Sex, Suicide, Drugs, and the Good Life.* New York: Basic Books.

Ferenczi, S. (1988), *The Clinical Diary of Sandor Ferenczi*, ed. J. Dupont. Cambridge, MA: Harvard University Press.

Freud, S. (1940), An outline of psycho-analysis. *Standard Edition* 23:144–207. London: Hogarth Press, 1964.

Guntrip, H. (1969), *Schizoid Phenomena, Object Relations and the Self.* New York: International Universities Press.

Harris, A. (1991), Gender as contradiction. *Psychoanal. Dial.*, 1:197–224.

Khan, M. M. R. (1963), *The Privacy of the Self.* New York: International Universities Press.

Kohut, H. (1977), *The Restoration of the Self.* New York: International Universities Press.

Lakoff, G. & Johnson, M. (1980), *Metaphors We Live By.* Chicago: University of Chicago Press.

Little, M. (1985), Winnicott working in areas where psychotic anxieties predominate: A personal record. *Free Associations*, 3:9–42.

Loewald, H. (1960), On the therapeutic action of psychoanalysis. *Internat. J. Psycho-Anal.*, 58:463–472.

_____ (1978), The waning of the oedipus complex. In: *Papers on Psychoanalysis.* New Haven, CT: Yale University Press, 1980.

Mitchell, S. (1988), *Relational Concepts in Psychoanalysis.* Cambridge, MA: Harvard University Press.

Ogden, T. (1986), *The Matrix of the Mind.* New York: Aronson.

_____ (1989), *The Primitive Edge of Experience.* New York: Aronson.

Person, E. (1980), Sexuality as the mainstay of identity: Psychoanalytic perspectives. *Sigma*, 5:605–630.

Rapaport, D. (1957), A theoretical analysis of the superego concept. In: *The Collected Papers of David Rapaport*, ed. M. Gill. New York: Basic Books, pp. 685–709.

Ryle, G. (1949), *The Concept of Mind.* Chicago: University of Chicago Press.

Sartre, J. (1953), *Existential Psychoanalysis.* Chicago: Gateway.

Schafer, R. (1976), *A New Language for Psychoanalysis.* New Haven, CT: Yale University Press.

_____ (1983), *The Analytic Attitude.* New York: Basic Books.

Simon, J. & Gagnon, W. (1973), *Sexual Conduct.* Chicago: Aldine.

Slavin, M. & Kreigman, D. (1990), Toward a new paradigm: An evolutionary/biological perspective on the classical-relational dialectic. *Psychoanal. Psychol.*, 7(suppl.):5–31.

Stern, D. (1985), *The Interpersonal World of the Infant.* New York: Basic Books.

Sullivan, H. S. (1953), *The Interpersonal Theory of Psychiatry.* New York: Norton.

Waelder, R. (1960), *The Basic Theory of Psychoanalysis.* New York: International Universities Press.

Winnicott, D. W. (1960), Ego distortion in terms of true and false self. In: *The Maturational Process and the Facilitating Environment.* New York: International Universities Press, 1965, pp. 140–152.

_____ (1963), Communicating and not communicating leading to a study of certain opposites. In: *The Maturational Process and the Facilitating Environment.* New York: International Universities Press, pp. 179–192.

_____ (1968), The use of an object and relating through identifications. In: *Playing and Reality.* Middlesex, Eng.: Penguin, 1974, pp. 101–111.

2

Self Psychology
The Self and Its Vicissitudes
Within a Relational Matrix

JAMES L. FOSSHAGE

A well-documented shift from a one-person to a two-person psychology (Rickman, 1957; Balint, 1968; Greenberg and Mitchell, 1983; Modell, 1984; Mitchell, 1988; Ghent, 1989) cuts across a number of psychoanalytic theoretical developments, including the British school of object relations, self psychology, interpersonal psychoanalysis, and currents within Freudian ego psychology. Because of its pervasiveness, it has led to the use of the term "relational perspectives" (Greenberg and Mitchell, 1983; Mitchell, 1988), the subject matter of this book. This shift from an intrapsychic to a field perspective can be likened to the Copernican revolution, in that the individual, like planet earth, does not exist alone but can be understood only in relation to the "gravitational forces" of the universe at large.

SHIFT IN OBSERVATIONAL STANCES

Fundamental shifts in theoretical perspectives within the domain of science often entail basic changes in both observational and conceptual stances. The shift from an intrapsychic to a field model within psychoanalysis is in part based on the on-going, far-reaching change from the positivistic science of the 19th century, wherein so-called "facts" were "objectively" observed, to the relativistic science of the 20th century, marked by Heisenberg's Uncertainty

Principle, wherein the "observed" is recognized as always shaped by the observer.[1]

The shift from positivistic to relativistic (or perspectivistic) science is apparent in the psychoanalytic observational stances of the "objective" observer versus the subsequent formulation of the "empathic mode of observation." A breakthrough in Freud's work was his investigation of the patient's intrapsychic world, implicitly using the yet unformulated empathic mode of observation. The positivistic science of the day, however, significantly influenced the investigation of the patient's inner life. The analyst's observations and interpretations tended to be, and often still are (particularly in clinical discussions), viewed as "objective."[2] Recognizing from a relativistic scientific position that the analyst always affects what is observed, Kohut (1959, 1982) clarified and proposed the *consistent* use of the empathic mode of observation namely, to attempt to understand from *within* the vantage point of the analysand. Placing the analysand's perspective and experience in the foreground *militates* against imposing the analyst's point of view onto the analysand. Although this listening stance is designed "to hear" as well as possible from within the vantage point of the analysand, this is clearly a relative matter, for what is heard is always *variably* shaped by the analyst.[3] To refer to this

---

[1]This shift to a relativistic science is both reflected and further developed in Piaget's theory of constructionism.

[2]We can surmise that Freud did not formulate the "empathic mode of observation" principally because of the positivistic science of the day. Although he seldom used the term empathy, Freud (1921) did address its fundamental importance in referring to it as "the mechanism by means of which we are enabled to take up any attitude at all towards another mental life" (p. 110). Empathy has generally referred to affective resonance with the other (see Greenson, 1960). As a data-gathering stance (Kohut, 1959), empathy enables us to feel into and to "vicariously introspect" about the other's subjective experience—a complex affective and cognitive process (see Lichtenberg, 1981).

[3]In his critical assessment of self psychology, Bromberg (1989) erroneously links the empathic mode of observation with "dedication to full empathic responsiveness" (p. 282). Kohut (1959, 1982) conceptualized the empathic mode of observation as a data-gathering stance, distinct from ensuing interventions. The confusion may partially emanate from Kohut's (1982) noting that this data-gathering activity of the analyst (which the patient experiences as a response from the analyst) in itself may be experienced by the patient as "empathic" and "therapeutic" and his use of the word "empathy" also to refer to a "powerful emotional bond between people." Referring to the *responses* of the analyst based on empathically-gathered data, Kohut (1977) also noted the need for an "average empathic responsiveness" (p. 253). Contrasting empathic responsiveness with the "neutrality" of the classical stance, Kohut used the term to address the requisite affective involvement of the analyst. What is meant by empathic responsiveness is a far too complex subject to approach here, but it is to be differentiated from the empathic mode of observation.

listening stance as a mode of "observation" reflects the ongoing shift from positivistic to relativistic science, for "observation" conveys a sense of an "outside" observer. A more relativistic description is to identify this mode as the empathic mode of *perception*, referring to the analyst's perceptual process (Lichtenberg, 1981, for example, uses this latter term). The analyst's perceptions, understandings, and explanations are subsequently offered to the analysand for his or her experiential assessment (Schwaber, 1984, has further delineated this stance).

When the analyst's observations and interpretations are no longer viewed as "objective" facts but as "subjective" organizations, the analytic field shifts immeasurably as the analyst is "dethroned" from the position of the "objective" observer and becomes a coparticipant in perceiving and constructing the analytic process. The perceptual-affective-cognitive organizing principles or schemas of the analyst variably shape the analyst's experience and reading of the analysand's experience, just as the analysand's schemas variably shape his or her experience of the analyst. This fundamental shift from positivistic to relativistic science and paradigmatic change in observational stances underscores that the *analytic arena* involves an interaction between two persons (and their respective subjectivities) and, therein, is a relational or intersubjective field.[4]

ONE-PERSON AND TWO-PERSON PSYCHOLOGIES: A NEW SYNTHESIS

In understanding a person (personality theory), a one-person psychology model emphasizes biologically determined developmental unfolding and conflictual experience and views psychopathology as primarily intrapsychically generated. A two-person psychology model emphasizes development and conflict emergent within a relational field and views psychopathology primarily as emergent

---

[4]The terms relational (Greenberg and Mitchell, 1983) and intersubjective (Atwood and Stolorow, 1984) are used here interchangeably. The term relational directly refers to (internal and external) relationships and is easily recognizable and also broadly applicable outside the analytic context; the term intersubjective, in emphasizing the interaction of two subjective worlds (to be distinguished from Stern's (1985) use of the term intersubjective, which refers to a distinctive form of relatedness), includes more easily, when applied to the analytic arena, the full range of self experience in which the relational dimension shifts between foreground and background. Both terms refer to a field model in which the individual is viewed as developing and living within a relational matrix.

within and generated by the relational field. Because these theories of development and pathogenesis reflect an intrapsychic and relational emphasis respectively, a one-person psychology model *applied* to the analytic arena tends to support the classical view of transference as a displacement and projection onto the blank screen of the analyst wherein the contribution of the analyst is considered minimal, that is, transference as distortion (for a review, see Fosshage, 1990a). Interpretation and insight, and not the relational experience, tend to be viewed as the central agents of therapeutic action. Correspondingly, a two-person psychology model supports the view that both patient and analyst variably contribute to the transference (for a review, see Fosshage, 1990a). Conceptualizing the analytic scene as a two-person psychology opens the door to including, if not emphasizing, the new relational experience, in addition to interpretation and insight, as important agents in therapeutic action.

As Modell (1984) and Mitchell (1988) point out, considerable overlap exists between these two theoretical perspectives. The one-person perspective is not "naively solipsistic" and the two-person perspective is not "naively environmental" (Mitchell, 1988, p. 4). Environmental influences are included within a one-person perspective, but the *action* in development, pathogenesis, transference, and therapy tends to be intrapsychic. Conversely, biological determinants are included within a two-person perspective (for example, primary motivations in all psychoanalytic theories are biologically anchored or prewired), but the *action* in development, pathogenesis, transference and therapy tends to be relational. All theories have elements of both, although most theories emphasize, as evidenced in interpretive constructions, one side or the other. Moreover, the elements in the various monadic and dyadic models significantly vary *in content*. For example, all theories of primary motivation assume that motivation is inherent to the organism, but differ as to what the specific motivational strivings are.

Although Freud (1896) in his seduction theory began with a two-person emphasis, his theory evolved primarily into an intrapsychic model. The reemergence of a field perspective in psychoanalysis, the Hegelian "antithesis," has prepared the way, initially, for the use of complementary models (Modell, 1984) and, now, for a possible new synthesis through the integration of the one-person and two-person perspectives (Modell, 1984; Ghent, 1989).[5] As Ghent (1989)

---

[5]Similarly, the developmental arrest (self) theory was initially juxtaposed with the conflict/defense model (Kohut, 1971) as a complementary model in the 1970s and early 80s (see Stolorow and Lachmann, 1980). As the theory evolved a new synthesis

points out, one emergent synthesis, guided by the overlapping work of Winnicott, Guntrip, and Kohut, involves the concept of the self "as the center of activity of the psyche," within a relational field.[6]

With the central focus on the development, consolidation, and maintenance of the self, self psychology is viewed by some advocates (for example, Goldberg, 1986, and Wolf, 1988) and critics (for example, Bromberg, 1989, and, as relating to transference, Hoffman, 1983, and Mitchell, 1988, 1990) as fundamentally a one-person psychology. This assessment, I believe, is based principally on Kohut's initial separation of the narcissistic and object relational lines of development, a separation that he never fully resolved, and on his early notion of merger between self and object when the object serves archaic selfobject functions. To separate conceptually two lines of development implies erroneously that self-development does not occur within a relational field, a theoretical contradiction (to be developed) in the light of the emphasis on the self-selfobject matrix. This separation also erroneously implies that the state of the self does not affect one's object relations and that one's object relations, in turn, do not affect the sense of self. Although Kohut legitimized self-concerns by focusing on the development of the self (in contrast to classical theory wherein the developmental pathway is from infantile narcissism to object relatedness), initially he inadvertently repeated the error in classical theory of dichotomizing self and object relational concerns. Although Kohut (1984) never fully extricated himself from this dichotomization, his description of "self-selfobject relationships" became more relational in that it typically involved two separate persons (see pp. 49–52). Subsequently, other authors (for example, Modell, 1984; Stolorow, Brandchaft, and Atwood, 1987; Bacal, 1990; Bacal and Newman, 1990; Fosshage, 1990c) have more forcefully set forth that the self-selfobject matrix is a relational matrix; they, therefore, consider self psychology, in part, to be fundamentally a two-person field model.

My thesis is that the evolving theory of self psychology, a direction Kohut (1984) provided especially in his last book, newly synthesizes monadic and dyadic features and that a new synthesis is required to

---

emerged in an overarching self psychological theory in which conflict was readily included through a redefinition of the primary ingredients of conflict. A primary model of conflict, in Stolorow's (1985) words, is that "conflict states often arise when central strivings and affective qualities of the person are believed to be inimical to the maintenance of an important selfobject bond" (p. 200). (This model corresponds with Winnicott's, 1960, notion of the formation of "a false self on a compliant basis.")

[6]The concept of self as a guiding center was also central for Jung (1953), but without a corresponding emphasis on the relational field.

provide a comprehensive understanding of an individual and the analytic process. My purpose here is to illustrate this emergent synthesis by examining some of the one-person and two-person features of self psychology in the conceptualizations of psychological development, pathogenesis, transference, and therapeutic action. Self-psychological psychoanalysis, like all psychoanalytic orientations, continues to be an evolving theory and includes a wide range of theoretical and clinical variations and differences. The ensuing discussion, of course, emphasizes my perspective.

PSYCHOLOGICAL DEVELOPMENT

All developmental models posit that human beings are prewired to follow general developmental patterns. The specificity, content, and emphasis of these patterns differ considerably. *How* and *the degree to which development requires* a relational field and *the degree to which the relational field shapes* the person point up the one-person and two-person distinction.

Kohut (1984) placed at the center of psychological development the *self as striving "to realize" "its intrinsic program of action" within a self-selfobject matrix.* Kohut's "nuclear self" refers, in part, to an innate or prewired general developmental program (Goldberg, 1986) involving mirroring, idealizing, and twinship selfobject needs that provides an overall direction to the development of the self.[7] In addition, the nuclear self includes the unique talents through which the emergent ambitions and ideals are expressed. Although Kohut described various experientially accessible features of the self as "vigor," "vitality," "harmoniousness," and an "independent center of initiative," he avoided defining the concept of the self precisely, because of concern that it was premature to reach closure on so new a concept. The "intrinsic program of action" refers to an inbuilt overall developmental "program" or "guiding" principle unique to each person. This notion of a unique guiding center of the person varies in emphasis but has been recognized and described by several psycho-analytic authors. For example, Loewald (1960) writes:

> If the analyst keeps his central focus on this emerging core, he avoids moulding the patient in the analysts's own image or imposing on the

---

[7]These selfobject needs exist throughout one's life (Kohut, 1977) and are not viewed as only infantile needs. While developmental lines are delineated for each selfobject realm, the full range of selfobject experience is always potentially accessible and shaped by immediate needs, stresses, and psychic structure.

patient his own concept of what the patient should become. It requires an objectivity and neutrality the essence of which is love and respect for the individual and for individual development [p. 229].

The conceptualization of an inner "core" emerges in Winnicott's (1960) idea of a "true self" as distinct from a "false self," in Guntrip's (1971) concept of self, and in Jung's (1953) overarching concept of self wherein the self is viewed as a "guiding" center (Whitmont, 1987).[8]

Evidence of an unique inner "core" for each individual and inherent developmental strivings continues to accrue. The concept of self-righting (Tolpin, 1986; Lichtenberg, 1989) has recently been appropriated from the embryologist Waddington (1947), who proposed a genetically programmed self-organizing and self-righting tendency inherent in all organisms. Lichtenberg (1989) posits "an inherent tendency to rebound from a deficit with a developmental advance when a positive change in an inhibiting external condition occurs" (p. 328). Tolpin (1986) observes that the frustrated baby spontaneously revives and insists on getting the "mother to act right!" (p. 121). A deprivation of REM leads to a self-righting or "rebound effect" (see Fiss, 1986, for a review).[9] Self-state dreams (Kohut, 1977) are seen as attempts to restore a failing sense of self. And on the basis of clinical evidence, REM and dream content research, I (Fosshage, 1983, 1987) have postulated that, pertaining to psychological organization, dreaming mentation fundamentally serves developmental, maintenance, and restorative (or self-righting) functions.[10] Regarding the many constitutional givens, Thomas and Chess (1977) have provided us with a powerful research demonstration of basic temperamental differences existent at

---

[8]Comparing interpersonal psychoanalysis and self psychology, Bromberg (1989) suggests that crucial to analysis is our "need to find out who the patient is rather than believing you know in advance what he needs" (p. 283); he ascribes the latter stance to self psychology. Bromberg's analysis may partially rest on Kohut's posited nuclear self, which is unique for each individual; but, it is to be hoped, no analyst, self psychologists included, believes that he or she "know[s] in advance what a patient needs." Bromberg states, and I concur, that we need to discover "who the patient is." Interestingly, his formulation, "who the patient is," implies a "core" self. This "core" self emerges within a relational matrix and within the analytic relationship. Actual theoretical differences probably lie between the degree of emphasis on an intrinsic "nuclear" (Kohut) or "true" (Winnicott) self and the degree to which the self is shaped by the relational matrix.

[9]At the microbiological level, the self-righting tendency is reflected in the discoveries of DNA's complex genetic instructions for damage reparation.

[10]My positing that dreaming, just as waking mentation, can further developmental processes somewhat overlaps with Jung's concept of the compensatory function of dreams. For Jung, when "ego consciousness" deviates from the self, a predominately unconscious developmentally guiding center of personality, the dream attempts to compensate or self-right the person.

birth and continuous throughout life. And based on infant research, Stern (1985) presents an array of hard-wired givens in the developmental unfolding and structuring of a sense of self within an "interpersonal" field. Stern's description of "a continuous unfolding of an intrinsically determined social nature" (p. 234) makes relationships a built-in feature of the self.

The postulation of developmental strivings and of a "nuclear" core, however specified, provides the *motivation for* and the *overall direction* of an analysis. *A person who seeks analytic treatment hopes for the developmentally requisite experiences* (termed, within a self-psychological perspective, the selfobject dimension of the transference or analytic relationship; see Ornstein, 1974, on the search for the new beginning), *expects the old to reoccur and tends to organize and construct the analytic experience according to the well-established schemas (transference), and tends to connect in those characteristic ways established in past relationships.* These various processes are intricately interwoven and are the focus of the analysis. If developmental strivings are not postulated, the analysand tends to be viewed as exclusively invested in the "old," whether conceptualized as infantile fixations or repetitious relational configurations (the latter, for purposes of attachment, psychological organization, or both). Under these circumstances, the overall momentum for analytic change, rather than being buoyed by the analysand's developmental striving to change, can subtly shift to the analyst and potentiate the analysand's accommodation or aversiveness to what then becomes the analyst's agenda for change.

To posit and include developmental strivings, in addition to problematic schemas (transference), profoundly affects the analyst's listening to and organization of clinical material. For example, in a recent case presentation (Fosshage, 1990b) the discussants and the analyst viewed the analysand's incessant demands to feel cared for and "careable" quite differently. Some viewed the analysand's "demandingness" as a remnant of infantile (narcissistic) omnipotence; others, as the repetition of "bad" object relational patterns. Those analysts (including the author) who posit developmental strivings viewed demandingness as partially an expression of both the patient's difficulty with maintaining (due to problematic schemas) and the patient's striving to consolidate a feeling of being cared for and "careable" (Kohut referred to the latter as the "leading edge" of the material [Miller, 1985]; and Guntrip, 1971, as the "cry" within the hysteric).[11]

---

[11]In my view the patient suffered *both* from a deficiency in a positive, cohesive self-structure (namely, an arrest in the development of sense of self as cared for and "careable" and of self-esteem regulatory capacities) *and* from pathological structures,

The emphasis on a prewired general developmental program of the self, primary in self psychology, is a one-person psychology feature. Infant and developmental research and clinical evidence, however, clearly indicate that self-development does not occur in a vacuum. Self-development not only includes relationships as central but *requires* a relational field. Kohut's most important clinical finding focused on the ways that patients make use of their analysts to develop, consolidate, and maintain a positive cohesive sense of self. He conceptualized this dimension of analytic experience as the selfobject transference and gradually etched out a developmental model based on the self-selfobject matrix.[12] Lichtenberg (1991) writes, "In agreement with much infant research, Kohut conceptualizes a constant interrelationship between *motive*, to achieve and restore self cohesion, and *environment*, the empathic responsiveness" (pp. 4–5). Kohut (1984) considered this self-selfobject matrix as a life-giving and -preserving relational matrix:

> Self psychology holds that self-selfobject relationships form the essence of psychological life from birth to death, that a move from dependence (symbiosis) to independence (autonomy) in the psychological sphere is no more possible, let alone desirable, than a corresponding move from a life dependent on oxygen to a life independent of it in the biological spheres [p. 47].

The development of the self *within* a self-selfobject matrix is central to the developmental model and is an emergent theoretical synthesis of one- and two-person psychologies.

Are Self-Selfobject Relationships Relational?

Much confusion surrounds the question whether the self-selfobject matrix is a relational matrix. The confusion emanates, I believe, from

---

namely, a negatively valenced self-schema in relation to problematic schemas of the other. At those times when "normal" development is arrested, resulting in *specific deficiencies* in self-structure, *specific problematic* (or pathological) *structures* are formed (for example, problematic schemas of self and other). Deficiencies and pathological structures are complexly interwoven, further negating the earlier theoretical and clinical dichotomization of developmental arrest and conflict/defense models. (Eagle, 1984, makes the same point, although he retains the notion of conflict as defined within the conflict/defense model.) Psychopathology always includes both arrests in development and conflict, the latter *as redefined* within self psychology (refer to footnote 5). Structural deficiencies and their corresponding developmental needs as well as pathological structures must be addressed analytically.

[12]The concept of the selfobject emphasizes development rather than repetition of the past and, therefore, in my judgment, does not fit properly under the concept of transference. This dimension is more accurately viewed as the selfobject dimension of the analytic relationship (Bacal and Newman, 1990; Fosshage, 1990a).

two sources, namely, the merger concept as applied to self-selfobject connections and the original differentiation between narcissistic and object relational lines of development.

Kohut (1971) initially conceived the self and object to be merged when a person uses the other to provide self-maintenance or self-restorative functions. Without self and object differentiation, so the argument goes, a person cannot "relate" to the other.[13] Therefore, the self-selfobject matrix is not relational. (This line of reasoning is based on a conceptualization of "relating" as requiring self and object differentiation.) Subsequently, Kohut (1977, 1984) suggested that selfobject relationships had developmental lines and only the most "archaic" involved a merger between self and object. Stern's (1985) more recent conception, based on infant research, that self and object differentiation is most probably present at birth requires a reconceptualization of even the earliest self-selfobject relationships.

Kohut (1984) came to view a selfobject "as that *dimension of our experience of another person* that relates to this person's function in shoring up our self" (p. 49; italics added), firmly anchoring the conceptualization of selfobject in a relational matrix. The selfobject dimension is *one* dimension of object relationships that comes to the foreground and recedes into the background depending on self needs (Lichtenberg, 1983; Stolorow, 1986) and the particular relationship. *Self experience is central in the theory and analytic focus, and the many dimensions of object relationships are a major aspect of self experience.* With the selfobject dimension of relationships crucial in development, pathogenesis, transference, and therapeutic action, self psychology becomes fundamentally a relational model (Modell, 1984; Bacal, 1990; Bacal and Newman, 1990; Fosshage, 1990c).

The second source of confusion about whether or not the self-selfobject matrix is relational emanates from Kohut's original division between the narcissistic and object relational lines of development. This division was made, in part, to create a place for the new theory equal in importance to, and without tampering with, the old. His initial postulation of two independent lines of development, to reiterate, inadvertently repeated the error in classical theory of dichotomizing self and object relational concerns. The division implies that how we feel about ourselves does not affect our feelings toward others and vice versa. This theoretical conundrum is resolved

---

[13]Hoffman, 1983, used the argument to support his thesis that Kohut's conception of selfobject transference was not a "social" or two-person model. I believe, as I have spelled out in detail elsewhere (Fosshage, 1990a), that this is an inaccurate assessment, for it is based on Kohut's initial theory of selfobjects involving an archaic merger.

if it is understood that self-development occurs within and requires a relational matrix.

Consistent reference to the self-selfobject matrix within self psychology implies that the selfobject dimension of relationships is primary in development, pathogenesis, transference, and therapeutic action. Because the term self-selfobject matrix inadequately reflects other dimensions of relational experience, Stolorow and his colleagues (Atwood and Stolorow, 1984; Stolorow, Brandchaft, and Atwood, 1987) have introduced the concept of intersubjectivity to encompass the full range of psychological life and the interaction of two subjectivities within the analytic relationship. The complex multidimensions of self-experience and object relations (for example, sexual, aversive, affiliative—see Lichtenberg, 1989) and corresponding schemas are included with greater facility under the rubric of intersubjectivity. Analysis requires focus on *both* the selfobject or developmental dimension of the analytic relationship (Kohut's selfobject transference) *and* on the problematic schemas (transference). The schemas and the selfobject dimension are often intricately interwoven, shifting from background to foreground in a complex interplay. Other self psychologists attempt to include this full range of experience under the rubric of the self-selfobject matrix (P. Ornstein, personal communication).

Lichtenberg (1991) recently shifted the conceptual focus from selfobjects to *selfobject experiences* to maintain the focus on the analysand's experience. Selfobject experience refers to "an affective state of vitality and invigoration, of needs being met and of intactness of self" (p. 478). More precisely, the selfobject experience refers to the dimension of experience that pertains to a vital and invigorated sense of self (Fosshage, 1990c). Kohut's emphasis that a consolidated, vital experience of self can fully occur only when there is an internal sense of empathic resonance with actual or symbolic others is still retained. Even when the activity is solitary and is not relationally dominated, an empathic resonance with others is a necessary ingredient and backdrop for a fully vitalized sense of self.

PATHOGENESIS

Kohut's thesis was that consistently faulty self-selfobject relationships during the formative years were the principal cause for derailments in self-development. Faulty selfobject relationships entail insufficient developmentally required selfobject availability and responsiveness, which disrupts the development and maintenance of a positive cohesive sense of self. Additionally, these ruptures gradually form pathological structures or schemas of self and other, based in part on accommodation to the other to maintain some, albeit limited, selfobject tie (corresponding with Winnicott's, 1960, notion of the "false self"). Originally applied to the narcissistic personality disorder, this basic model of pathogenesis has become applicable to all disorders (viewed as disorders of the self) as the theory has expanded into a supraordinate theory of the psychology of the self. Psychoanalytic self psychology has emphasized developmental derailments *due to relational deficiencies*. For example, Kohut (1977) posited that unresolvable oedipal difficulties were related not to biologically determined oedipal conflict, but to failures in the self and oedipal-selfobject matrix, namely, that the oedipal selfobject had failed to respond adequately to either the sexual or the competitive strivings of the child. Whereas the concept of self, with its "program of action," is a one-person feature, pathogenic derailments, occurring within a two-person matrix, are clearly a two-person feature. Containing both monadic and dyadic features has, ironically, led to contradictory critiques of self psychology: on one hand, as an "asocial," intrapsychic model and, on the other, as a "parent blaming," two-person model.

The combination of monadic and dyadic features is built into the interactional patterns between mother and infant that are currently viewed as the building blocks of psychic structure formation (Stern, 1985; Beebe and Lachmann, 1988). These interactional patterns are based on the temperament of the infant and his or her shifting priority of needs and motivational systems (Lichtenberg, 1989) in conjunction with the attunement of the mother, determined, in part, by her temperament and shifting priority of needs and motivational systems. These interactional patterns gradually build perceptual-affective-cognitive schemas with which subsequent life experience is organized and constructed. A consistent mismatch serves as a basis for developmental derailment *and* formation of pathological structures. The constitutional factors and the shifting needs and motivations of both participants, and the interactions between the participants, are all intricately interwoven and required for understanding the complex developmental or structure formation scenario. This general theory of pathogenesis represents an emergent synthesis of monadic and dyadic features.

TRANSFERENCE

Pivotal to Kohut's contribution was his observation of patients striving to use the analyst for self-restorative and developmental functions, what he came to term *selfobject transferences*. Analysis might focus for some time on self-protective measures and conflicts surrounding the emergence of particular selfobject needs, conflicts principally related to the dread of the repetition of the traumatogenic occurrences of the past (Ornstein, 1974). Working through these conflicts and related protective operations gradually enables the selfobject needs to come to the foreground.

The establishment of selfobject transferences does not depend solely on the selfobject needs, conflicts, schemas, and protective operations of the analysand, but also requires a sufficient availability of the analyst. Kohut (1977) referred to the latter as the requisite "average expectable responsiveness." The selfobject transference is a relational matrix to which *both* analysand and analyst contribute. The conceptualization of the selfobject transference, therefore, is a two-person psychology model. (It can be seen, incorrectly in my judgment, as "asocial" only when the selfobject is not viewed as a relational dimension.)

Recognition of a necessary responsiveness from the analyst implicitly places a new emphasis on the *relational experience* within analysis. Interpretation is one, and certainly not the only, type of response from the analyst which contributes to the relational experience of the patient. Within this complex interactional field, the term optimal responsiveness (Bacal, 1985) more adequately reflects the broad range of analytic interventions that facilitate the analytic process. Without this overarching technical concept, interventions other than interpretation often go unrecognized or are denigrated as nonanalytic. While verbal exploration and interpretation is often optimal, at times nonverbal communication, for example, a facial expression, is the optimal response (see Balint, 1968).

Notwithstanding that the selfobject dimension of the analytic relationship is central from a self psychological perspective, are there other dimensions of the relationship and of self experience that need to be brought into the analysis? Kohut (1984), never completely resolving his dichotomizing narcissistic and object relational concerns, confusingly noted that the object relational transferences, that is, transferences related to object relational conflicts (as if these did not involve the selfobject dimension and were essentially different) also required analysis. According to Kohut, object relational transferences frequently served as needed-to-be-analyzed impediments to the emergence of selfobject needs and the establishment of selfobject transferences. The principal structure-building process, for Kohut, occurred through the establishment and analysis of the selfobject transferences.

A new, albeit not unitary, model of transference has subsequently emerged, which I have termed the organization model (for a review of the model and the contributions of Gill and Hoffman, Stolorow and Lachmann, Wachtel, and myself, see Fosshage, 1990a). In this model transference refers to perceptual-affective-cognitive organizing principles or schemas (generated out of interactional patterns and thematic experiences) with which the analysand perceives, organizes and constructs the analytic experience.[14] These schemas include a successful or failing selfobject feature, namely, the feature that enhances or depletes a vital sense of self. For example, an analysand's expectation (schema) of an abusive other based on past experience involves a particular view of the other that incorporates a selfobject failure. Analysis focuses principally on the illumination of the problematic schemas (that is, schemas that involve arrested development and render conflict unresolvable) as they are activated in the analytic relationship and on the selfobject dimension of the analytic relationship as the analysand uses the analyst for self-development and self-maintenance.

Both analysand and analyst *variably* contribute to the analytic relationship. When entering analysis, the analysand hopes for the new (that is, the selfobject need or developmental striving is in the forefront), expects the old (according to the schemas), and organizes and interacts in ways (based on schemas) that tend to elicit new and old repetitious relational experiences. As part of this two-person conception of transference, or, more accurately, the analytic relationship, the analyst attempts to understand and explain the analysand's experience through organizing the experience with his or her schemas.

Understanding transference as variably shaped by both analysand and analyst within a two-person field model enables us to recognize that the degree to which the analyst contributes to the activation of the analysand's schema will determine whether the schema can be illuminated or the schema is reinforced through a replication of the relational pattern. For example, if the analysand fearfully expects the analyst to be removed and emotionally unresponsive, the degree to

---

[14] As I have delineated, the conceptualization of transference as an organizing activity nullifies the dichotomy between distorted and realistic perceptions and the use of this dichotomy to differentiate transference from nontransference (Fosshage, 1990a, pp. 12–15). Schemas vary quantitatively along a number of dimensions, for example, frequency of use, modifiability, conscious awareness, and self-enhancing versus self-depleting, that prevent a dichotomization between transference and nontransference. For these reasons, I have proposed the use of the term schemas. The term transference is used to refer to those schemas and to typically problematic schemas activated within the analytic relationship.

which the analyst's behavior and presence corresponds with this schema will determine whether the schema is reinforced or illuminated. "The patient will only be able to observe and identify a particular organizing principle when the contribution of the analyst is sufficiently minimal that alternative interpretations, from the patient's vantage point, are feasible" (Fosshage, 1990a, p. 26).

Terminologically, "countertransference" places the emphasis on the analyst's reactions to the transference and does not adequately reflect the totality of the analyst's subjectivity participating in the analytic encounter.[15] "Both patient and analyst shape the countertransference and, as with transference, the contribution of each can range from minimal to extreme" (p. 18). For example, the analyst, like the patient, may selectively attend to minimal cues in experiencing the patient. The analyst's activated schemas and reactions may or may not facilitate the analysis, depending on the respective patient and analyst contributions to the analyst's experience and on the subsequent analysis of the intersubjective scenario. Discrepancies between analyst and patient experiences can be useful in understanding and analyzing the intersubjective encounters (Wolf, 1988). The recognition of the interaction of two subjectivities occurring within the analytic arena makes this a more complete field model.

The complex intersubjective nature of the patient–analyst encounter precludes so-called inevitable countertransferences, namely, specific countertransferences that all analysts would predictably experience in reaction to specific transferences. For example, what one analyst might experience as hostility, another might experience as assertiveness.

The analyst is often portrayed as inevitably "pulled into" the transference, but within a field model it becomes clear that the analyst also shapes *how* he or she is pulled in (Fosshage, 1990a). Similarly, the analyst must be sufficiently available to the developmental "pull" of the selfobject dimension of the analytic relationship, but that response too is shaped by the analyst.

The complex interaction of analysand and analyst and their respective subjectivities reflected in the evolving organization model of transference synthesizes one- and two-person elements.

---

[15]In viewing countertransference as encumbering or distorting the analyst's view, Kohut never extricated himself from the "classical" view of countertransference. In contrast, his recognition of the importance of the "personal presence" of the analyst, the need for the analyst to be sufficiently available ("average expectable responsiveness") and the formulation and emphasis on the self-selfobject matrix in the analytic arena, all underscored the profound participation of the analyst and the analyst's subjectivity in the analytic process.

THERAPEUTIC ACTION

Fundamental ingredients of therapeutic action are: (1) an ongoing, sufficiently consistent and reliable experience of selfobject (idealizing, mirroring, and twinship) components within the analytic relationship; (2) the subsequent analysis and consequent management of the self-selfobject ruptures; (3) the illumination, within the current context, of primary problematic experiential themes and schemas and their geneses (that is, analysis of transference); and (4) the fundamentally new relational experience (that is, self with other) that in large measure is created by the previously mentioned components of the analytic process. These processes bring about psychological organization, an increase in regulatory and management capacities (structure building), and modification of problematic schemas (structural change).

An Ongoing Selfobject Experience

Kohut (1982) recognized (somewhat reluctantly) that the use of the empathic mode of observation, by providing an ongoing experience of being acknowledged and understood, could be therapeutic. This realization opened the door to recognizing the potentially curative value of the relational experience within the analytic arena, a major departure from the traditional emphasis on interpretation and insight (resonating with the work of Ferenczi, Balint, Winnicott, Guntrip, and others). By 1984, Kohut had acknowledged without hesitation the curative or developmental value of an ongoing selfobject experience (see p. 78). He was well aware that this experience could be called an "emotionally corrective experience," but unlike Alexander (1956), he stipulated that the analyst should not *sharply* deviate from the analytic stance. Yet, Kohut (1977) recognized that the analyst had to be sufficiently available for the selfobject or developmental "pull" and referred to it, as previously noted, as the "average expectable responsiveness."

> Although this average empathic responsiveness lies within a broad band in the spectrum of possibilities and allows many individual variations, it is not—*in principle*—an approximation of the functions of a psychologically programmed computer that restricts its activities to giving correct and accurate interpretations. The conclusion that it is "in principle" true that the analyst must not try to function like a well-programmed computer rests on two premises: that the *analyst's responses require the participation of the deep layers of his personality* and . . .

that the responses of a computer would not constitute an average expectable environment for the analysand [p. 252; second italics added].

The "human presence" (Kohut, 1984) is crucially important and is basic to therapeutic action. The relationship within which the analysand can develop (partially created by but certainly not limited to interpretation and insight) makes clear that the model of therapeutic action represents, once again, a new synthesis of one- and two-person psychology features.

Whereas some self psychologists are still reluctant to speak of the new relational experiences in psychoanalysis and still emphasize interpretation as the primary mode of intervention (see Wallerstein, 1985), others are not (see Bacal, 1985; Stolorow et al., 1987; Wolf, 1988; Fosshage, 1990a, c). The *interpretive sequence* is crucially important in psychoanalysis and often central, but it needs to be viewed, in addition to its insight-increasing aim, as *a response of the analyst* that contributes to the analysand's experience of the relationship. Often the interpretive sequence is optimal in facilitating the analytic and developmental processes, and at times other actions are necessary (for example, see Bacal's, 1985, discussion of Kohut's well-known offering of his "two fingers" to be held by a deeply depressed patient).

The Subsequent Analysis and Consequent Management of the Self-Selfobject Ruptures

With the emergence of a selfobject connection, often following analysis of protective measures (defenses), Kohut emphasized as central to therapeutic action the repair of the inevitable self-selfobject ruptures through interpretation. These self-selfobject ruptures are ruptures in the relational (understanding the selfobject dimension to be a component of relationships) connection between patient and analyst that negatively affect the patient's sense of self. During a so-called optimal rupture, the patient may be able to "stretch" and provide the necessary self-regulatory function without, or in spite of, the analyst. And following the repair of ruptures (by understanding the patient's experience), optimal and not, the patient incrementally learns that ruptures are manageable and thus increases overall regulatory capacity.

Self-selfobject ruptures are inevitable because no analyst can understand perfectly or always be sufficiently available for the necessary selfobject functions and because a analysand will tend to perceive, organize, and construct the analytic experience by using problematic schemas that entail selfobject failures. Yet, analysts contribute more or less to ruptures (a two-person field model). Specific ruptures (with regard to content) may or may not occur, depending in part on the contribution of the analyst.

Recognizing that analysts contribute more or less to self-selfobject ruptures raises a thorny question: Do analysts, or should analysts, ever attempt to avoid selfobject ruptures? Deviating from the "standard" analytic stance is typically viewed as a momentarily necessary parameter or more often as a countertransferentially acting in (an example is how some discussants viewed my answering an analysand's question [Fosshage, 1990b]). To view the analytic stance as static is a remnant of a one-person psychology and positivistic science. Ornstein (1990) recently noted:

> Any entry into a psychoanalysis—as well as the full journey through it—is always highly idiosyncratic for both participants, no matter how we may generalize about these entries. On this microscopic level there is nothing "standard" or "well defined" about the precise conduct of an analysis, because no two analyses are ever alike, even if they are not haphazard and have their definite, well-articulated general "rules" [p. 478].

Ruptures are inevitable and, indeed, through repair enable structure-building and structure-changing (reorganization). Yet, when the analyst contributes "too much" to the rupture, or when the patient is feeling particularly fragile, or in the beginning phase of treatment when the analytic connection is still unreliable, the rupture can prove to be retraumatizing and unanalyzable. If we are not sufficiently "pliable" (Balint, 1968) (for example, to avoid, if only temporarily, certain behaviors that are particularly traumatic to the analysand), the analysand, at the least, may not feel understood or, at the worst, may experience the analyst as not caring to understand. A field model enables recognition that the analyst is a full participant in the analytic relationship. This recognition, the ramifications of which are still emerging, is central in self psychology and, indeed, in all relational perspectives.

The Illumination Within the Current Context of Primary Problematic Schemas and Their Geneses (the Analysis of Transference)

The analysis of the schemas or transference is vital to facilitating psychological reorganization. As primary problematic schemas are illuminated within the analytic and extraanalytic relationships and their geneses understood, the analysand gradually becomes able to suspend and even to transform these schemas and develops new ways of experiencing and organizing his or her sense of self, others, and the world.

The analysand's use of particular schemas results in selective attention to, and at times behaviors that elicit specific cues or responses. Because both participants contribute to the analysand's experience, it is the degree of contribution from the analyst that will in large measure determine whether or not the schema is illuminated or the experiential pattern on which the schema is based is repeated and the schema is reinforced. Although the analyst's contribution is usually inevitable (for something the analyst does will usually activate a patient's primary schema), the analyst's contribution can vary widely. Other factors that affect whether a schema is analyzable or is reinforced are the history of the analytic relationship, including the previous illumination of the particular schema, the rigidity of the schema, and frequency of its use.

The Fundamentally New Relational Experience (That Is, Self with Other) That in Large Measure Is Created by the Components of the Analytic Process

Within a self-psychological field model, the process of understanding and explaining selfobject needs, ruptures, and schemas substantially provides a *new relational experience*. To consider this new relational experience as an overriding central change agent (in contrast to insight, which is only one, albeit very important, aspect of the relational experience) facilitates inclusion of the vast array of complex and subtle verbal and nonverbal communications and experiences that go on within the analytic situation. The experience of this process, discussed and not discussed, ultimately provides new interactional patterns that are the basis for new schemas of self and other, and self with other. Within a field model, new relational experiences, within which interpretation (that is, understanding and explaining) and insight are often central ingredients, are fundamental to psychological organization and reorganization.

CONCLUSION

Self psychology, with its emphasis on the unique "program of action" of the nuclear self, a one-person psychology, and its emphasis on the self-selfobject matrix, a two-person psychology, is providing an emergent synthesis of monadic and dyadic features for the understanding of development, pathogenesis, transference and therapeutic action.

REFERENCES

Alexander, F. (1956), *Psychoanalysis and Psychotherapy*. New York: Norton.

Atwood, G. & Stolorow, R. (1984), *Structures of Subjectivity*. Hillsdale, NJ: The Analytic Press.

Bacal, H. (1985), Optimal responsiveness and the therapeutic process. In: *Progress in Self Psychology, Vol. 1*, ed. A. Goldberg. New York: Guilford Press, pp. 202–227.

_____ (1990), Does an object relations theory exist in self psychology? *Psychoanal. Inq.*, 2:197–220.

_____ & Newman, K. (1990), *Theories of Object Relations*. New York: Columbia University Press.

Balint, M. (1968), *The Basic Fault*. London: Tavistock.

Beebe, B. & Lachmann, F. (1988), Mother–infant mutual influence and precursors of psychic structure. In: *Frontiers of Self Psychology: Progress in Self Psychology, Vol. 3*, ed. A. Goldberg. Hillsdale, NJ: The Analytic Press, pp. 3–26.

Bromberg, P. (1989), Interpersonal psychoanalysis and self psychology: A clinical comparison. In: *Self Psychology*, ed. D. Detrick & S. Detrick. Hillsdale, NJ: The Analytic Press, pp. 275–292.

Eagle, M. (1984), *Recent Developments in Psychoanalysis*. New York: McGraw-Hill.

Fiss, H. (1986), An empirical foundation for a self psychology of dreaming. *J. Mind & Beh.*, 7:161–191.

Fosshage, J. (1983), The psychological function of dreams: A revised psychoanalytic perspective. *Psychoanal. Contemp. Thought*, 6:4:641–669.

_____ (1990a), Toward reconceptualizing transference: Theoretical and clinical considerations. Presented at American Psychological Association Division 39 meeting, April 5, New York City.

_____ (1990b), Clinical protocol and the analyst's reply. *Psychoanal. Inq.*, 4:461–477, 601–622.

_____ (1990c), The latest word: A discussion with the authors of three major contributions to self psychology. Presented at the 13th Annual Conference on the Psychology of the Self, Oct. 21, New York City.

_____ (1987), A revised psychoanalytic approach. In: *Dream Interpretation* (rev. ed.), ed. J. Fosshage & C. Loew. Costa Mesa, CA: PMA.

Freud, S. (1896), The aetiology of hysteria. *Standard Edition*, 3:187–221. London: Hogarth Press, 1955.

_____ (1921), Group psychology and the analysis of the ego. *Standard Edition*, 18:69–143. London: Hogarth Press, 1955.

Ghent, E. (1989), Credo: The dialectics of one-person and two-person psychologies. *Contemp. Psychoanal.*, 2:169–211.

Goldberg, A. (1986), Reply to Philip M. Bromberg's discussion of "The Wishy-Washy Personality" by Arnold Goldberg. *Contemp. Psychoanal.*, 22:387–388.

Greenberg, J. & Mitchell, S. (1983), *Object Relations in Psychoanalytic Theory*. Cambridge, MA: Harvard University Press.

Greenson, R. (1960), Empathy and its vicissitudes. *Internat. J. Psycho-Anal.*, 41:418–424.

Guntrip, H. (1971), *Psychoanalytic Theory, Therapy, and the Self*. New York: Basic Books.

Hoffman, I. Z. (1983), The patient as interpreter of the analyst's experience. *Contemp. Psychoanal.*, 3:389–422.

Jung, C. (1953), *Two Essays on Analytical Psychology: The Collected Works of C. G. Jung*, Vol. 7, New York: Pantheon.

Kohut, H. (1959), Introspection, empathy and psychoanalysis. *J. Amer. Psychoanal. Assn.*, 7:459–483.

_____ (1971), *The Analysis of the Self*. New York: International Universities Press.

_____ (1977), *The Restoration of the Self*. New York: International Universities Press.

_____ (1982), Introspection, empathy, and the semicircle of mental health. *Internat. J. Psycho-Anal.*, 63:395–408.

_____ (1984), *How Does Analysis Cure?* ed. A. Goldberg & P. Stepansky. Chicago: University of Chicago Press.

Lichtenberg, J. (1981), The empathic mode of perception and alternative vantage points for psychoanalytic work. *Psychoanal. Inq.*, 3:329–356.

_____ (1983), *Psychoanalysis and Infant Research*. Hillsdale, NJ: The Analytic Press.

_____ (1989), *Psychoanalysis and Motivation*. Hillsdale, NJ: The Analytic Press.

_____ (1991), What is a selfobject? *Psychoanal. Dial.*, 1:455–479.

Loewald, H. (1960), On the therapeutic action of psychoanalysis. *Internat. J. Psycho-Anal.*, 58:463–472.

Miller, J. (1985), How Kohut actually worked. In *Progress in Self Psychology, Vol. 1*, ed. A. Goldberg. New York: Guilford Press, pp. 13–30.

Mitchell, S. (1988), *Relational Concepts in Psychoanalysis*. Cambridge, MA: Harvard University Press.

_____ (1990), A relational view. *Psychoanal. Inq.*, 10:523–540.

Modell, A. (1984), *Psychoanalysis in a New Context*. New York: International Universities Press.

Ornstein, A. (1974), The dread to repeat and the new beginning. The *Annual of Psychoanalysis*, 2:231–248, New York: International Universities Press.

Ornstein, P. (1990), How to "enter" a psychoanalytic process conducted by another analyst: A self psychology view. *Psychoanal. Inq.*, 10:478–497.

Rickman, J. (1951), Number and the human sciences. In: *Psychoanalysis and Culture*. New York: International Universities Press. (Reprinted in *Selected Contributions on Psychoanalysis*. London: Hogarth Press, 1957).

Schwaber, E. (1984), Empathy, a mode of analytic listening. In: *Empathy II*, ed. J. Lichtenberg, M. Bornstein & D. Silver. Hillsdale, NJ: The Analytic Press, pp. 143–172.

Stern, D. (1985), *The Interpersonal World of the Infant*. New York: Basic Books.

Stolorow, R. (1985), Toward a pure psychology of inner conflict. In: *Progress in Self Psychology, Vol. 1*, ed. A. Goldberg. New York: Guilford Press, pp. 193–201.

_____ (1986), On experiencing an object: A multidimensional perspective. In: *Progress in Self Psychology, Vol. 2*, ed. A. Goldberg. New York: Guilford Press, pp. 273–279.

_____ & Lachmann, F. (1980), *Psychoanalysis of Developmental Arrests*. New York: International Universities Press.

_____ Brandchaft, B. & Atwood, G. (1987), *Psychoanalytic Treatment*. Hillsdale, NJ: The Analytic Press.

Thomas, A. & Chess, S. (1977), *Temperament and Development*. New York: Brunner/Mazel.

Tolpin, M. (1986), The self and its selfobjects: A different baby. In: *Progress in Self Psychology, Vol. 2*, ed. A. Goldberg. New York: Guilford Press, pp. 115–128.

Waddington, C. (1947), *Organizers and Genes*. Cambridge, UK: The University Press.

Wallerstein, R. (1985), How does self psychology differ in practice? *Internat. J. Psycho-Anal.*, 66:391–404.

Whitmont, E. (1987), Jungian approach. In *Dream Interpretation* (rev. ed.), ed. J. Fosshage & C. Loew. Costa Mesa, CA: PMA, pp. 53–78.

Winnicott, D. W. (1960), Ego distortion in terms of true and false self. In: *The Maturational Processes and the Facilitating Environment*. London: Hogarth Press, 1965, pp. 56–63.

Wolf, E. (1988), *Treating the Self.* New York: Guilford Press.

3

Recognition and Destruction
An Outline of Intersubjectivity

JESSICA BENJAMIN

We are all of us born in moral stupidity, taking the world as an udder
to feed our supreme selves: Dorothea had early begun to emerge from
that stupidity, but yet it had been easier to her to imagine how she
would . . . become wise and strong in his strength and wisdom, than
to conceive with that distinctness which is no longer reflection but
feeling . . . that he had an equivalent center of self, whence the lights
and shadows must always fall with a certain difference.

George Eliot, *Middlemarch*, p. 243.

In recent years analysts from diverse psychoanalytic schools have
converged in the effort to formulate relational theories of the self
(Eagle, 1984; Mitchell, 1988). What these approaches share is the belief
that the human mind is interactive rather than monadic, that the
psychoanalytic process should be understood as occurring between
subjects rather than within the individual (Atwood and Stolorow,
1984; Mitchell, 1988). Mental life is seen from an intersubjective perspective. Although this perspective has transformed our theory and
our practice in important ways, such transformations create new problems. A theory in which the individual subject no longer reigns absolute must confront the difficulty that each subject has in recognizing
the other as an equivalent center of experience (Benjamin, 1988).

The problem of recognizing the other emerges the moment we

An earlier version of this chapter appeared in *Psychoanalytic Psychology*, 1990,
7(suppl.):33–47.

consider that troublesome legacy of intrapsychic theory, the term "object." In the original usage, still common in self psychology and object relations theories, the concept of object relations refers to the psychic internalization and representation of interactions between self and objects. While such theories ascribe a considerable role to the early environment and parental objects—"real" others—they have taken us only to the point of recognizing that "where ego is, objects must be." For example, neither Fairbairn's insistence on the need for the whole object nor Kohut's declaration that selfobjects remain important throughout life addresses directly the difference between object and other. Perhaps the elision between "real" others and their internal representation is so widely tolerated because the epistemological question of what is reality and what is representation appears to us, in our justifiable humility, too ecumenical and lofty for our parochial craft. Or perhaps, because we are psychoanalysts, the question of reality does not really trouble us.

But the unfortunate tendency to collapse other subjects into objects cannot simply be ascribed to this irresoluteness with regard to reality. Nor can it be dismissed as a terminological embarrassment that could be dissolved by greater linguistic precision (see Kohut, 1984). It is instead a symptom of the very problems in psychoanalysis that a relational theory should aim to cure. An inquiry into the intersubjective dimension of the analytic encounter would aim to change our theory and practice so that "where objects were, subjects must be."

What does such a change mean? A beginning has been made with the introduction of the term intersubjectivity for the analytic situation (Atwood and Stolorow, 1984; Stolorow, Brandchaft, and Atwood, 1987), defining intersubjectivity as the field of intersection between two subjectivities, the interplay between two different subjective worlds. But how is the meeting of two subjects different from one in which a subject meets object? Once we have acknowledged that the object makes an important contribution to the life of the subject, what is added by deciding to call this object another subject? And what are the impediments to the meeting of two minds?

To begin our inquiry, we must address this question: what difference does the other make, the other who is perceived as truly outside, not within our mental field of operations? Isn't there a dramatic difference between the experience with the other perceived as outside the self and the subjectively conceived object? Winnicott (1971) formulated the basic outlines of this distinction in what may well be considered his most daring and radical statement, "The Use of an Object and Relating Through Identifications." Since then, with a few exceptions (Eigen, 1981; Modell, 1984; Ghent, 1989), there has been little effort to elaborate Winnicott's juxtaposition of the two possible relationships of the subject to the object. Yet, as I show here, the difference between the other as subject and the other as object is crucial for a relational psychoanalysis.

The distinction between the two types of relationships to the other can emerge clearly only if we acknowledge that both are endemic to psychic experience and hence both valid areas of psychoanalytic inquiry. If there is a contradiction between the two modes of experience, then we ought to probe it as a condition of knowledge rather than assume it to be a fork in the road. Other theoretical grids that have bifurcated psychoanalytic thought—drive theory vs. object relations theory, ego vs. id psychology, intrapsychic vs. interpersonal theory—insisted on a choice between the two opposing perspectives. I am proposing, instead, that the two dimensions of experience with the object/other are complementary, even though they sometimes stand in an oppositional relationship. By encompassing both dimensions, we can fulfill the intention of relational theories: to account both for the pervasive effects of human relationships on psychic development and for the equally ubiquitous effects of internal psychic mechanisms and fantasies in shaping psychological life and interaction.

I refer to the two categories of experience as the intrapsychic and the intersubjective dimensions (Benjamin, 1988). The idea of intersubjectivity, which has been brought into psychoanalysis from philosophy (Habermas, 1970, 1971), is useful because it specifically addresses the problem of defining the other as object. Intersubjectivity was deliberately formulated in contrast to the logic of subject and object that predominates in Western philosophy and science. It refers to that zone of experience or theory in which the other is not merely the object of the ego's need/drive or cognition/perception, but has a separate and equivalent center of self.

Intersubjective theory postulates that the other must be recognized as another subject in order for the self to fully experience his or her subjectivity in the other's presence. This means, first, that we have a need for recognition and second, a capacity to recognize others in return—mutual recognition. But recognition is a capacity of individual development that is only unevenly realized—in a sense, the point of a relational psychoanalysis is to explain this fact. In Freudian metapsychology the process of recognizing the other "with that distinctness which is no longer reflection but feeling" would appear, at best, as a background effect of the relationship between ego and external reality. Feminist critics of psychoanalysis have suggested that the conceptualization of the first other, the mother, as an object underlies this theoretical lacuna: cultural antithesis between male subject and female object contributed much to the failure to take into account the subjectivity of the other. The denial of the mother's subjectivity, in theory and in practice, profoundly impedes our ability to see the world as inhabited by equal subjects. My purposes are to show that, in fact, the capacity to recognize the mother as a subject is an important part of early development; and to bring the process of recognition into the foreground of our thinking.

I suggest some preliminary outlines of the development of the capacity for recognition. In particular I focus on separation-individuation theory, showing how much more it can reveal when it is viewed through the intersubjective lens, especially in the light of the contributions of both Stern and Winnicott. Because separation-individuation theory is formulated in terms of ego and object, it does not fully realize its own contribution. In the ego-object perspective the child is the individual, seen as moving in a progression toward autonomy and separateness. The telos of this process is the creation of psychic structure through internalization of the object in the service of greater independence.

As a result, separation-individuation theory focuses on the structural residue of the child's interaction with the mother as object; it leaves the aspects of engagement, connection, and active assertion that occur with the mother as other in the unexamined background. This perspective is infantocentric: Typical studies of mother–child interaction will formulate the mother's acts of independence as a contribution to the child's self-regulation but not to the child's recognition of her subjectivity. (see, e.g., Settlage et al., 1991) This perspective also misses the *pleasure* of the evolving relationship with a partner from whom one knows how to elicit a response, but whose responses are not entirely predictable and assimilable to internal fantasy. The idea of pleasure was lost when ego psychology put the id on the backburner, but it might be restored by recognizing the subjectivity of the other.

An intersubjective perspective helps to transcend the infantocentric viewpoint of intrapsychic theory by asking how a person becomes capable of enjoying recognition with an other. Logically, recognizing the parent as subject cannot simply be the result of internalizing the parent as mental object. This is a developmental process that has barely begun to be explicated. How does a child develop into a person who, as a parent, is able to recognize her or his own child? What are the internal processes, the psychic landmarks, of such development? Where is the theory that tracks the development of the child's responsiveness, empathy, and concern, and not just the parent's sufficiency or failure?

It is in regard to these questions that most theories of the self have fallen short. Even self psychology, which has placed such emphasis on attunement and empathy and has focused on the intersubjectivity of the analytic encounter, has been tacitly one-sided in its understanding of the parent–child relationship and the development of intersubjective relatedness. Perhaps in reaction against the oedipal reality principle, Kohut (1977, 1984) defined the necessary confrontation with the other's needs or with limits in a self-referential way — optimal failures in empathy (parallel to analysts' errors) — as if there were nothing for children to learn about the other's rights or feelings. Although the goal of self psychology was to enable individuals to open "new channels of empathy" and "in-tuneness between self and selfobject" (Kohut, 1984, p. 66), the self was always the recipient, not the giver of empathy. The responsiveness of the selfobject, by definition, serves the function of "shoring up our self" throughout life; but at what point does it become the responsiveness of the outside other whom we love? The occasionally mentioned (perhaps more frequently assumed) "love object," who would presumably hold the place of outside other, has no articulated place in the theory. Thus, once again the pleasure in mutuality between two subjects is reduced to its function of stabilizing the self, not of enlarging our awareness of the outside, nor of recognizing others as animated by independent though similar feelings.[1]

In this essay I outline some crucial points in the development of recognition. It is certainly true that recognition begins with the other's confirming response that tells us we have created meaning, had an impact, revealed an intention. But very early on we find that recognition between persons — understanding and being understood, being in attunement — begins to be an end in itself. Recognition between persons is essentially mutual. By our very enjoyment of the other's confirming response, we recognize her in return. I think that what the research on mother–infant interaction has uncovered about early reciprocity and mutual influence is best conceptualized as the development of the capacity for mutual recognition. The frame-by-frame studies of face-to-face play at three to four months have given us a kind of early history of recognition.

The pathbreaking work of Stern (1974, 1977, 1985) and the more recent contributions of Beebe (1977, 1985, 1988) have illuminated how crucial the relationship of mutual influence is for early self-

---

[1]My remarks may be more apt for Kohut than for self psychology as a whole, which has recently shown an impetus to correct this one-sidedness and to include the evolution of difference in relation to the other (e.g., Lachmann, 1986) as well as the relationship to the "true" object (Stolorow, 1986).

development. They have also shown that self-regulation at this point is achieved through regulating the other: I can change my own mental state by causing the other to be more or less stimulating. Mother's recognition is the basis for the baby's sense of agency. Equally important, although less emphasized, is the other side of this play interaction: the mother is dependent to some degree on the baby's recognition. A baby who is less responsive is a less "recognizing" baby, and the mother who reacts to her apathetic or fussy baby by overstimulation or withdrawal is a mother feeling despair that the baby does not recognize her.

In Stern's (1985) view, however, early play does not yet constitute intersubjective relatedness. He instead designates the next phase, when affective attunement develops at eight or nine months, as intersubjectivity proper. This is the moment when we discover "there are other minds out there!" and that separate minds can share a similar state. I would agree that this phase constitutes an advance in recognition of the other, but I think the earlier interaction can be considered an antecedent, in the form of concrete affective sharing. Certainly, from the standpoint of the mother whose infant returns her smile, affective sharing is already the beginning of reciprocal recognition. Therefore, rather than designate the later phase as intersubjective relatedness, I would rather conceptualize a development of intersubjectivity in which there are key moments of transformation.

In this phase, as Stern (1985) emphasizes, the new thing is the sharing of the inner world. The infant begins to check out how the parent feels when he is discovering a new toy and the parent demonstrates attunement by responding in another medium. By translating the same affective level into another modality—for instance, from kinetic to vocal—the adult conveys the crucial fact that it is the *inner* experience that is congruent. The difference in form makes the element of similarity or sharing clear. I would add that the parent is not literally sharing the same state, since the parent is (usually) excited by the infant's reaction, not the toy itself. The parent is in fact taking pleasure in *contacting the child's mind.*

Here is a good point to consider the contrast between intersubjective theory and ego psychology, a contrast Stern makes much of. The phase of discovering other minds coincides roughly with Mahler's differentiation and practicing subphases, but there is an important difference in emphasis. In the intersubjective view, the infant's greater separation, which Mahler emphasizes in this period, actually proceeds in tandem with, and enhances the felt connection with, the other. The joy of intersubjective attunement is: This *other* can share my feeling. According to Mahler (Mahler, Pine, and Bergman, 1975),.

though, the infant of ten months is primarily involved in exploring, in the "love affair with the world." The checking back to look at mother is not about sharing the experience, but about safety/anxiety issues, "refueling." It is a phase in which Mahler sees the mother not as contacting the child's mind, but giving him a push from the nest.

While Stern emphasizes his differences with Mahler, I think the two models are complementary, not mutually exclusive. It seems to me that here intersubjective theory amplifies separation-individuation theory by focusing on the affective exchange between parent and child and by stressing the simultaneity of connection and separation. Instead of opposite endpoints of a longitudinal trajectory, connection and separation form a tension, which requires the equal magnetism of both sides.

Now it is this tension between connection and separation that I suggest we track beyond the period of affective attunement. If we follow it into the second year of life, we can see a tension developing between assertion of self and recognition of the other. Translating Mahler's rapprochement crisis into the terms of intersubjectivity, we can say that in this crisis the tension between asserting self and recognizing the other breaks down and is manifested as a conflict between self and other.

My analysis of this crisis derives, in part, from philosophy, from Hegel's (1807) formulation of the problem of recognition in *The Phenomenology of Spirit*. In his discussion of the conflict between "the independence and dependence of self-consciousness" Hegel showed how the self's wish for absolute independence conflicts with the self's need for recognition. In trying to establish itself as an independent entity, the self must yet recognize the other as a subject like itself in order to be recognized by the self, immediately compromising the self's absoluteness and posing the problem that the other could be equally absolute and independent. Each self wants to be recognized and yet maintain his absolute identity: the self says, I want to affect you, but I want nothing you do or say to affect me, I am who I am. In its encounter with the other, the self wishes to affirm its absolute independence, even though its need for the other and the other's similar wish give the lie to it.

This description of the self's absoluteness covers approximately the same territory as narcissism in Freudian theory, particularly its manifestation as omnipotence: the insistence on being one (everyone is identical to me) and all alone (there is nothing outside of me that I do not control). Freud's (1911, 1915) conception of the earliest ego with its hostility to the outside, or its incorporation of everything good into itself, is not unlike Hegel's absolute self. Hegel's notion of the conflict between independence and dependence meshes with the classic psychoanalytic view in which the self does not wish to give up omnipotence.

But even if we reject the Freudian view of the ego, the confrontation with the other's subjectivity and the limits of self-assertion is a difficult one to negotiate. The need for recognition entails this fundamental paradox: in the very moment of realizing our own independent will, we are dependent upon another to recognize it. At the very moment we come to understanding the meaning of I, myself, we are forced to see the limitations of that self. At the moment when we understand that separate minds can share similar feelings, we begin to find out that these minds can also disagree.

Let us return to Mahler and her associates' (1975) description of rapprochement, and see how it illustrates the paradox of recognition and how the infant is supposed to get out of it. Prior to rapprochement, in the self-assertion of the practicing phase, the infant still takes herself for granted, and her mother as well. She does not make a sharp discrimination between doing things with mother's help and without it. She is too excited by *what* she is doing to reflect on who is doing it. Beginning about 14 months a conflict emerges between the infant's grandiose aspirations and the perceived reality of her or his limitations and dependency. Although now able to do more, the toddler is aware of what she or he can't do and what she or he can't make mother do—for example, stay with her or him instead of going out. Many of the power struggles that begin here (wanting the whole pear, not a slice) can be summed up as a demand: "recognize my intent!" The child will insist that mother share everything, participate in all her or his deeds, acquiesce to all her or his demands. The toddler is also up against the increased awareness of separateness, and, consequently, of vulnerability: she or he can move away from mother—but mother can also move away from her or him.

If we reframe this description from the intersubjective perspective, the infant now knows that different minds can feel differently, that he or she is dependent as well as independent. In this sense, rapprochement is the crisis of recognizing the other, specifically of confronting mother's independence. It is no accident that mother's leaving becomes a focal point here, for it confronts the child not only with separation but with mother's independent aims. For similar reasons, the mother may experience conflict at this point; the child's demands are now threatening, no longer simply needs, but expressions of his or her independent (tyrannical) will. The child is different from *her* mental fantasy, no longer *her* object. He may switch places with her: from passive to active. He, not she, is now the repository of omnipotence once attributed to the "good" all-giving mother. How she responds to her child's and her own aggression depends on her ability to mitigate such fantasies with a sense of real agency and separate selfhood, on her confidence in her child's ability to survive conflict, loss, imperfection. The mother has to be able to both set clear boundaries for her child and to recognize the child's will, to both insist on her own independence and respect that of the child—in short, to balance assertion and recognition. If she cannot do this, omnipotence continues, attributed either to the mother or the self; in neither case can we say that the development of mutual recognition has been furthered.

From the standpoint of intersubjective theory, the ideal "resolu-" tion" of the paradox of recognition is for it to continue as a *constant tension* between recognizing the other and asserting the self. However, in Mahler's (1975) theory the rapprochement conflict appears to be resolved through internalization, the achievement of object constancy—when the child can separate from mother or be angry at her and still be able to contact her presence or goodness. In a sense, this sets the goal of development too low: it is difficult and therefore sufficient for the child to accomplish the realistic integration of good and bad object representations (Kernberg, 1980). The sparse formulation of the end of the rapprochement conflict is, shall we say, anticlimactic, leaving us to wonder, is this all? In this picture, the child has only to accept mother's disappointing her; she or he does not begin to shift her or his center of gravity to recognize that mother does this because she has her own center.

The breakdown and recreation of the tension between asserting one's own reality and accepting the other's is a neglected aspect of the crisis, but it is equally important. This aspect emerges when we superimpose Winnicott's (1971) idea of destroying the object over Mahler's rapprochement crisis. It is destruction—negation in Hegel's sense—that enables the subject to go beyond relating to the object through identification, projection, and other intrapsychic processes having to do with the subjectively conceived object. It enables the transition from relating (intrapsychic) to using the object, carrying on a relationship with an other who is objectively perceived as existing outside the self, an entity in her own right. That is, in the mental act of negating or obliterating the object, which may be expressed in the real effort to attack the other, we find out whether the real other survives. If she survives without retaliating or withdrawing under the attack, then we know her to exist outside ourselves, not just as our mental product.

Winnicott's scheme can be expanded to postulate not a sequential relationship but rather a basic tension between denial and affirmation of the other (between omnipotence and recognition of reality). Another way to understand the conflicts that occur in rapprochement is through the concepts of destruction and survival: the wish to absolutely assert the self and deny everything outside one's own mental omnipotence must sometimes crash against the implacable reality of the other. The collision Winnicott (1971) has in mind, however, is not one in which aggression occurs "reactive to the encounter with the reality principle," but one in which aggression "creates the quality of externality" (p. 110). When the destructiveness damages neither the parent nor the self, external reality comes into view as a sharp, distinct contrast to the inner fantasy world. The outcome of this process is not simply reparation or restoration of the good object, but love, the sense of discovering the other (Eigen, 1981; Ghent, 1990).

The flipside of Winnicott's analysis would be that when destruction is not countered with survival, when the other's reality does not come into view, a defensive process of internalization takes place. Aggression becomes a problem—how to dispose of the bad feeling. What cannot be worked through and dissolved with the outside other is transposed into a drama of internal objects, shifting from the domain of the intersubjective into the domain of the intrapsychic. In real life, even when the other's response dissipates aggression, there is no perfect process of destruction and survival; there is always also internalization. All experience is elaborated intrapsychically, we might venture to say, but when the other does not survive and aggression is not dissipated it becomes almost exclusively intrapsychic. It therefore seems to me fallacious to see internalization processes only as breakdown products or defenses; I would see them rather as a kind of underlying substratum of our mental activity—a constant symbolic digestion process that constitutes an important part of the cycle of exchange between the individual and the outside. It is the loss of balance between the intrapsychic and the intersubjective, between fantasy and reality, that is the problem.

Indeed, the problem in psychoanalytic theory has been that internalization—either the defensive or the structure-building aspects (depending on which object relations theory one favors)—has obscured the component of destruction that Winnicott (1964, p. 62) emphasizes: discovering "that fantasy and fact, both important, are nevertheless different from each other." The complementarity of the intrapsychic and intersubjective modalities is important here: as Winnicott makes clear, it is in contrast to the *fantasy* of destruction that the *reality* of survival is so satisfying and authentic.

Winnicott thus offers a notion of a reality that can be loved, something beyond the integration of good and bad. While the intrapsychic ego has reality imposed from the outside, the intersubjective ego discovers reality. This reality principle does not represent a detour to wish fulfillment, a modification of the pleasure principle. Nor is it the acceptance of a false life of adaptation. Rather it is a continuation under more complex conditions of the infant's original fascination with and love of what is outside, his appreciation of difference and novelty. This appreciation is the element in differentiation that gives separation its positive, rather than simply hostile, coloring: love of the world, not merely leaving or distance from mother. To the extent that mother herself is placed outside, she can be loved; separation is then truly the other side of connection to the other.

It is this appreciation of the other's reality that completes the picture of separation and explains what there is beyond internalization—the establishment of shared reality. First (1988) provided some very germane observations of how the toddler does begin to apprehend mutuality as a concomitant of separateness, specifically in relation to the mother's leaving. The vehicle of this resolution is, to expand Winnicott's notion, cross-identification: the capacity to put oneself in the place of the other based on empathic understanding of similarities of inner experience. The two-year-old's initial role-playing imitation of the departing mother is characterized by the spirit of pure retaliation and reversal—"I'll do to you what you do to me." But gradually the child begins to identify with the mother's subjective experience and realizes that "I could miss you as you miss me," and, therefore, that "I know that you could wish to have your own life as I wish to have mine." First shows how, by recognizing such shared experience, the child actually moves from a retaliatory world of control to a world of mutual understanding and shared feeling. This analysis adds to the idea of object constancy, in which the good object survives the bad experience, the idea of recognizing that the leaving mother is not bad but independent, a person like me. By accepting this, the child gains not only her own independence (as traditionally emphasized) but also the pleasure of shared understanding.

Looking backward, we can trace the outlines of a developmental trajectory of intersubjective relatedness up to this point. Its core feature is recognizing similarity of *inner* experience in tandem with difference. We could say that it begins with "We are feeling this feeling," and then moves to "I know that you, who are an other mind, share this same feeling." In rapprochement, however, a crisis occurs as the child begins to confront difference—"you and I don't want or feel the same thing." The initial response to this discovery is a breakdown of recognition between self and other: I insist on my way, I refuse to recognize you, I begin to try to coerce you, and therefore I experience your refusal as a reversal: you are coercing me. As in earlier phases, the capacity for mutual recognition must stretch to accommodate the tension of difference, in this case to accept the knowledge of conflicting feelings.

In the third year of life this tension can be expressed in symbolic play. The early play at retaliatory reversal may now be a kind of empowerment in which the child feels "I can do to you what you do to me." But then the play expands to include the emotional identification with the other's position, and becomes reflexive so that, as First puts it, "I know you know what I feel." In this sense, the medium of shared feeling remains as important to intersubjectivity in later phases as in early ones. But it is now extended to symbolic understanding of feeling so that "you know what I feel, even when I want or feel the opposite of what you want or feel." This advance in differentiation means that "we can share feelings without my fearing that my feelings are simply your feelings."

The child who can imaginatively entertain both roles—leaving and being left—begins to transcend the complementary form of the mother-child relationship. The complementary structure organizes the relationship of giver and taker, doer and done to, powerful and powerless. It allows one to reverse roles, but not to alter them. In the reversible relationship, each person can play only one role at a time: one person is recognized, the other negated; one subject, the other object. This complementarity does not dissolve omnipotence, but shifts it from one partner to the other. The movement out of the world of complementary power relations into the world of mutual understanding thus shows us an important step in the dismantling of omnipotence: power is dissolved, rather than transferred back and forth in an endless cycle between child and mother. Again, this movement refers not to a one-time sequence or final accomplishment, but an ongoing tension between complementarity and mutuality.

When mutual recognition is not restored, when shared reality does not survive destruction, complementary structures and "relating" to the inner object predominate. Because this occurs commonly enough, the intrapsychic, subject-object concept of the mind actually fits with the dominant mode of internal experience. This is why—notwithstanding our intersubjective potential—the reversible complementarity of subject and object conceptualized by intrapsychic theory illuminates so much of the internal world. The principles of mind Freud first analyzed—reversal of opposites like active and passive, the exchangeability or displacement of objects—thus remain indispensable guides to the inner world of objects.

But even when the capacity for recognition is well-developed, when the subject can use shared reality and receive the nourishment of "other-than-me substance," the intrapsychic capacities remain. The mind's ability to manipulate, to displace, to reverse, to turn one thing into another is not a mere negation of reality, but the source of mental creativity. Furthermore, when things go well, complementarity is a step on the road to mutuality. The toddler's insistent reciprocity, his or her efforts to reverse the relationship with the mother, to play at feeding, grooming, and leaving her, is one step in the process of identification that ultimately leads to understanding. It is only when this process is disrupted, when the complementary form of the relationship is not balanced by mutual activity, that reversal becomes entrenched and the relationship becomes a struggle for power.

The attempt to reverse the mother's omnipotence within the context of complementary structures may shed light on the problem of male dominance. One important mental structure that has perpetuated male power is the complementarity in which male = subject and female = object. As feminist theory has repeatedly pointed out, the failure of psychoanalysis to formulate a perspective in which the mother appears as subject limits our understanding of the infant as well. Insofar as the mother–infant relationship postulated by much psychoanalytic thinking was framed in terms of subject-object complementarity, the theory reproduced the prevalent cultural stance toward woman as mother. In other words, there is both a formal fit and a dynamic relationship between subject–object relations and male-female relations. Formally, the reversible, complementary structure of the mother–infant dyad dovetails with later representations of self-other relations as power relationships. Dynamically, the omnipotent mother of this dyad becomes the basis for the dread and retaliation that inform men's exercise of power over women. Thus the adult relation between men and women becomes the locus of the great reversal, turning the tables on the omnipotent mother of infancy.

The intersubjective view of development offers a contrast that throws this reversal into bold relief. It shows that within the maternal dyad mutuality exists alongside complementarity, and the child engages in the first struggles for recognition. This is in direct contrast to the implicit assumption, from Freud up to the current work of Chasseguet-Smirgel (1986), that the acceptance of reality and the separation from the mother are brought about through the intervention and internalization of the oedipal father. In this view, the mother remains archaic and omnipotent in the child's mind and omnipotence must be counteracted by power of the oedipal father. The underlying premise is that the problem of recognition (that is, narcissism) cannot be worked on or resolved within the relationship to the primary other; it requires the intercession of an outside other, a third term, the "Name of the Father" as Lacan (1977) explicitly proposed. In other words, two subjects alone can never confront each other without merging, one being subordinated and assimilated by the other. This position justifies a split in which the mother's power is displaced onto the father, and he serves as the independent other whom the (boy) child recognizes and with whom he struggles.

But, according to the intersubjective theory of destruction and recognition, differentiation does take place within the maternal dyad. Omnipotence can be counterbalanced and in this sense overcome. For it is not necessary that the fantasy of maternal omnipotence be dispelled, only that it be modified by the existence of another dimension—mutual recognition. From this perspective, the problem lies not in the unconscious fantasy of maternal omnipotence per se. Rather, the dread of the mother that has been linked to domination in the masculine stance toward women (Horney 1932; Stoller, 1975) becomes problematic when not counterbalanced by the development of intersubjectivity.

Horney's (1932) remarks on male dread of woman illustrate how the loss of intersubjectivity affects the subject as well as the object: " 'It is not,' he says, 'that I dread her; it is that she herself is malignant, capable of any crime, a beast of prey, a vampire, a witch, insatiable in her desires. She is the very personification of what is sinister' " (p. 135). The projective power of this fantasy reflects the predominance of the intrapsychic over the intersubjective: "she is that thing I feel." The lack of intersubjectivity in this psychic situation can be conceptualized as the assimilation of the subject to the object, as the lack of the space in between subjects. As Ogden (1986) puts it, the existence of potential space between mother and child allows the establishment of the distinction between the symbol and the symbolized. The subject who can begin to make this distinction now has access to a triangular field—symbol, symbolized, and interpreting subject. The space between self and other can exist and facilitate the distinction, let us say, between the real mother and the symbolic mother; this triangle is created without a literal third person.[2] Lacking

---

[2]Of course, the satisfactory development of this space may generate or become associated with the intrapsychic representation of the third person, even in children with one parent. The point here is not to disqualify oedipal representations, but to say

that space, the mother becomes the dreaded but tempting object; the subject is overwhelmed by that object since it really is "the thing in itself" (Ogden, 1986). In the denial of the other's subjectivity the exercise of power begins.

The creation of this space within the relationship between infant and mother is an important dimension of intersubjectivity, a concomitant of mutual understanding. This space is not only a function, as Winnicott emphasized, of the child's play alone in the presence of the mother, but also of play between mother and child, beginning with the earliest play of mutual gaze. As we see in First's (1988) analysis of play with identification with the leaving mother, the transitional space also evolves within the communicative interaction between mother and child. Within this play, the mother is simultaneously "related to" in fantasy, but "used" to establish mutual understanding, a pattern that parallels transference play in the analytic situation. In the elaboration of this play the mother can appear as the child's fantasy object as well as other subject without threatening the child's subjectivity.

The existence of this space is ultimately what makes the intrapsychic capacities creative rather than destructive; perhaps it is another way of referring to the tension between using and relating. Using, that is recognizing, implies the capacity to transcend complementary structures, but not the absence of them. It does not mean the disappearance of fantasy or of negation but that "destruction becomes the unconscious backcloth for love of a real object." (Winnicott, 1971, p. 111) It means a balance of destruction with recognition. In the broadest sense, internal fantasy is always eating up or negating external reality—"While I am loving you I am all the time destroying you in (unconscious) fantasy" (p. 106). The loved one is being continually destroyed but its survival means that we can eat our reality and have it too. From the intersubjective standpoint, all fantasy is the negation of the real other, whether the fantasy's content is negative or idealized; just as, from the intrapsychic view, external reality is simply that which is internalized as fantasy. The ongoing interplay of destruction and recognition is a dialectic between fantasy and external reality.

---

that the oedipal father is not the way out of an otherwise engulfing maternal dyad. More likely, the traditional formulation of the oedipal relationship, which has emphasized identification with an idealized male power as the payoff for renouncing the mother, represents a fantasy "solution." But when the symbolic father does substitute for the space between mother and child, the mother's existence as an object of desire remains terrifying; the oedipal repudiation of femininity, with its disparagement of women, then becomes a further obstacle to the creation of intersubjective space.

In the analytic process, the effort to share the productions of fantasy changes the status of fantasy itself, moving it from inner reality to intersubjective communication. The fantasy object who is being related to or destroyed and the usable other who is there to receive the communication and be loved complement each other. What we find in the good hour is a momentary balance between intrapsychic and intersubjective dimensions, a sustained tension or rapid movement between the patient's experience of us as inner material and as the recognizing other. This suspension of the conflict between the two experiences reflects the successful establishment of a transitional space in which the otherness of the analyst can be ignored as well as recognized. The experience of a space that allows both creative exploration within omnipotence and aknowledgment of an understanding other is, in part, what is therapeutic about the relationship.

The restoration of balance between intrapsychic and intersubjective in the psychoanalytic process should not be construed as an adaptation that reduces fantasy to reality, but rather as practice in the sustaining of contradiction. When the tension of sustaining contradiction breaks down, as it frequently does, the intersubjective structures—mutuality, simultaneity and paradox—are subordinated in favor of complementary structures. The breakdown of tension between self and other in favor of relating as subject and object is a common fact of mental life. For that matter, breakdown is a common feature within intersubjective relatedness—what counts is the ability to restore or repair the relationship. As Beebe and Lachmann (1988) have proposed, one of the main principles of the early dyad is that relatedness is characterized not by continuous harmony but by continuous disruption and repair (Beebe and Lachmann, 1991; Tronick, 1989).

Thus an intersubjective theory can explore the development of mutual recognition without equating breakdown with pathology. It does not require a normative ideal of balance which decrees that breakdown reflects failure, and that the accompanying phenomena—internalization/fantasy/aggression—are pathological. If the clash of two wills is an inherent part of intersubjective relations, then no perfect environment can take the sting from the encounter with otherness. The question becomes how the inevitable elements of negation are processed. It is "good enough" that the inward movement of negating reality and creating fantasy should eventually be counterbalanced by an outward movement of recognizing the outside. To claim anything more for intersubjectivity would invite a triumph of the external, a terrifying psychic vacuity, an end to creativity altogether. A relational psychoanalysis should leave room for the messy, intrapsychic side of creativity and aggression; it is the contribution of the intersubjective view that may give these elements a more hopeful cast, showing destruction to be the "other" of recognition.

REFERENCES

Atwood, G. & Stolorow, R. (1984), *Structures of Subjectivity*. Hillsdale, NJ: The Analytic Press.

Beebe, B. (1985), Mother–infant mutual influence and precursors of self and object representations. In: *Empirical Studies of Psychoanalytic Theories, Vol. 2*, ed. J. Masling. Hillsdale, NJ: The Analytic Press, pp. 27–48.

_____ & Lachmann, F. (1988), Mother–infant mutual influence and precursors of psychic structure. In: *Frontiers in Self Psychology: Progress in Self Psychology, Vol. 3*, ed. A. Goldberg. Hillsdale NJ: The Analytic Press, pp. 3–25.

_____ & Lachmann, F. (1991), The organization of representation in infancy: Three principles. Unpublished manuscript.

_____ & Stern, D. (1977), Engagement-disengagement and early object experiences. In: *Communicative Structures and Psychic Structures*, ed. N. Freedman & S. Grand. New York: Plenum Press.

Benjamin, J. (1988), *The Bonds of Love*. New York: Pantheon.

Chasseguet-Smirgel, J. (1986), *Sexuality and Mind*. New York: New York University Press.

Eagle, M. (1984), *Recent Developments in Psychoanalysis*. Cambridge, MA: Harvard University Press.

Eigen, M. (1981), The area of faith in Winnicott, Lacan and Bion. *Internat. J. Psychoanal.*, 62, 413–433.

Eliot, George. (1871), *Middlemarch*. Harmondsworth, Eng.: Penguin, 1965.

Fairbairn, W. R. D. (1952), *Psychoanalytic Studies of the Personality*. London: Routledge & Kegan Paul.

First, E. (1988), The leaving game: I'll play you and you'll play me: The emergence of the capacity for dramatic role play in two-year-olds. In: *Modes of Meaning*, ed. A. Slade & D. Wolfe. New York: Oxford University Press, pp. 132–166.

Freud, S. (1911), Formulation on the two principles in mental functioning. *Standard Edition*, 12:213–226. London: Hogarth Press, 1958.

_____ (1915), Instincts and their vicissitudes. *Standard Edition*, 14:11–140. London: Hogarth Press, 1957.

Ghent, E. (1989), Credo: The dialectics of one-person and two-person psychologies. *Contemp. Psychoanal.*, 25:169–211.

_____ (1990), Masochism, submission, surrender. *Contemp. Psychoanal.*, 26:108–136.

Habermas, J. (1970), A theory of communicative competence. In: *Recent Sociology, No. 2*, ed. H. P. Dreitzel. New York: Macmillan.

_____ (1971), *Knowledge and Human Interests*. Boston: Beacon.

Hegel, G. W. F. (1807), *Phenomenologie des Geistes*. Hamburg: Felix Meiner, 1952.

Horney, K. (1932), The dread of women. In: *Feminine Psychology*. New York: Norton, 1967.

Kernberg, O. (1980), *Object Relations Theory and Clinical Psychoanalysis*. New York: Aronson.

Kohut, H. (1977), *The restoration of the self*. New York: International Universities Press.
_____ (1984), *How Does Analysis Cure?* ed. A. Goldberg & P. Stepansky. Chicago: University of Chicago Press.
Lacan, J. (1977), *Ecrits, A Selection*. New York: Norton.
Lachmann, F. (1986), Interpretation of psychic conflict and adversarial relationships: A self psychological perspective. *Psychoanal. Psychol.*, 3:341–355.
Mahler, M., Pine, F. & Bergman, A. (1975), *The Psychological Birth of the Human Infant*. New York: Basic Books.
Mitchell, S. (1988), *Relational Concepts in Psychoanalysis*. Cambridge, MA: Harvard University Press.
Modell, A. (1984), *Psychoanalysis in a New Context*. New York: International Universities Press.
Ogden, T. (1986), *The Matrix of the Mind*. New York: Aronson.
Settlage, C. F., Bemesderfer, S. J., Rosenthal, J., Afterman, J. & Spielman, P. M. (1991), The appeal cycle in early mother–child interaction: Nature and implications of a finding from developmental research. *J. Amer. Psychoanal. Assn.*, 39:987–1014.
Stern, D. (1974), The goal and structure of mother–infant play. *J. Amer. Acad. Child Psychiat.*, 13:402–421.
_____ (1977), *The First Relationship*. Cambridge, MA: Harvard University Press.
_____ (1985), *The Interpersonal World of the Infant*. New York: Basic Books.
Stoller, R. (1975), *Perversion*. New York: Pantheon.
Stolorow, R. (1986), On experiencing an object: A multidimensional perspective. In: *Progress in Self Psychology, Vol. 2*, ed. A. Goldberg. New York: Guilford, pp. 273–279.
_____ Brandchaft, B. & Atwood, G. (1987), *Psychoanalytic Treatment*. Hillsdale, NJ: The Analytic Press.
Tronick, E. (1989), Emotions and emotional communication. *Amer. Psychol.*, 44:112–119.
Winnicott, D. W. (1964), *The Child, the Family and the Outside World*. Harmondsworth, Eng.: Penguin.
_____ (1971), The use of an object and relating through identifications. In: *Playing and Reality*. London: Tavistock.

4

A Dyadic Systems View
of Communication

BEATRICE BEEBE
JOSEPH JAFFE
FRANK M. LACHMANN

Although psychoanalysis has developed a rich understanding of the self and the object, we suggest that the dyad as a system of communication is less well conceptualized. The dyad has always been of interest to psychoanalysis, but not until recently has it begun to be recognized as central to an understanding of development and of psychoanalytic theory and practice. A dyadic systems view of communication can elucidate the nature of interpersonal process and interactive regulation in the dyad. It has implications for our concepts of psychic structure and its formation and can facilitate an integration of one-person and two-person psychology models.

Historically, dyadic systems and the process of interpersonal influence have been of major concern to psychoanalysts (Sullivan, 1953), social psychologists (Cottrell, 1942), cognitive psychologists (Vygotsky, 1978), philosophers (Simmel, 1950; Mead, 1934), biological systems theorists (von Bertalanffy, 1952; Weiss, 1973) and ethologically oriented observers (Blurton Jones, 1972; McGrew, 1972; Bowlby, 1980). Much of the early work was programmatic, even poetic, and devoid of operational definitions that might enable quantitative studies. In the time domain, the analysis of dyadic systems has been given methodological sophistication by researchers employing the method of "interaction chronometry" (Chapple, 1970, 1971; Jaffe and Feldstein,

The authors wish to thank Stanley Feldstein, Ph.D., Cynthia Crown, Ph.D., Michael Jasnow, Ph.D., Kenneth Feiner, Psy.D., Sarah Hahn-Burke, Nancy Freeman, and Marina Koulomzin.

1970; Matarazzo and Wiens, 1972; Condon and Sander, 1974; Warner, 1987; Cappella, 1991a). Interpersonal process in the dyadic system has also been a central theme in the literature on mother–infant interaction that has burgeoned in the last 20 years.

We use Bloom's (1983) distinctions to define communication in two senses. One refers to the linguistic content of messages, including wishes and fantasies. This chapter does not address communication in this sense. The second refers to the way communication has most often been studied in infant social interactions: "a framing of the interaction—a 'getting into sync'—that involves a process in which persons act in ways that are responsive to the actions of those with whom they are in communication" (p. 84). This aspect of communication, often out of awareness, conveys "the affective quality of the relationship, . . . through observation of rhythm sharing, body movement, timing of speech, and silences" (p. 84). Although psychoanalysis tends to focus on the linguistic content of communication, it is important to note that the paralinguistic aspect of communication is a "necessary frame . . . for communication with language" to occur (p. 84).

Altmann (1967) defines social communication as "a process by which the behavior of an individual affects the behavior of others" (p. 326). We conceive of communication as the mutual modification of two ongoing streams of behavior of two persons. Each person has his own likelihood (probability) of behaving. At any particular moment, the behavior of an individual is not a determined process. Communication occurs when each person affects the probability distribution of the other's behavior. We believe that when such communication occurs, cognitive and affective changes also occur.

HISTORICAL BACKGROUND OF DYADIC SYSTEMS

In describing the interactive model informing much of infant research, Tronick (1980) reviewed the contributions of a number of philosophers and scientists who all, in various ways, articulated a dyadic systems view of communication (Mead, 1934; Lashley, 1951; Habermas, 1969; Ryan, 1974; Bruner, 1977). He noted that, using such terms as a system of mutuality, a system of reciprocal relations and reciprocal obligations, mutual recognition, and a shared set of rules, they converged in their views regarding how interactions are structured. Exemplifying a profoundly dyadic view of communication, Habermas (1969) suggested that the primary task in communication is to understand the messages of the other while at the same time modifying one's own action in accord both with the other's intentions and with one's own (see also Tronick, 1980). This formulation implicitly takes into account both the self-regulatory and the interactive dimensions of interaction that we spell out later.

Vygotsky (1978) proposed the dyad as the irreducible unit of study. He considered that all higher functions originate as actual relations between individuals. He wrote, "Any function in the child's development appears . . . first on the social level, and later on the individual level; first between people . . . and then inside the child . . . (p. 57). Ruesch and Bateson (1951) also used the term mutual influence and emphasized the dyadic nature of communication:

> The mutual recognition of having entered into each other's field of perception equals the establishment of a system of communication. . . . The perception of the perception . . . is the sign that a silent agreement has been reached by the participants, to the effect that mutual influence is to be expected [p. 23].

Purely verbal conversation, as on the telephone, requires turntaking, since it is difficult to speak and listen at the same time (Jaffe, 1977). When two people smile at each other, however, they are simultaneously sending and receiving information. In a face-to-face dyadic system, unlike in telephone communication, there can be simultaneous transmission of information between continuously adjusting organisms. Such nonverbal communication provides the most extreme example of simultaneous transmission of information where the information-processing limitations of verbal exchange are absent. It requires a continuous control model, where sending and receiving are concurrent and reciprocally evoked (Jaffe, 1962). In his conceptualizations of the evolution of dialogue and the derailment of dialogue, Spitz (1983) also conceptualized a process where sending and receiving were simultaneous.

BIDIRECTIONAL MODEL OF INFLUENCE

Although the ideas underlying a dyadic systems view have been conceptually influential for decades, only more recently have they been operationalized sufficiently for quantitative research to be done. This quantitative emphasis has been particularly strong in the research on mother–infant interaction where bidirectional influences have now been extensively documented and a systems model of the dyad has been richly elaborated. In his study of adaptation in the early weeks of life, Sander (1977, 1985) has suggested that the organization of behavior be viewed primarily as a property of the mother–infant system rather than as a property of the individual. The dyad, rather than the individual, is treated as the system. Nevertheless, the individuals are the components, each with his or her own range of self-regulatory capacities. Within this model, mother and infant should no longer be studied as two isolated entities, each sending the other discrete messages as if one person provided the "stimulus" and the other the "response" (Condon and Sander, 1974). Rather, they should be studied as a system of "shared organizational forms," such as shared rhythms, or shared affective directions. Using this model, it is also no longer possible to conceptualize either partner as "activated by the other." Rather, each brings to the exchange his or her own intrinsic motivation (Piaget, 1937; Hunt, 1965; Berlyne, 1966) and primary endogenous activity. Sander (1977) emphasized the primary activity characteristic of all living organisms:

> In the process of adaptation between the components (organism and environment), one is not activated by the other, but the two, already complexly organized and actively generating behavior, must be interfaced with each other to reach an enduringly harmonious coordination. . . . That is, both mother and infant are seen as inherently in states of readiness or reactivity; these become synchronized or coordinated one with each other [p. 136].

A remarkable body of research, both experimental and naturalistic, now exists with which to further define Sander's claim that the infant brings an inherent readiness to the interactive exchange. A body of research on perceptual capacities documents the infant's ability to detect and expect order in the environment and to react with distress to violations of expected order (DeCasper and Carstens, 1980; Spelke and Cortelyou, 1981; Fagen et al., 1984; Watson, 1985). Haith (cited in Emde, 1988) suggests that "the infant is biologically prepared to engage in visual activity in order to stimulate its own brain" and is "self-motivated to detect regularity, to generate expectancies, and to act upon these expectancies" (p. 29). The work on perturbations of naturalistic exchanges extends the conclusions of the experimental perception work into the naturalistic domain (Tronick et al., 1978; Cohn and Tronick, 1983; Murray and Trevarthen, 1985). These studies all demonstrate that in the naturalistic social exchange infants bring a similar inherent readiness to behave. They have the capacity to detect order and to react with distress to violated expectancies. Finally, Sander's (1977) suggestion that these inherent states of reactivity in both partners must become coordinated has been borne out by two decades of work on the naturalistic social exchange documenting many patterns of mutually regulated coordination to be described further later.

These dyadic systems concepts have influenced infant researchers and helped to generate a bidirectional model of mutual influence. In his seminal paper, Bell (1968) opened the question of direction of influence. He argued that most of the literature to date had emphasized parental influence on children, a one-way influence model, to the relative exclusion of the child's influence on the parent.

Interest in the contribution of the infant was paralleled by a growing body of evidence that infants are both active and socially effective (Lewis and Rosenblum, 1974). With increasing recognition of the infant's social competence, researchers became interested in a bidirectional, or mutual, model of influence. Informally, the most romantic extremes of this theorizing seemed to verge on a notion of adult–infant symmetry. The mutual influence model, however, does not assume that each partner influences the other in equal measure or like manner. The mother obviously has a greater range, control, and flexibility of behavior than the infant. Rather, the basic assumption is that each partner's behavior can be shown to be predictable from that of the other, regardless of the particular content of the behavior, which may indeed be age- or experientially specific. Thus, when we speak of dyadic symmetry, we mean something more abstract, in the sense that both partners actively contribute to the regulation of the exchange. This notion is beautifully illustrated by the analyses of communicative timing using the method of interaction chronometry and time-series analysis to be discussed.

There is a dynamic interplay between mother and infant, and each affects the other's actions, perception, affect, and proprioceptions to create a great variety of mutual regulatory patterns. With development, both infant and caretaker are continuously influenced and altered by the other in systematic ways. Although the bidirectional model of influence points to the importance of the dyad in conceptualizing the organization of individual behavior, this model is incomplete without the additional specification of the individual's self-regulatory contribution.

The Integration of Mutual Regulation and Self-Regulation

Various research traditions, each with its own methods and literature spanning development across the lifespan, have tended to focus either on self-regulation or interactive regulation to the relative exclusion of the other. Such traditions as psychophysiology, cybernetic models, endocrinology, and maturational approaches to development have examined self-regulation by addressing such issues as arousal; rhythmicity; organization of cycles of sleep–wake, REM sleep, breathing, and feeding; and various pathological patterns of autonomic reactivity. In contrast, ethology and social psychology have focused on dyadic regulation and examined such issues as eye contact, proxemics, conversational rhythms, games, and signaling. These approaches to dyadic regulation construe the dyad as the critical unit of organization. The dyad is seen as a system of joint participation in shared organizational forms, such as shared rhythms or affective displays (Condon and Sander, 1974). Some research approaches, however, have explicitly integrated the self-regulatory and the interactive approaches (see, e.g., Brazelton, Kozlowski, and Main, 1974; Sander, 1977, 1985; Lichtenberg, 1983; Hofer, 1984, 1987; Gianino and Tronick, 1988).

Similarly, in the infant literature on the development of psychic structure and the self some authors emphasize self-regulation as the key organizing principle (see, e.g., Stechler and Kaplan, 1980; Emde, 1981). Others emphasize mutual interactive regulation (Stern, 1971, 1977; Beebe and Lachmann, 1988) or an integration of the two (Sander, 1977, 1985; Demos, 1983, 1984; Lichtenberg, 1983; Hofer, 1984, 1987; Gianino and Tronick, 1988; Beebe and Lachmann, 1990; Lachmann and Beebe, 1992). Sander's view that organization is a property of the dyadic system, rather than solely of the individual, explicitly integrates the simultaneous influences of self and mutual regulation. A theory of interactive behavior must specify how each person is affected by his own behavior—self-regulation—as well as that of the partner—interactive regulation (Thomas and Martin, 1976).

The study of self regulation can begin with the fetus. Brazelton (1973) has shown that the fetus regulates its level of arousal and responsivity as a function of the nature of the stimulation provided. For example, when the experimenter shone a very bright light on the mother's belly, the fetus changed its state, dampened its arousal, and eventually put itself to sleep to cope with aversive stimulation. When the light was changed to a more moderate level, the fetus again changed state and now showed patterns of approaching the stimulus. Thus, the fetus continued to monitor the nature of incoming stimulation and regulate its own state in relation to the nature of this stimulation.

Newborns differ in temperament and in their capacity to regulate their states, modulate their arousal levels, and in general to organize their behaviors predictably. The importance of the initial intactness of the organism's capacity to tolerate and use stimulation alerts us to the enormous contribution of normal self-regulatory capacities that are prerequisite to engaging with the environment. This capacity can be compromised to varying degrees, for example, in premature infants or in autistic children. The Brazelton (1973) Neonatal Assessment Scale was specifically designed to evaluate the joint contribution of self- and mutual regulation. It assesses the infant's self-regulatory capacity, for example, to dampen his state in response to aversive stimuli. At the same time, it assesses how much help from the partner is required and can be utilized by the infant to stabilize his state after stress and to maintain engagement with the environment.

The integration of mutual and self-regulation has a direct bearing on the development of representations and psychic structure as organized through the dyad. The current concept that self and object and their representations are rooted in relationship structures (Fast, 1985, 1987; Kegan, 1982; Stern, 1985; Wilson and Malatesta, 1989) holds true only so long as relationship structures are broadly construed to include an integration of self-regulatory with mutual regulatory processes. To posit the dyadic interaction alone as the source of psychic structure formation omits the crucial contribution of the organism's own self-regulatory capacities (Beebe and Lachmann, 1990).

Individual Stability of Responsivity Versus Emergent Properties of the Dyad

To what degree can interpersonal responsivity be conceptualized as a stable characteristic of a person, and to what degree can a person's responsivity be conceptualized as unique to a particular partner? These two factors always operate, but the balance between them may shift in different dyadic systems. For example, in a pathological mother–infant dyad, the difficulty may be seen as a relatively stable characteristic of either partner. That is, the baby may be intrinsically hard to reach, or the adult partner may actually be producing difficulty in the baby. Alternatively, the nature of relatedness may be seen as an emergent property of the unique dyadic system, that is, unique to this particular dyad, and not attributable to stable characteristics of either partner. An integration of these factors provides a view of the dyadic system as organized *both* by stable characteristics of the participants (a one-person psychology model) and by emergent dyadic properties (a two-person psychology model).

Consistency of responsiveness across partners is one way of

defining the degree to which a person's responsivity is a stable characteristic. This question is ideally addressed using a "round-robin" design, in which each person interacts with every other person, yielding interactions between all possible dyads in the group. For each individual in the round-robin design, a range of interpersonal environments can be studied, and each person can be evaluated both as actor and as partner. For example, if persons A, B, C, and D interact, it is possible to evaluate whether person A (the actor) is consistent in responding to partners B, C and D. This is known as the "actor effect" (B→A, C→A, D→A). It is also possible to evaluate whether A is consistent in eliciting responsivity from partners B, C, and D. This is known as the "partner effect" (A→B, A→C, A→D). The same procedure can be followed with each of B, C, and D as the target person. Finally, it is possible to evaluate the degree to which each dyad matches level of responsivity, that is, whether A's responsivity to B is similar to B's responsivity to A. This is known as the "relationship effect."

Cappella (1991b) used this round-robin design to evaluate the coordination of vocal timing in eight adults. He did not find much consistency in either actor effects or partner effects. He did, however, find high relationship effects. Each dyad reached some kind of match of responsivity specific to that particular interaction. Although this work needs to be replicated with a larger sample, it suggests that each person does not necessarily have a generalized level of responsivity or stimulus value that he carries with him into various interactions. Instead, each dyad generates its own unique system in which both participants adjust their level of responsivity to each other in ways they do not necessarily display with other partners.

Transactional approaches propose that systems that function together are changed by their mutual activity; that is, they generate emergent properties (Sameroff, 1983). Cappella's (1991b) findings illustrate the concept that the dyad is a system with emergent properties, with its own tendency to match level of responsivity, which is not easily predictable from knowing either partner separately. This work suggests that a one-person psychology model, in which each person "has" a relatively stable or consistent personality, measured here as the disposition to respond in a predictable way, does not do justice to the complexity of human relatedness. Nevertheless, stable characteristics of the person (see Ryle, 1949), the contribution of the one-person model, still play a role.

It is possible that the concept of emergent properties of the dyad may help conceptualize the nature of therapeutic action in psychoanalysis. What emerges from the therapeutic dyad is something generative that cannot be completely predicted from the patient alone or from the analyst alone. Transference and countertransference can also be conceptualized as emergent dyadic properties. That is, knowing both the patient's and the analyst's self-regulatory and interactive patterns prior to the analysis will not completely or even adequately predict the specific nature of the match that the dyad will generate. This view of transference differs from that of a one-person model, in which transference is defined as a pattern that the patient brings to the interaction, as a stable characteristic of the individual. Rather, we conceptualize transference as a complex product of the stable characteristics of both the patient and the analyst individually, as well as of the emergent properties of the dyad (see also, e.g., Racker, 1968; Gill, 1982; Atwood and Stolorow, 1984; Lachmann and Beebe, 1990, 1992).

More generally, in attempting to conceptualize the dyadic system, we suggest that there is always a complex integration between some part of the variance that is accounted for by the stability of each individual's behavior and some that is accounted for by the particular nature of the interactive regulatory match. Still remaining for empirical investigation are which aspects of behavior and representations are more stable and which are more subject to interpersonal influence, under what conditions, and their respective relevance to structure formation and transformation.

DYADIC RULES OF REGULATION

A basic empirical concern in a dyadic systems approach to communication is to discern the structure of the mutual regulatory system. What are the dyadic rules that create order? What are the potential shared organizational forms? What are the ways of conceptualizing and measuring dyadic regulation? Stern (1971, 1977) addresses this issue by documenting the rules for initiating, maintaining, terminating, or avoiding dyadic states. Tronick (1980, 1982) discusses the regulation of joint exchanges as a shared set of generative communicative rules. These rules generate predictions in each partner about the other's behavior. The rules are probabilistic, in the sense that particular dyadic sequences are significantly different from chance (Ryle, 1949). These dyadic sequences are defined by the predictability of one partner's behavior from that of the other. That is, each partner's behavior is contingent on that of the other. Tronick (1980) considers the basis of joint regulation to be the mutual matching of communicative acts and predictions, that is, the continuous confirmation and disconfirmation of predictions of the partner's behavior. In a well-coordinated interaction, each participant's communicative act conforms to the partner's prediction.

Perhaps the central contribution of infant research to the structure of social interaction has been the rich documentation of many patterns of rules for the regulation of joint action, thus defining the complexity of early dyadic communication. We refer to these patterns of rules as "interaction structures" (Beebe and Lachmann, 1988). These rules have been shown to be mutually regulated by both mother and infant. The rules begin to define the ways in which the dyad jointly constructs patterns of order, variously termed resonance, synchrony, coordination, or relatedness. Using experimental perturbations of ongoing interactions, research has also begun to demonstrate ways in which these patterns can be disrupted and repaired (Tronick et al., 1978; Cohn and Tronick, 1983; Beebe and Lachmann, 1990; Murray, 1991). Researchers have documented various phenomena of mutual regulation that have been variously termed synchronization (Stern, 1971, 1977), behavioral dialogue (Bakeman and Brown, 1977), echo (Trevarthan, 1979, 1979), tracking (Kronen, 1982), protoconversation (Beebe, Stern, and Jaffe, 1979), accommodation (Jasnow and Feldstein, 1986), reciprocity (Brazelton et al., 1975), mutual dialogues (Tronick, Als, and Brazelton, 1980), reciprocal and compensatory mutual influence (Cappella, 1981), and coordinated interpersonal timing (Beebe et al., 1985; Crown, 1991; Jaffe et al., 1991). These researchers share a method of quantitative analysis of the organization of two ongoing naturalistic streams of behavior (one for mother, one for infant) and their interrelation. However, the behavioral categories used, the statistical methods that document the interrelation of the two streams of behavior, and the metaphors used to describe these interrelations differ widely from study to study.

The Measurement of Dyadic Rules of Regulation

The problem of how to conceptualize interpersonal process and dyadic regulation sufficiently well to measure it has plagued infant research for the last two decades. Generous borrowing from other fields, such as econometrics, has given us a kit of statistical tools that yield quantitative statements about interpersonal influence and self-regulation. At the root of all these measures is the prediction of the behavior of each partner in the dyad from that of the other.

Time series regression techniques are one approach to the analysis of interaction structures (Gottman, 1981; Gottman and Ringland,

1981). Time series regression (TSR) addresses the central issues that have preoccupied infancy research in its attempt to define the organization of interpersonal process in mother–infant interactions. This method preserves the entire moment-to-moment behavioral stream; statistically controls for "autocorrelation," a self-regulatory component; determines, by lag correlation, who influences whom; and identifies the sign of the influence. A positive sign indicates that the behaviors of the two partners are similar; for instance, when one partner elongates the duration of a vocalization, the other partner does also. A negative sign indicates that the behaviors of the two partners are systematically dissimilar; when one person elongates the duration of vocalization, the other parter shortens the duration.

To demonstrate that an infant and caregiver may influence, or be influenced by, each other, autocorrelational effects must first be identified and statistically "removed" (Gottman and Ringland, 1981). Autocorrelation refers to the influence of each partner's past behavior on his own current behavior and has been termed "self-influence" (Thomas and Martin, 1976). Large cross-covariances can be totally spurious; that is, the apparent covariation of two processes that are actually uncorrelated may be the result of a large autocorrelation within each process (Gottman and Ringland, 1981). Once autocorrelation is controlled, time series regression provides separate indices of each interactant's influence on the other ("lag correlation"). Influence is defined by the degree to which either partner's behavior can be predicted by the other's. By separately addressing the effects of autocorrelation and lagged correlation, TSR explicitly integrates the contributions of a self-regulatory component with interactive regulation in its strategy of analysis.

For example, if we find that the daily closing prices on the Tokyo and Wall Street stock exchanges are correlated, we have no idea of which is influencing the other. But if we realize that the closing is earlier in Tokyo than in New York, we can infer that the influence is going from Tokyo to New York. The lag in time defines the direction of influence. Similarly, TSR first lags one person's stream of behavior relative to that of the other and then reverses this procedure. Thus, the possibility that either person influences the other can be assessed. These assessments are lag correlations. This model does not yield causality but does imply that one stream of behavior can predict the other. In bidirectional influence, where each partner's behavior predicts that of the other, neither has "caused" the other. Rather, both are seen as jointly constructing the pattern of regulation.

The time series regression model has been used to demonstrate bidirectional influence in the mother–infant facial-visual exchange, with each partner matching the direction of affective change second-by-second (Cohn and Tronick, 1988), and fraction-of-second-by-fraction-of-second (Cohn and Beebe, 1990). Time series regression has demonstrated bidirectional influence in the timing of vocal exchanges between mother and infant and between stranger and infant (Jaffe et al., 1991), with each partner tracking and matching the durations of vocalizations and pauses of the other. This vocal dialogue model was translated into the mother–infant kinesic system, where time series analysis demonstrated a similar bidirectional tracking of the durations of "movements" and "holds" in the changes of facial expression and direction of gaze (Beebe et al., 1985). Time series regression has also been used to investigate the affective exchange between depressed mothers and their infants. In some samples, the bilateral influence process was shown to be intact (Cohn et al., 1990) and in other samples it broke down (Cohn and Tronick, 1989). This same time series regression model has been used to demonstrate bilateral influence in the timing of adult vocal interactions (Warner, 1987; Crown, 1991; Capella, 1991a,b; Jaffe et al., 1991).

Interpersonal involvement and empathy are associated with similarity or matching of adult communicative behaviors (Feldstein and Jaffe, 1963; Jaffe and Feldstein, 1970; Feldstein and Welkowitz, 1978). In adult conversation, to the degree that the partners match timing patterns of their speech, they rate each other as warmer and more similar (Welkowitz and Kuc, 1973; Feldstein and Welkowitz, 1978). In mother–infant interaction, the various findings of time series analysis documenting bilateral influence show that each partner is sensitive to the affective direction or temporal pattern of the other's behavior. These findings provide a behavioral basis for each partner to perceive and enter into the temporal world and feeling state of the other (Beebe et al., 1985; Beebe and Lachmann, 1988).

We now have evidence that the timing of the adult communicative process is very similar to that of the infant–adult process. For example, in both the durations of vocal pauses are matched, the degree of control of various vocal rhythms is matched, and there is bidirectional influence where each partner's vocal durations are predictable from the other's (Beebe et al., 1985; Crown, 1991; Jaffe et al., 1991). These striking similarities suggest that there are important continuities in the timing of the communicative process across the life span. The timing of the communicative process affects what it feels like to be with the other and contributes to the representation of self and other at every developmental level. Although much of our own work has focused on the timing of communication, similar organizational coherence has been documented in other communicative modalities, such as the facial-visual exchange (Stern, 1971, 1977, 1983; Kronen, 1982; Cohn and Tronick, 1988; Cohn and Beebe, 1990).

The Representation of Interaction Structures

The dyad provides the route to predictability in development (Sameroff and Chandler, 1976; Sroufe, 1979; Sameroff, 1983; Sander, 1983, 1985; Sroufe and Fleeson, 1986; Emde, 1988a,b; Zeanah et al., 1990). Many authors note the relative failure of predicting development from the individual alone. Sameroff argues that difficulty in prediction stems from using oversimplified models of development. It is not possible to predict from the organism alone, nor from the environment alone. Prediction is based on the transaction between organism and environment and the transaction's regular restructurings (Sameroff, 1976). Zeanah et al. (1990) argue that continuity in development as documented in the empirical infant literature is at the level of relationship structures. Stern (1989) argues that a relationship pattern resides in the interaction, in the dyad, not in the individual.

Thus, our concept of the interactive organization of experience and of psychic structure is based on a dyadic systems view of communication. Mother and infant jointly construct the rules of negotiating social relatedness. These rules guide the management of attention, turntaking, participating in discourse, and affect sharing. These rules are represented, are "internalized," and define the initial organization of psychic structure (Beebe and Stern, 1977; Beebe and Lachmann, 1988, 1990).

The model of representation that we employ is a process model. We claim that it is an interactive process, or a patterned sequence of movements between two people, that is represented by the infant (Beebe, 1986). Stern (1977, 1983; Beebe and Stern, 1977) employs a similar process model, which defines representation in the social sphere as the internalization of an intercoordination of dynamic interpersonal schemas of action. A schema of being with another person is a memory of a dynamic series of events. We conceptualize these as "interactive representations" in which the pattern of interplay of the interactive behaviors is represented.

In Piaget's (1937) framework, action schemas provide the infant with a way of knowing about the object. These action schemas are interiorized in the first mental representations. We suggest that the detailed knowledge of infant action schemas in relation to the mother's and their interactive regulation provide a way of assessing the nature of the object relation that is constructed and represented. The dominant modes of the ongoing relationship, based on detailed analysis of the mutual regulation of the dyadic system and of self-regulation processes, will prevail in the representation of the relationship. Piaget has shown that the internalization of the object does not proceed independently of the child's actions with reference to the object. We suggest, then, that what is initially represented is not an object per se, but an object relation: actions of self in relation to actions of partner and their pattern of dyadic regulation (Beebe and Stern, 1977; Beebe and Lachmann, 1988). These representations of self and object are simultaneously constructed in relation to each other. Thus, what is represented by the infant is an emergent dyadic phenomenon not residing in either partner alone. This initial representation will proceed through the nonverbal representation system and may or may not be later translated into the verbal representation system. Bucci (1985) suggests that such a translation is one task of adult psychoanalysis.

Modell (1992) has recently reviewed the use of the terms self- and object representations in psychoanalysis. He points out that the origins of these terms in the work of 18th-century philosophers such as Locke and Mill have influenced their usage in psychoanalysis toward a discrete, static, atomistic image of self and object. He notes that Sandler and Rosenblatt (1962) did not view representations as passive or atomistic. Instead, they influenced the usage of the terms toward a more fluid creation by the child. The idea of the representation of the interactive process emerging out of the infant research further elaborates Sandler and Rosenblatt's formulations and substantially changes the use of the terms away from their discrete, atomistic origins. The interaction is represented in relation to the self-regulatory system as each alters the other. Zelnick and Buchholz (1990), reviewing the concept of mental representations in the light of recent infant research, come to a conclusion similar to that of Modell, that these early interactions constitute unconscious organizing structures or unconscious memory structures.

THERAPEUTIC ACTION AND TRANSFERENCE

The mutual and self-regulation processes documented in the infant literature can provide analogues to two-person and one-person psychology perspectives. A one-person psychology model emphasizes the intrapsychic organization of experience as primary. Experience is shaped initially according to one's needs, one's biologically based urges, and, later, by wishes, although certainly the environment plays a role. A two-person psychology view emphasizes the original interactive organization of experience. Psychoanalysis has tended to use one or the other of these models in addressing the question of the primary organizational principles structuring experience. One- and two-person psychology perspectives are presented as though they were dichotomies, as though either endogenously organized and elaborated structures *or* relational, interactively organized structures were primary. The considerable polarization around these "mutually exclusive" theories in adult analysis has been detailed by Greenberg and Mitchell (1983). Similar polarizations exist in the infant literature.

Both self- and mutual regulation are organized at birth and play a crucial role from the beginning of life. The necessity for integrating these two regulatory organizations in infancy argues for integrating them in a psychoanalytic theory of adult treatment as well (see Lichtenberg, 1983; Gianino and Tronick, 1988; Ghent, 1989; Tronick, 1989; Beebe and Lachmann, 1990; Lachmann and Beebe, 1990; Stolorow and Atwood, 1992). Both the one- and the two-person psychology views, each without recognition of the other, contain serious drawbacks. If one takes an exclusively two-person view of structure formation, how can one distill a sense of individuality, a sense of one's own self, as distinct from the dyad? If one takes an exclusively one-person view, the contributions of the partner and the environment are underestimated. The research we have cited in illustrating a dyadic systems model depicts the dyad as a more complex organization than is usually recognized by either the one- or the two-person psychology view.

The contrasts between one- and two-person psychologies are nowhere more evident than in our understandings of the transference. Is the analyst required to function as a "screen" upon which the patient displays his life, past and present? Or is the analyst an active participant in the construction of the treatment relationship and the transference? We propose a model of transference and structuralization in adult treatment that integrates the simultaneous contributions of the patient–analyst interaction (the two-person psychology perspective) with the enduring structures from the patient's past that the patient has retained, rigidified, or diminished through his own subjective, personal elaborations (the one-person psychology perspective). Both sources operate interactively and concurrently throughout treatment, regardless of the origins of the pathology (Lachmann and Beebe, 1990, 1992). A consideration of both perspectives opens many more paths for intervention.

Our overview of the research documenting the negotiation of mother–infant interaction suggests two consequences for our understanding of the analytic dyad. First, the "rules" that the patient has internalized through the experiences of joint constructions between patient and analyst will contribute to the organizing principles in the transference. Second, the manner in which the relatedness is constructed will bear the stamp of both participants. Each influences the process through his own self-regulatory range, as well as through specific contributions to the pattern of interaction.

In development, the organizing principles of psychic structure are an emergent dyadic phenomenon. In the adult, the capacity to generate these principles, their availability, and their specific content is both generalized from past relationships and also partially specific to the particular current dyadic system. In this sense, the psychic structure of an individual may only be completely definable in the context of a specific dyad.

The dyadic systems view of communication presented here provides a theoretical background for the research described in the next chapter, on the origins of self- and object representations in infancy.

REFERENCES

Altmann, S. (1967), The structure of primate communication. In: *Social Communication Among Primates*, ed. S. Altmann. Chicago: University of Chicago Press, pp. 325–362.

Atwood, G. & Stolorow, R. (1984), *Structures of Subjectivity*. Hillsdale, NJ: The Analytic Press.

Bakeman, R. & Brown, J. V. (1977), Behavioral dialogues: An approach to the assessment of the mother–infant interaction. *Child Devel.*, 48:195–203.

Beebe, B. (1986), Mother–infant mutual influence and precursors of self- and object representations. In: *Empirical Studies of Psychoanalytic Theories, Vol. 2*, ed. J. Masling. Hillsdale, NJ: The Analytic Press, pp. 27–48.

_____ Jaffe, J., Feldstein, S., Mays, K. & Alson, D. (1985), Interpersonal timing: The application of an adult dialogue model to mother–infant vocal and kinesic interactions. In: *Social Perception in Infants*, ed. T. Field & N. Fox. Norwood, NJ: Ablex, pp. 217–247.

_____ & Lachmann, F. (1988), Mother–infant mutual influence and precursors of psychic structure. In: *Frontiers in Self Psychology: Progress in Self Psychology, Vol. 3*, ed. A. Goldberg. Hillsdale, NJ: The Analytic Press, pp. 3–26.

_____ & _____ (1990), The organization of representations in infancy: Three principles of salience. Paper presented at the 10th annual meeting, American Psychological Association, Division of Psychoanalysis, New York City.

_____ & Stern, D. (1977), Engagement-disengagement and early object experiences. In: *Communicative Structures and Psychic Structures*, ed. N. Freedman & S. Grand. New York: Plenum, pp. 35–55.

_____ _____ & Jaffe, J. (1979), The kinesic rhythm of mother–infant interactions. In: *Of Speech and Time*, ed. A. W. Siegman & S. Feldstein. Hillsdale, NJ: Lawrence Erlbaum Associates, pp. 23–34.

Bell, R. Q. (1968), A reinterpretation of the direction of effects in studies of socialization. *Psycholog. Rev.*, 75:81–95.

Berlyne, D. (1966), Curiosity and exploration. *Science*, 153:25–33.
Bertalanffy, L. von (1952), *Problems of Life*. New York: Wiley.
Bloom, L. (1983), Of continuity and discontinuity and the magic of language develop-
ment. In: *The Transition from Prelinguistic to Linguistic Communication*, ed. R. Gol-
linkoff. Hillsdale, NJ: Lawrence Erlbaum Associates, pp. 79–92.
Blurton-Jones, N. (1972), *Ethological Studies of Child Behavior*. Cambridge: Cambridge
University Press.
Bowlby, J. (1980), *Attachment and Loss* (Vol. 3). New York: Basic Books.
Brazelton, T. B. (1973), Neonatal behavioral assessment scale. *Clinics in Behavioral
Medicine*, 50. Spastics International Medical Publications. London: Heinemann
Medical Books.
_____ Kozlowski, B. & Main, M. (1974), The origins of reciprocity. In: *The Effect of the
Infant on Its Caregiver*, ed. M. Lewis & L. Rosenblum. New York: Wiley-Interscience,
pp. 49–76.
_____ Tronick, E., Adamson, L., Als, H. & Wise, S. (1975), Early mother–infant
reciprocity. In: *The Parent-Infant Relationship*, ed. M. A. Hofer. New York: Elsevier,
pp. 137–154.
_____ (1992), Touch and the fetus. Presented at Touch Research Institute, Miami, FL,
May.
Bruner, J. (1977), Early social interaction and language acquisition. In: *Studies in
Mother–Infant Interaction*, ed. H. R. Schaffer. New York: Norton, pp. 271–289.
Bucci, W. (1985), Dual coding: A cognitive model for psychoanalytic research. *J. Amer.
Psychoanal. Assn.*, 33:571–608.
Cappella, J. N. (1981), Mutual influence in expressive behavior: Adult and infant-adult
dyadic interaction. *Psycholog. Bull.*, 89:101–132.
_____ (1991a), The biological origins of automated patterns of human interaction.
Communicat. Theory, 1:4–35.
_____ (1991b), Individual consistency in temporal adaptation in nonverbal behavior in
conversations: High and low expressive dyads. Paper delivered at meeting of
International Communication Association.
Chapple, E. (1970), *Culture and Biological Man*. New York: Holt, Rinehart & Winston.
_____ (1971), Toward a mathematical model of interaction: Some preliminary consid-
erations. In: *Explorations in Mathematical Anthropology*, ed. P. Kay. Cambridge, MA:
MIT Press, pp. 141–178.
Cohn, J. & Beebe, B. (1990), Sampling interval affects time-series regression estimates
of mother–infant influence. *Infant. Beh. & Devel.*, 13:317.
_____ Campbell, S., Matias, R. & Hopkins, J. (1990), Face-to-face interactions of
postpartum depressed and nondepressed mother–infant pairs at 2 months. *Devel.
Psychol.*, 26:15–13.
_____ & Tronick, E. (1983), Three-month-old infants' reaction to simulated maternal
depression. *Child Devel.*, 54:185–193.
_____ & _____ (1988), Mother–infant face-to-face interaction: Influence is bidirectional and unrelated to periodic cycles in either partner's behavior. *Devel. Psychol.*,
24:386–392.
_____ & _____ (1989), Specificity of infants' response to mothers' affective behavior.
J. Amer. Acad. Child & Adolesc. Psychiat., 28:242–248.
Condon, W. & Sander, L. (1974), Synchrony demonstrated between movements of the
neonate and adult speech. *Child Devel.*, 45:456–462.
Cottrell, L. S. (1942), The analysis of situational fields in social psychology. *Amer. Soc.
Rev.*, 7:370–382.
Crown, C. (1991), Coordinated interpersonal timing of vision and voice as a function of
interpersonal attraction. *J. Social Psychol.*, 10:29–46.

DeCasper, A. & Carstens, A. (1980), Contingencies of stimulation: Effects on learning and emotion in neonates. *Infant Beh. & Devel.*, 4:19–36.

Demos, V. (1983), Discussion of papers by Drs. Sander and Stern. In: *Reflections on Self Psychology*, ed. J. Lichtenberg & S. Kaplan. Hillsdale, NJ: The Analytic Press, pp. 105–112.

_____ (1984), Empathy and affect: Reflections on infant experience. In: *Empathy, Vol. 2*, ed. J. Lichtenberg, M. Bornstein & D. Silver. Hillsdale, NJ: The Analytic Press, pp. 9–34.

Emde, R. (1981), The prerepresentational self and its affective core. *The Psychoanalytic Study of the Child*, 36:165–192. New Haven, CT: Yale University Press.

_____ (1988a), Development terminable and interminable. I. Innate and motivational factors. *Internat. J. Psycho-Anal.*, 69:23–43.

_____ (1988b), Development terminable and interminable. II. Recent psychoanalytic theory and therapeutic considerations. *Internat. J. Psycho-Anal.*, 69:283–296.

Fagen, J. W., Morrongiello, B. A., Rovee-Collier, C. & Gekoski, M. J. (1984), Expectancies and memory retrieval in three-month-old infants. *Child Devel.*, 55:936–943.

Fast, I. (1985), *Event Theory*. Hillsdale, NJ: Lawrence Erlbaum Associates.

_____ (1987), Interaction schemes in the establishment of psychic structure and therapeutic change. Unpublished manuscript.

Feldstein, S. & Welkowitz, J. (1978), A chronography of conversation: In defense of an objective approach. In: *Nonverbal Behavior and Communication*, ed. A. W. Siegman & S. Feldstein. Hillsdale, NJ: Lawrence Erlbaum Associates, pp. 329–377.

Ghent, E. (1989), Credo: The dialectics of one-person and two-person psychologies. *Contemp. Psychoanal.*, 25:169–211.

Gianino, A. & Tronick, E. (1988), The mutual regulation model: The infant's self and interactive regulation and coping and defensive capacities. In: *Stress and Coping*, ed. T. Field, P. McCabe & N. Schneiderman. Hillsdale, NJ: Lawrence Erlbaum Associates, pp. 47–68.

Gill, M. (1982), *The Analysis of Transference, Vol. 1. Psychological Issues*, Monogr. 53. New York: International Universities Press.

Gottman, J. (1981), *Time Series Analysis*. Cambridge: Cambridge University Press.

_____ & Ringland, J. (1981), Analysis of dominance and bidirectionality in social development. *Child Devel.*, 52:393–412.

Greenberg, J. & Mitchell, S. (1983), *Object Relations in Psychoanalytic Theory*. Cambridge, MA: Harvard University Press.

Habermas, J. (1979), *Communication and the Evolution of Society*. Boston, MA: Beacon Press.

Haith, M. (1980), *Rules that Babies Look By*. Hillsdale, NJ: Lawrence Erlbaum Associates.

_____ Hazan, C. & Goodman, G. (1988), Expectation and anticipation of dynamic visual events by 3.5 month old babies. *Child Devel.*, 59:467–79.

Hofer, M. (1984), Relationships as regulators: A psychobiological perspective on bereavement. *Psychosom. Med.*, 46:183–197.

_____ (1987), Early social relations: A psychobiologist's view. *Child Devel.*, 58:633–647.

Hunt, U. McV. (1965), Intrinsic motivation and its role in psychological development. In: *Nebraska Symposium on Motivation, Vol. 13*, ed. D. Levine. Lincoln: University of Nebraska Press, pp. 189–282.

Jaffe, J. (1962), *Dyadic Analysis*. Unpublished manuscript.

_____ (1977), Parliamentary procedure and the brain. In: *Nonverbal Behavior and Communication*, ed. A. Siegman and S. Feldstein. Hillsdale, NJ: Lawrence Erlbaum Associates.

_____ & Feldstein, S. (1970), *Rhythms of Dialogue*. New York: Academic Press.

_____ _____ Beebe, B., Crown, C. L., Jasnow, M., Fox, H. Anderson, S. W. &

Gordon, S. (1991), *Interpersonal Training and Infant Social Development*. Final report for NIMH Grant No. MH41675.

Jasnow, M. & Feldstein, S. (1987), Adult-like temporal characteristics of mother–infant vocal interactions. *Child Devel.*, 57:754–61.

Kegan, R. (1982), *The Evolving Self*. Cambridge, MA: Harvard University Press.

Kronen, J. (1982), Maternal facial mirroring at four months. Doctoral dissertation, Yeshiva University, New York.

Lachmann, F. L. & Beebe, B. (1990), On the formation of psychic structure: Transference. Presented at meeting of American Psychological Association, Div. of Psychoanalysis, New York.

—— —— (1992), Reformulations of early development and transference: Implications for psychic structure. In: *Psychoanalysis and Psychology*, ed. D. Wolitzky, M. Eagle & J. Barron. Hillsdale, NJ: Lawrence Erlbaum Associates.

Lashley, K. S. (1951), The problem of serial order in behavior. In: *Cerebral Mechanisms in Behavior*, New York: Wiley, pp. 112–146.

Lewis, M. & Rosenbaum, L., ed. (1974), *The Effect of the Infant on Its Caregivers*. New York: Wiley.

Lichtenberg, J. D. (1983), *Psychoanalysis and Infant Research*. Hillsdale, NJ: The Analytic Press.

Matarazzo, J. D. & Wiens, A. N. (1972), *The Interview*. Chicago: Aldine-Atherton.

Mead, G. H. (1934), *Mind, Self and Society*. Chicago: University of Chicago Press.

McGrew, W. C. (1972), *An Ethological Study of Children's Behavior*. New York: Academic Press.

Modell, A. (1992), *The Private Self in Public Space*. Harvard University Press.

Murray, L. (1991), Intersubjectivity, object relations theory, and empirical evidence from mother–infant interactions. *Infant Ment. Health J.*, 12:219–232.

—— & Trevarthen, C. (1985), Emotion regulation of interactions between 2 month old infants and their mothers. In: *Social Perception in Infants*, ed. T. Field & N. Fox. N.J.: Ablex, pp. 137–154.

Piaget, J. (1937), *The Construction of Reality in the Child* (M. Ccok, trans.). New York: Basic Books, 1954.

Racker, H. (1968), *Transference and Countertransference*. New York: International Universities Press.

Ruesch, J. & Bateson, G. (1951), *Communication*. New York: Norton.

Ryan, J. (1974), Early language development. In: *The Integration of a Child into a Social World*, ed. M. P. M. Richards. Cambridge: Cambridge University Press.

Ryle, G. (1949), *The Concept of Mind*. London: Hutchinson.

Sameroff, A. (1983), Developmental systems: Contexts and evolution. In: *Mussen's Handbook of Child Psychology, Vol. 1*, ed. W. Kessen. New York: Wiley, pp. 237–294.

—— & Chandler, M. (1976), Reproductive risk and the continuum of caretaking casualty. In: *Review of Child Development Research, Vol. 4.*, ed. F. D. Horowitz. Chicago, IL: University of Chicago Press, pp. 187–244.

Sander, L. (1977), The regulation of exchange in the infant-caretaker system and some aspects of the context-content relationship. In: *Interaction, Conversation, and the Development of Language*, ed. M. Lewis & L. Rosenblum. New York: Wiley, pp. 133–156.

—— (1983), Polarity paradox, and the organizing process in development. In: *Frontiers of Infant Psychiatry*, ed. J. D. Call, E. Galenson & R. Tyson. New York: Basic Books, pp. 315–327.

—— (1985), Toward a logic of organization in psycho-biological development. In: *Biologic Response Styles*, ed. K. Klar & L. Siever. Washington, DC: American Psychiatric Press.

Sandler, J. & Rosenblatt, B. (1962), The concept of the representational world. The *Psychoanalytic Study of the Child*, 17:128–145. New York: International Universities Press.

Simmel, G. (1950), *The Sociology of Georg Simmel* (K. H. Wolff, trans. & ed.). Glencoe, IL: Free Press.

Spelke, E. S. & Cortelyou, A. (1981), Perceptual aspects of social knowing. In: *Infant Social Cognition*, ed. M. Lamb & L. Sherrod. Hillsdale, NJ: Lawrence Erlbaum Associates, pp. 61–84.

Spitz, R. (1983), The evolution of dialogue. In: *Rene A. Spitz*, ed. R. Emde. New York: International Universities Press, pp. 179–195.

Sroufe, L. A. (1979), The ontogenesis of emotion. In: *Handbook of Infant Development*, ed. J. Osofsky. New York: Wiley, pp. 462–516.

_____ & Fleeson, J. (1986), Attachment and the construction of relationships. In: *Relationships and Development*, ed. W. Hartup & Z. Rubin. New York: Cambridge University Press, pp. 51–71.

Stechler, G. & Kaplan, S. (1980), The development of the self. The *Psychoanalytic Study of the Child*, 35:85–105. New Haven, CT: Yale University Press.

Stern, D. (1971), A microanalysis of the mother–infant interaction. *J. Amer. Acad. Child Psychiat.*, 10:501–507.

_____ (1977), *The First Relationship*. Cambridge, MA: Harvard University Press.

_____ (1983), The early development of schemas of self, of other, and of "self with other." In: *Reflections on Self Psychology*, ed. J. Lichtenberg & S. Kaplan. Hillsdale, NJ: The Analytic Press, pp. 49–84.

_____ (1985), *The Interpersonal World of the Infant*. New York: Basic Books.

_____ (1989), The representation of relational patterns: Developmental considerations. In: *Relationship Disturbances in Early Childhood*, ed. A. Sameroff & R. Emde. pp. 52–69. New York: Basic Books.

Stolorow, R. & Atwood, G. (1992), *Contexts of Being*. Hillsdale, NJ: The Analytic Press.

Sullivan, H. S. (1953), *The Interpersonal Theory of Psychiatry*. New York: Norton.

Thomas, E. A. C. & Martin, J. (1976), Analyses of parent-infant interaction. *Psychol. Review*, 83:141–155.

Trevarthen, C. (1979), Communication and cooperation in early infancy. In: *Before Speech*, ed. M. Bullowa. New York: Cambridge University Press, pp. 321–347.

Tronick, E. (1980), The primacy of social skills in infancy. In *Exceptional Infant, Vol. 4.* D. Sawin, R. Hawkins, L. Walker, & J. Penticuff (Eds.) New York: Brunner Mazel, 144–158.

_____ (1982), Affectivity and sharing. In: *Social Interchange in Infancy*, ed. E. Tronick. Baltimore, MD: University Park Press, pp. 1–8.

_____ (1989), Emotions and emotional communication in infants. *Amer. Psychol.*, 44:112–119.

_____ Als, H., Adamson, L., Wise, S. & Brazelton, T. B. (1978), The infant's response to entrapment between contradictory messages in face-to-face interaction. *J. Amer. Acad. Child Psychiat.*, 17:1–13.

_____ Als, H. & Brazelton (1980), Monadic phases: A structural descriptive analysis of infant–mother face-to-face interaction. *Merrill Palmer Quart.*, 26:3–24.

Vygotsky, L. S. (1978), *Mind In Society*. Cambridge, MA: Harvard University Press.

Warner, R. (1987), Rhythmic organization of social interaction and observer ratings of positive affect and involvement. *J. Nonverb. Beh.*, 11:57–74.

Watson, J. (1985), Contingency perception in early social development. In: *Social Perception in Infants*, ed. T. Field & N. Fox. Norwood, NJ: Ablex, pp. 157–176.

Weiss, P. (1973), *The Science of Life*. Mt. Kisco, NY: Futura.

Welkowitz, J. & Kuc, M. (1973), Interrelationships among warmth, genuineness, empathy and temporal speech pattern in interpersonal attraction. *J. Consult. Clin. Psychol.*, 41:472–73.

Wilson, A. & Malatesta, C. (1989), Affect and the compulsion to repeat: Freud's repetition compulsion revisited. *Psychoanal. Contemp. Thought*, 12:243–290.

Zeanah, C., Anders, T., Seifer, R. & Stern, D. (1990), Implications of research on infant development for psychodynamic theory and practice. *J. Amer. Acad. Child Psychiat.*, 28:657–668.

Zelnick, L. & Bucholz, E. (1990), The concept of mental representations in light of recent infant research. *Psychoanal. Psychol.*, 7:29–58.

5

The Contribution of Mother–Infant Mutual Influence to the Origins of Self- and Object Representations

BEATRICE BEEBE
FRANK M. LACHMANN

Research on mother–infant interaction in the first year of life can contribute to conceptualizing the development of self- and object representations and the emerging organization of infant experience. Numerous authors have suggested that the early internal models of self, object, and their relationship evolve out of the patterns of interaction experienced by the infant (Sullivan, 1953; Fairbairn, 1954; Beebe and Stern, 1977; Stern, 1977, 1983, 1985; Stechler and Kaplan, 1980; Emde, 1981; Sander, 1983a,b; Demos, 1984; Main, Kaplan, and Cassidy, 1985; Beebe, 1986). Nevertheless, this proposition remains vague unless amplified by detailed descriptions of these patterns and their implications for representation. Empirical infant research is increasingly in a position to describe numerous patterns of interactive regulation between parent and infant in exquisite detail (e.g., Brazelton, Kozlowski, and Main, 1974; Sander, 1977, 1983b; Stern, 1977, 1985; Kaye, 1982; Tronick, 1982; Cohn and Tronick, 1988). In addition, recent evidence for early infant presymbolic representational capacity allows us to conceptualize how patterns of interactive regulation are represented in the first year of life and how they

An earlier version of this chapter appeared in *Psychoanalytic Psychology* (1988), 5:305–337

The contributions of Daniel Stern, M.D., Michael Basch, M.D., Jeffrey Fagen, Ph.D., Thomas Horner, Ph.D., Fred Pine, Ph.D., Sidney Blatt, Ph.D., Wendy Olesker, Ph.D., Robert Stolorow, Ph.D., and Joseph Jaffe, M.D., are gratefully acknowledged. This research was partially supported by National Institute of Mental Health Grant R01-MH41675.

provide the basis for emerging symbolic forms of self- and object representations. We relate two different empirical infant literatures to the psychoanalytic theory of self- and object representations: patterns of interactive regulation during social play and evidence for a presymbolic representational capacity.

In previous publications, we proposed a central role for mother–infant mutual influence in the development of precursors of psychic structure (Beebe and Stern, 1977; Beebe, 1986; Beebe and Lachmann, 1988). Our basic proposal is that early interaction structures provide an important basis for the organization of infant experience and emerging self- and object representations. Interaction structures are characteristic patterns of mutual regulations in which both infant and caretaker influence each other. The infant comes to recognize, remember, and expect these recurring interaction structures.

There are two bases from which we infer the relevance of early interactions for self- and object representations. The first is a large empirical literature documenting that variations in social interactions in the first six months of life predict aspects of later social and cognitive development. The second, evidence from recent research on the nature of the representational process, suggests that, prior to the emergence of symbolic forms of representations, a representational world is being organized. We describe evidence for this presymbolic representational capacity in the early months of life by means of which the infant stores distinctive features of stimuli, creating models against which he can match his own behavior. We suggest that, prior to the development of symbolic capacities, the infant is able to represent expected, characteristic interaction structures, including their distinctive temporal, spatial, and affective features. Toward the end of the first year, representations of expected interaction structures are abstracted into generalized prototypes, which become the basis for later symbolic forms of self- and object representations. The dynamic, mutually regulated interplay between infant and caretaker creates a wide variety of potential patterns of interaction structures from which prototypes are abstracted.

Several empirical studies of early interactive regulation are reviewed in detail to illustrate how various patterns of interrelatedness may be represented. A study of derailment contrasts with matching interactions to illustrate qualitative variations in the emerging organization of infant experience. Finally, we attempt to capture the infant's subjective experience by offering translations from the behavioral interaction patterns to initial symbolic, or "verbalizable," experiences.

We focus on purely social exchanges and specifically do not address such issues as self-regulation and the management of alone states that, because of their importance for the organization of infant experience, require detailed consideration beyond the present scope (see Sander, 1983a,b; Pine, 1985; Gianino and Tronick, 1988). We also assume that, throughout the period of forming representations, interaction patterns continue to shape representations. However, our discussion is limited to the contribution of the first year's interactive experiences to the formation of self- and object representations.

In using patterns of mutual influence as a link to the organization of infant experience, we draw on systems concepts. Organization of experience is viewed not solely as a property of the individual, but also as a property of the dyadic system (Sander, 1977). This interactionist perspective, which emphasizes patterns of mutual influence or fitting together, is derived from biological systems theorists (Waddington, 1940; von Bertalanffy, 1952; Weiss, 1973). Its influence can be noted in psychoanalytic theories as well (e.g., Erikson, 1950; Sullivan, 1953; Spitz, 1959; Winnicott, 1974; Atwood and Stolorow, 1984).

SELF- AND OBJECT REPRESENTATIONS

Self- and object representations are typically discussed within the context of symbolic capacity (see, e.g., Lichtenberg, 1983). There has, however, been continuing psychoanalytic interest in the origins of self- and object representations before symbolic capacity is established (see e.g., Fraiberg, 1969; Horowitz, 1972; McDevitt, 1975). Several investigators of mother–infant interaction have suggested that the origins of self and representations of self and object can be meaningfully addressed prior to the emergence of symbolic capacity (Emde, 1981; Sander, 1983a,b; Horner, 1985; Stern, 1985; Beebe and Lachmann, 1988). Recent evidence on infant perception and memory is changing our views of early infant representational capacity. This research supports the attempt to conceptualize the origins of self- and object representations in the first year of life, prior to the emergence of symbolic capacity.

Historically, a distinction has been made between representational and prerepresentational processes (Piaget, 1937; Church, 1961; Werner and Kaplan, 1963; Schimek, 1975; Emde, 1981). According to Piaget's timetable, representational processes begin at approximately 7 to 9 months, undergo major reorganization at 16 to 18 months, and are considered symbolic by the third year. A number of students of infant perception and memory, however, consider representation to be a more general capacity, probably present at birth. In this view, symbol formation occurs as a later development in a system that already possesses rudimentary representational features. Evidence for some basic form of representation in the early months of life comes from experiments on recognition memory (Fagan, 1974), cued recall tasks (Fagen et al., 1984), early imitation (Meltzoff, 1985), and, later in the first year, the creation of prototypes (Strauss, 1979). This early representational capacity can be defined generally as the storage of distinctive features of stimuli (Cohen, 1973; Fagan, 1974; J. Fagen, personal communication, January 15, 1988).

INFANT CAPACITIES AND EARLY REPRESENTATION

A number of capacities underlie an early general representational ability. In the early months of life, the infant is able to detect and analyze features of stimuli through several modalities, such as brightness and hue of color, and pattern and contrasts of form. The infant actively seeks differences, selects similarities, and induces relationships among these perceptual features (see, e.g., Fantz, Fagan, and Miranda, 1975; Bornstein, 1979, 1985; Eimas and Miller, 1980; Kuhl and Meltzoff, 1984; Eimas, 1985; Kuhl, 1985; Mehler, 1985; Meltzoff, 1985). The infant's capacity to extract these features enables him to perceive rudimentary aspects of order, stability, and invariance, in short, to organize the world. As Bornstein (1979) noted, the importance of such a capacity for communication can hardly be overestimated.

Memory is also a critical capacity that underlies an early representational ability. Some form of memory and learning in utero can be inferred from the work of DeCasper and his coworkers (DeCasper and Carstens, 1980; DeCasper and Fifer, 1980; DeCasper and Spence, 1986). He asked pregnant women to read a Dr. Seuss book, *The Cat in the Hat*, to their fetuses during the last trimester of pregnancy. At birth, the babies preferred to hear a tape recording of their mothers reading the story they had heard in utero, rather than to hear their mothers reading another Dr. Seuss story.

Extensive work on infant visual recognition memory (Fagan, 1974; Cohen and Gelber, 1975; Fantz et al., 1975) has shown that infants can recognize and remember patterns over extended periods of time. For example, five-month-old infants can recognize multidimensional patterns after a delay of 48 hours and can recognize photographs of faces after a delay of two weeks (Fagan, 1974; Cohen and Gelber, 1975). At four to five months, a stimulus exposed for only one to two minutes is recognized two weeks later (Cohen and Gelber, 1975). Most of these authors assume that while the infant watches a stimulus, a model is being stored, so that later presentations of the stimulus can be compared to the model.

Recent work by Greco et al. (1986) showed evidence of longer recall in two- and three-month-olds if the infant was given a "reminder cue." Infants were trained for 18 minutes over a two-day period to learn that a foot-kick produced movement in a mobile. The infants remembered the foot-kick-mobile contingency for one week. Even after "forgetting," the infants could be reminded of the foot-kick-mobile contingency three weeks later, if they were briefly shown a "reminder cue." To cue the infant, the experimenter moved the mobile noncontingently at a rate equivalent to the infant's original responding (Greco et al., 1986). In a similar experiment, infants as young as two months were able to remember the specific objects in the training mobile and to detect minute changes in its composition after 24 hours (Hayne et al., 1986).

Hayne et al. argued that infants as young as two months are capable of encoding and maintaining a representation of the specific details of their training context for at least 24 hours. The traditional view of infant memory (see Kagan, 1978, 1979) is that not until approximately eight months to a year can an infant retrieve a representation of an earlier experience, hold it in memory, and compare it with a discrepant event in the immediate perceptual field. Hayne et al. suggest that their results contradict this view and that this capacity is already available by two months. A related study by Mast et al. (1980) also challenged the traditional view and argued that infants as young as three months can maintain a fairly detailed representation of a learning context, and that this representation can influence infant behavior for up to 24 hours.

Meltzoff's (1985; Meltzoff and Moore, 1977) work on neonatal imitation also argued for an early general representational ability, presumably part of the inherent feature-detection properties of the organism. Infants of two to three weeks match gestures of an adult model, such as mouth opening and tongue protrusion. Field et al. (1982) also had compatible findings. In explaining his findings, Meltzoff argued that infants can apprehend correspondences between body transformations they see (e.g., mouth opening of the model) and body transformations of their own that they do not see, but apprehend proprioceptively (their own imitative mouth opening). These correspondences operate cross-modally. Independent evidence for this position also comes from Bahrick and Watson (1985). Thus, in early behavioral matching, infants use correspondences as a basis for organizing their responses. Meltzoff argued that the infant's use of these correspondences indicates a representation of the actions. He suggested that the representation is not merely a visual mental image or iconic copy, but a nonmodality-specific description of the event, utilizing both visual and motor information. The representation constitutes a model against which the infant can match his own performance and guide his behavior.

THE REPRESENTATION OF SOCIAL EXPECTANCIES

This early representational ability can be used by the infant to represent early social interactions through the development of expectancies about how the interaction will go (see Lewis and Goldberg, 1969; Lamb, 1981; Stern, 1985; Beebe, 1986; Beebe and Lachmann, 1988). The neonate has a remarkable capacity to perceive time and temporal sequence, to detect contingencies between his behavior and environmental events, and to develop expectancies of when events occur (Lewis and Goldberg, 1969; Allen et al., 1977; Finkelstein and Ramey, 1977; Millar and Watson, 1979; Watson, 1985). When the neonate learns to expect that events occur contingent on his own behavior, such as that a particular sucking and pausing rhythm "produces" his mother's voice (by turning on a tape recorder), and when this expectancy is confirmed, affect is positive. The cessation or loss of expected consequences, on the other hand, leads to infant distress (Seligman, 1975; DeCasper and Carstens, 1980).

After only a minimum of two encounters, three-month-old infants can figure out whether an event will recur. Thus they generate "rules" that govern their expectancies. These "rules" are based on a determination that a pattern is the same or different and on the serial pattern in which events occur (Fagen et al., 1984). Similar serial pattern information is continuously available in social interactions. In the social interaction studies described later, where mutual influences are documented between infant and caretaker using time-series analyses, it can be inferred that the infant is using serial pattern information.

Using the definition of early representational capacity as the storage of distinctive features, we suggest that the infant represents the distinctive features of social interactions before they are abstracted and before they are symbolized. We must assume, however, that the same features demonstrated by the researcher as organizing social behavior are the features that the infant perceives as distinctive. As we describe in detail later, the features of social interactions demonstrated by researchers, which we suggest the infant will represent, are (1) the temporal patterning of the behavior of both partners (e.g., rate and rhythm and serial order), (2) the presence or absence of interpersonal contingencies and mutual influences, (3) the pattern of the movements of the two partners in space (e.g., approach-approach versus approach-withdrawal), and (4) the facial affective pattern. That is, "higher order" features, such as temporal, spatial, and affective organization, will be represented. "Lower order" features, such as who the partner is, the situation, and context, are represented as well. In addition, we suggest that what is stored goes beyond the features per se (J. Fagen, personal communication, January 15, 1988). The interaction structure itself is represented: patterns of mutual regulation, as they are organized by time, space, and affect.

This early representational capacity is elaborated by an increasing ability to abstract information. The infant constructs a prototype that is a composite of his experiences and transcends any particular specific instance (Lewis and Brooks, 1975). Evidence for abstraction is available by the end of the first year. Strauss (1979) showed 10-month-old infants a series of schematic drawings of faces, each slightly different. Through the use of a habituation paradigm, the infants were "asked" which drawing was "most similar," that is, most representative of the series. The infants chose a drawing they had never seen before, which averaged all the faces. The inference was that infants abstracted a general composite or prototype.

We suggest that the expectancies the infant has of characteristic interaction structures and their distinctive features summarize into generalized composites or prototypes at the point in the first year when the ability to abstract information develops. Stern (1985) made a similar argument for the infant's capacity to represent interactions that are generalized (RIG). It is these generalized, abstracted prototypes of interaction structures that become the basis for the symbolic level of the representation of self and object.

In summary, the storage of distinctive features of stimuli, in conjunction with specific capacities, such as cross-modal perception and detection of correspondences, and memory, constitutes an early representational system. Expectancies about how social interactions go are, in turn, represented through this system. These expectancies are abstracted into prototypes toward the end of the first year. These prototypes provide a crucial link to symbolic capacities, which also begin to emerge toward the end of the first year.

This description of an early representational ability differs from traditional accounts that propose the infant's own actions are the primary factor in the construction of representations (Piaget, 1937;

Werner, 1948; Church, 1961; Schilder, 1964). Piaget, for example, argued that there is no capacity for representation at birth, that action is originally the infant's only way of "knowing," and that representational ability grows out of sensorimotor action and imitation (Piaget, 1937; Meltzoff, 1985). Although the current account of an early representational ability contradicts the view that action is the infant's only way of constructing representations, action can still be considered to be another source of representational development, elaborating and solidifying representations and adding more detailed and distinctive features to them.

These studies are a brief sample of an emerging view that the various infant capacities for memory, cued recall, matching, cross-modal perception, and so on constitute an early representational system in the first year, prior to the development of symbolic functioning and language and prior to evocative recall independent of external experience. Some of this research is reviewed in further detail in Stern (1985). The argument for an early representational ability can alter our understanding of the origins of self- and object representations prior to the emergence of the symbolic forms of these representations. This "presymbolic" representational world is the basis for later symbolic forms of the representations and provides a crucial continuity in conceptualizing the origins of self- and object representations from birth.

Experiences of the first year are radically transformed with the onset of symbolic thought, which begins at the end of the first year, undergoes major reorganization at 16 to 18 months, and is constituted by approximately the third year. By using symbols, the child can refer to an object in a way that is "arbitrary," that is, not defined by its physical features. The child is now capable of imitating a model that is not physically present. With the ability to symbolize relationships between objects, the child can perceive himself as an objective entity (Kagan, 1979; McCall, 1979; Sroufe, 1979). This stage is the culmination of the process of constructing self- and object representations in the first three years of life, a process that continues in significant ways throughout life.

EMPIRICAL STUDIES OF EARLY INTERACTIVE REGULATION

At three to four months there is a flowering of the infant's social capacity. The infant's repertoire of interactive capacities is most clearly seen at this age during face-to-face play, where the only goals are mutual attention and delight (Brazelton et al., 1974; Stern, 1977). This situation elicits the infant's greatest communicative skill (Brazelton et al., 1975). Furthermore, the patterns of regulation of this face-to-face exchange in the first six months predict cognitive and social development at one year (as we discuss later; see e.g., Blehar, Lieberman, and Ainsworth, 1977; Alper, 1982; Langhorst and Fogel, 1982). It is this face-to-face play paradigm that is used in the empirical studies to follow.

The infant's interactive capacity in face-to-face play is predicated on a visual system that is highly functional at birth and by approximately three months achieves adult maturational status (Cohen, DeLoache, and Strauss, 1979). The capacity for sustained mutual visual regard is present by approximately the second month. It is considered to be a fundamental paradigm of communication that is central to the developing relationship between mother and infant (Stern, 1977) and continues throughout life (Robson, 1967). Moreover, as Stern (1971, 1977) documented, mothers tend to gaze steadily; it is the infant who "makes" and "breaks" the visual contact. Infants have control over looking, looking away, and closing the eyes, which allows them by two to three months a "subtle instant-by-instant regulation of social contact" (Stern, 1977, p. 502).

Normal mothers and three- to four-month-old infants at play were studied. They were seated face-to-face, with the infant in an infant seat, in an otherwise bare room. Videotape cameras were placed unobtrusively in the walls. The mother was told that anything that happened was fine. Mother and infant were then left alone to interact. Two cameras, one on each partner's face and torso, produced a split-screen view of the interaction. This research paradigm specifically examined only the purely social exchanges during periods of alert attention.

By three to four months, an extensive range of interpersonal affective display is present. The videotapes were converted into 16-mm film and viewed in slow motion. Thus fleeting and subtle interactions were revealed that often are not visible to the naked eye. Observations of infants sustaining or disrupting the face-to-face play encounter led to the development of a scale describing the various ways infant combine their orientation to the mother, their visual attention to her, and subtle variations in their facial expressiveness (Beebe and Stern, 1977; Beebe and Gerstman, 1980). This scale was influenced by the concept that nuances of affective quality occur on a continuum of gradations, rather than only as discrete on-or-off categories (Marler, 1965; Tobach, 1970; Stern, 1981). Figure 5.1 illustrates two similar scales of increasing and decreasing affective

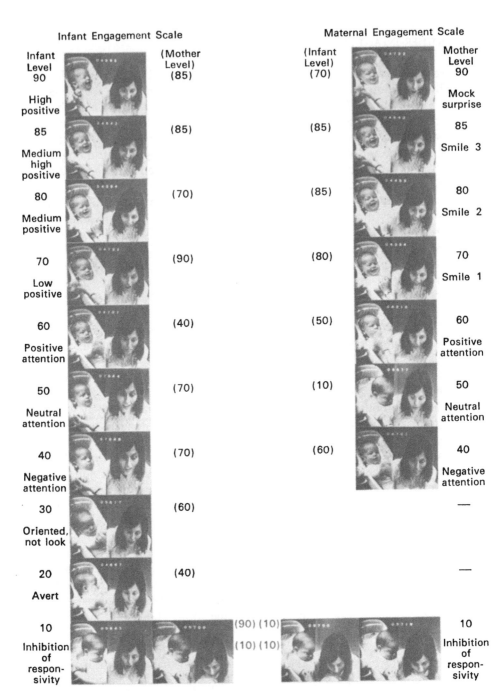

FIG. 5.1 Photographic Illustrations of Infant and Maternal Engagement Scales. From Beebe and Gerstman (1980, p. 328). Reprinted by permission.

engagement, one each for mother and infant. Although only the infant's scale is discussed in detail, the mother's scale operates in a similar fashion.

Considering first the upper half of the infant scale: At the neutral midpoint (50), the infant is oriented face-to-face with mother, visually engaging her face, with neutral expressiveness. In the upward direction of increasing engagement, orientation and attention remain constant, and the scale is ordered by increasing fullness of display of mouth opening and mouth widening, which may be accompanied by thrusts of the head upward toward mother and by positive vocalizations. At the highest level (90), termed the *gape smile*, the mouth is widened and opened to the utmost, the head thrust forward, accompanied by prolonged visual regard—giving the impression of an exhilarating moment of delight.

The multidimensional nature of the infant's positive expressiveness, based on head movements and mouth opening and closing as well as increments in the smile display (mouth widening and narrowing), potentially provide the infant with a remarkable ability to communicate slight changes in intensity and quality of mood without necessarily changing orientation or visual regard (Beebe, 1973). The facial mirroring study described later primarily illustrates regulations in the upper half of the scale.

We now turn to the lower half of the infant scale, moving in the direction of decreasing engagement (or increasing compromises in engagement). Below the neutral midpoint (50), there is a loss of neutral expressiveness to "negative attention" (40), a constellation of oriented face-to-face and visually attentive to mother, but with frown or grimace. The next level entails a loss of visual regard, although the infant remains oriented (30). This is followed by loss of face-to-face to mother orientation as well, into "avert" (20); that is, head and gaze averted away from mother. Finally, there is loss of responsivity altogether, termed *inhibition of responsivity* (10), in that the infant maintains a limp, motionless headhang, regardless of mother's attempts at engagement. The derailment study described later primarily illustrates regulations in the lower half of the scale.

The levels of engagement of this scale provide us with the data required to answer the following questions: (1) How can we know if these two partners are relating or influencing each other? (2) What is the nature of the responsivity? and (3) Is it mutual (bidirectional)? We briefly describe three patterns of interactive regulation: (a) facial mirroring, (b) matching of timing, and (c) derailment. These patterns all show mutual influence in which mother influences infant and infant influences mother. The patterns illustrate different interaction structures, that is, different ways the states of engagement are interactively organized (e.g., through the level, affective direction, or duration of engagement). All the patterns provide different ways in which each partner enters the other's state and affects and is affected by the other's state. From these patterns, different nuances of the infant's "experience" of being with the mother can be inferred.

FACIAL MIRRORING: MATCHING OF AFFECTIVE DIRECTION

Psychoanalytic writers have long appreciated the importance of mirroring in child development (Kohut, 1971, 1977; Mahler, Pine, and Bergman, 1975; Winnicott, 1974). For example, Winnicott (1974) described mirroring as follows: "[I]n individual development the precursor of the mirror is the mother's face; what does the infant see when he looks at his mother? He sees himself" (p. 131). A number of infant researchers also have suggested that some kind of mirroring (Papousek and Papousek, 1977, 1979), matching (Tronick, 1982), echo (Trevarthen, 1979), mimicry, imitation, and so on is a key aspect of the mother–infant face-to-face exchange in the early months of life. The exact nature of this match, however, has not been precisely defined. Furthermore, there is a difference of opinion as to whether this matching may primarily be a contribution of the adult partner (Schaffer, 1977; Kaye, 1982) can be considered to be mutually regulated (Stern, 1977; Cappella, 1981; Mayer and Tronick, 1985).

Several studies have considered the nature of matching in mother–infant play at four months and evaluated whether this matching is mutually regulated (Kronen, 1982; Beebe and Crown, 1988; Beebe and Kronen, 1988). The affective content, or levels of engagement, as defined in the scales previously discussed, were examined. Every movement of each partner can be assigned both a level on the scale (i.e., how engaged) and a direction on the scale (i.e., increasing or decreasing engagement).

Mothers and infants were found to match the direction of affective change, but to avoid an exact match of level on the scale. Thus, mother and infant both tend to increase engagement together or to decrease engagement together but are rarely at the same level of engagement.

The question of whether this matching is mutually regulated was investigated with a statistical technique (time-series analysis: see Gottman, 1981) that allows a determination of whether influence occurs at all and, if so, who is influencing whom. It was found that both mother and infant were mutually responsive. Mother influences infant and infant influences mother to follow or track the partner's direction of affective engagement change on a moment-to-moment basis. Similar findings have been reported by Cohn and Tronick (1988).

INTERPERSONAL TIMING: MATCHING OF TEMPORAL PATTERNS

Microanalyses of film have revealed that mother and infant live in a "split-second" world, where events with demonstrable significance in the interaction last approximately one-third to one-half sec (Stern, 1971; Beebe, 1973, 1982; Beebe and Stern, 1977; Beebe, 1985). These split-second mutual adjustments are so rapid that the temporal relations, and many of the fleeting behaviors themselves, cannot be fully grasped with the naked eye. Their rapidity suggests that they occur partially or fully out of conscious control (Sander, 1977, 1978; Beebe, 1982, 1986; Beebe and Lachmann, 1988). In the interlocking responsivity of the movements of one to the other, various temporal patterns are matched. Through this matching, a structure of "being with" another person is organized. We propose that the representation of self and object matched in the direction of affective change, and matched in various temporal patterns, is one prerequisite for the later ability to share subjective states with the object (see also Stern, 1985).

A perceptual basis for understanding the coordination and matching of temporal patterns of behavior in mother–infant social exchanges is provided by DeCasper's work (DeCasper and Carstens, 1980; DeCasper and Fifer, 1980). The infant can discriminate small differences in intervals of time, both in the environment and in his own behavior. The infant's capacity to alter the duration of intervals in his own behavior may provide the basis for subtle matching of the durations of behavior.

The concepts underlying the studies to be presented come from work on adult conversation by Jaffe and Feldstein (1970) and Feldstein and Welkowitz (1978), who have studied rhythms of verbal dialogue. They found a powerful phenomenon, which they termed *vocal congruence*, in which adult partners match pauses between vocalizations and match cycles of vocalizations and pauses. Most pertinent to the current work is the association they found between matching rhythms of dialogue and empathy and affect. When adult strangers in their studies matched pauses, they were found to like each other more, to perceive each other as warmer and more similar, and to choose each other as dinner partners. On the other hand, depressed and schizophrenic adults and autistic adolescents did not match rhythms of speech.

The adult dialogue model has been applied to the study of mother–infant interactions. Various temporal patterns of vocal and kinesic exchanges were found to match: vocal pauses, kinesic "turns," and kinesic "movements" and "holds." These patterns of interpersonal timing define an early mother–infant "dialogue."

Matching of Pauses in Mother–Infant Vocal Interactions

In everyday social conversation, people take turns speaking. During one speaker's turn, the other speaker listens. A turn can consist of many sequences of talking (vocalization) and pausing. Because the same speaker resumes after each pause, these are termed *intrapersonal pauses*. However, there are some pauses that signal the end of a speaker's turn and are followed by the other speaker's talking. At the moment the other speaker talks unilaterally, his turn begins. These *interpersonal* pauses are termed *switching pauses*, because they mark the boundary of the switch from the first to the second speaker's turn.

Switching pauses between mother and infant have been found to match at four months (Alson, 1982; Beebe et al., 1985; Beebe, 1988) and at nine months (Jasnow, 1983). Furthermore, Jasnow's nine-month findings show that the matching occurs as a result of mutual influence between the partners. That is, each partner influences the duration of the other's behavior to become more like his own.

In this switching-pause matching, mother and infant each pause for similar durations before the other takes a turn. Turn-taking can be considered the fundamental temporal structure of dialogue, and switching pauses mark the boundaries of the turn exchange. The function of switching-pause matching can be seen as regulating the exchange of turns at a similar pace. Because switching pauses are also characteristically matched in adult conversation, we conclude that a turn-taking, or dialogic, structure is already being regulated in the same way as seen in adult speech.

Although mothers and infants generally do not match intrapersonal pauses (Alson, 1982; Jasnow, 1983; Beebe et al., 1985), in those dyads where intrapersonal pauses are matched, infant affect is more positive (Alson, 1982). Intrapersonal pause matching may thus be a subtle index of attunement in the pair.

Matching of Temporal Patterns in Mother-Infant Kinesic Interaction

The term kinesic refers to movement, specifically to changes of orientation, gaze, and facial expression. Because these movements are all changes of level in the mother and infant affective engagement scales described previously, we are examining the interpersonal timing of affective exchanges. Although vocal interactions are a significant modality of exchange, kinesic interactions are far more frequent (Zelner, 1983) and are the dominant modality of interchange at four months. When the adult dialogue model is applied to kinesics, a vocalization is translated into a movement and a pause into a "hold," that is, the stationary posture between movements.

Matching of Kinesic Turns. A kinesic turn is comparable to a vocal turn. One partner gains the kinesic turn at the moment he moves unilaterally, and his turn lasts until the other partner moves unilaterally. These kinesic turns are generally composed of a single movement and an ensuing hold. A turn is thus the duration from the onset of one partner's behavior to the onset of the second partner's behavior as the partners alternate. Mothers and infants tend to match the average duration of these turns, which is one half sec (Beebe, Stern, and Jaffe, 1979; Kronen, 1982; Beebe et al., 1985). Because the turn is composed of a movement-hold cycle, this matching of turns can be interpreted to mean that mother and infant are sharing the same rhythm. Each alternatively enacts the rhythm, so that together they carry out one unbroken rhythm (Jaffe, Anderson, and Stern, 1979). To use a musical analogy, various instruments may take turns while others fall silent, but across all the instruments, the rhythm remains unbroken. Turn-matching in mother–infant exchanges parallels the rhythmic matching of phrase-pause cycles found in adult conversation (Natale, Dahlberg, and Jaffe, 1979).

Matching of Movements and Holds. A turn is composed of a movement and a hold. The durations of movements and holds were analyzed separately. Movements are defined as unilateral actions, such that one partner acts while the other is behaviorally "silent." Holds are defined as joint behavioral silences in which neither person moves. Mothers and infants tend to match the durations of movements and holds (Mays, 1984; Beebe et al., 1985). Time-series analysis was used to document that matching involved mutual influence to match. Unlike the previous findings, the type of matching demonstrated by these analyses was an inverse matching showing a negative correlation; as one partner's movement became longer, the other's became shorter and vice versa.

These findings of inverse matching of movement and hold duration can be interpreted as mother and infant each compensating for the other's change in activity level: The more active one partner is (in longer movement durations or shorter hold durations), the less active the other partner is (in shorter movement durations or longer hold durations). Thus, the two partners together maintain a fairly constant *dyadic* activity level. In this compensatory matching, mother and infant can be seen as participating in a "homeostatic negative feedback" system. Whereas a positive feedback system amplifies deviations, a negative feedback system counteracts deviations in the system. Because the sum of the dyadic activity level of mother and infant stays more or less constant in these data, extreme deviations in joint activity level are counteracted or modulated. This compensatory matching constitutes one type of attunement in the mother–infant dyad, where each sensitively tracks the durations of the behavior of the other, accomplishing the regulation of joint activity level within a relatively stable range.

In summary, various kinds of matching of temporal patterns are present in both the vocal and kinesic modalities. There is a mutual regulation of the timing of these interactions in which each partner is exquisitely sensitive to the duration of the other's behavior on a moment-to-moment basis.

IMPLICATIONS OF AFFECTIVE AND TEMPORAL MATCHING FOR THE ORGANIZATION OF INFANT EXPERIENCE

The Sharing of Subjective States

The translation of the findings of the regulation of action patterns into the language of experience always involves considerable inference and is difficult at best. Whereas psychoanalysis emphasizes how self and object are experienced, mother–infant interaction research measures what the two partners do. In making inferences from behavior to experience, it is assumed that at this age (in the first six months) the infant's observed actions closely parallel his experience. In later development, action and experience can be increasingly dissociated and even potentially contradictory. But the infant cannot hide his distress, pleasure, or fatigue.

The various ways in which mother and infant influence each other to match the timing and affective direction of behavior provide each a behavioral basis for knowing and entering into the partner's perception, temporal world, and feeling state (see Beebe et al., 1985). It is a common notion that when people empathize or "identify" with each other, their language and communicative behavior become more similar (see Feldstein and Welkowitz, 1978, for a review of this literature). The process of becoming related and better attuned to another involves, in part, becoming more similar because of presumably the increasing ability to predict the other's behavior. The implication is that similarity or symmetry in behavior is associated with a congruence of feeling states. What is the mechanism of this congruence?

We can identify three mechanisms in a dyadic process that link the feeling state of one person to another. The first occurs when subjective feeling states are expressed in behavior. In a social interaction, this expressive display is perceived by the partner, and there is a strong tendency to match the outward display in some way (in its timing, affect, direction, etc.). This matching is a second intermediate mechanism of transmission of a feeling state. The third way, as we previously suggested (Beebe and Lachmann, 1988), lies in the very act of matching, which generates a central emotional state in the receiving partner who matches. This concept is based on the work of Ekman (1983) and Zajonc (1985).

Ekman (1983) taught professional actors and scientists who study the face an exact set of muscle movements (e.g., contracting a particular forehead muscle in conjunction with particular eye and cheek muscles) which resulted in a series of facial expressions. In a second task, he taught the subjects to relive various emotions. During each task, autonomic indices, such as heart rate, temperature, and skin resistance, were recorded. Simply producing the facial muscle action patterns resulted in more clear-cut autonomic changes than actually reliving these emotions. Ekman concluded that contracting the facial muscles elicits the associated autonomic activity. His study thus suggests that the physiological state of the receiving partner who matches is very similar to the physiological state of the sending partner.

This experiment sheds light on the mechanism of empathy or the problem of how the feeling state of one person can be transmitted to another. Ekman suggested, for example, that the onlooker's contraction of the same facial muscles as he perceives on another's face enables the onlooker to feel the same autonomic sensations as the other person. Zajonc (1985) expressed a similar view:

If muscular movements of the face, by virtue of their effects on cerebral blood flow and on the release of particular neurotransmitters, are sufficient to induce changes in hedonic tone and result in changes of subjective states, then reproducing the expression of another may well produce in the onlooker a similar emotional state [p. 19].

We suggest that Ekman's and Zajonc's ideas apply more generally to a large range of matching phenomena, including matching of affective direction and temporal pattern as well as specific facial expressions. While reproducing the spatial or temporal pattern of another person's emotional display, one feels one's own face and body and an associated autonomic activity. This is a cross-modal transfer from the perception of an external image or temporal pattern to an internal proprioceptive experience. Such cross-modal transfer can be demonstrated in the first months of life (Rose, 1979; Lewkowicz and Turkewitz, 1980; Spelke and Cortelyou, 1981). Matching the spatial or temporal pattern of another person's display evokes a similar psychophysiological state in oneself. This mechanism may account for the emotional efficacy (for empathy, bonding, etc.) of matching phenomena that are so ubiquitous in social interactions. Although he had no data on the physiological correlates of matching, Byers (1975) made a similar argument for the matching of temporal patterns. He suggested that two interactants in tight synchrony are brought into the same state by virtue of their mutual entrainment.

We have suggested that, as mother and infant match each other's temporal and affective patterns, each recreates in himself or herself a psychophysiological state similar to that of the partner and thus participates in the subjective state of the other (Beebe and Lachmann, 1988). We hypothesize that, in the findings showing a positive correlation, each partner recreated in himself or herself the same subjective state that generated the temporal or affective pattern being matched. In the findings showing a negative correlation, such as the inverse matching of movement and hold durations, we hypothesize a re-creation of the subjective state of the other as the first of a two-stage empathic process. To do the opposite, the person must first match the other's state. In the second stage, this re-creation is used as a standard of reference for a further regulation in the opposite direction of the partner's behavior.

These mechanisms have specific relevance for the origins of empathy. For example, *empathy*, defined as "mental entering into the perception of another; motor mimicry" (*American College Dictionary*, 1962), relates a behavioral similarity, motor mimicry, to a subjective state. To behave in the same way or with the same temporal pattern is to enter into an aspect of the other's perception and provides a behavioral basis for knowing an important aspect of how the other feels. The findings of similar temporal patterns presented here suggest that when mother and infant time the durations of their behaviors in a similar way and each influences the other to match the timing, then this matching provides a mechanism for each to enter into an aspect of the other's temporal world and feeling state.

The matching of affective direction can be interpreted in a similar way. Each partner experiences similarities between what his or her face feels like and what the partner's face looks like. The findings of mutual influence to match and track affective direction, on a moment-to-moment basis, again suggest that mother and infant have remarkable access to each other's feeling states. Following our more general application of Ekman's (1983) work, as each matches the pattern (spatial or temporal) of the partner's emotional display, the matching evokes in each a proprioceptive experience that corresponds to that of the partner.

The Representation of Shared Subjective States

We suggest that the infant stores the experiences in which the timing and affect of his behavior are characteristically matched. Furthermore, the associated experiences of matching and participating in the partner's behavioral state are also stored. These experiences, when characteristic, result in an expectation of matching and being matched. This expectation is represented in a presymbolic form. These matching experiences can be assumed to be a ubiquitous aspect of daily social interactions for most infants (Fogel, 1977; Stern, 1977; Beebe et al., 1985; Crown et al., 1988).

Stern (1985) experimented with nine-month-old infants by asking mothers purposely to "mismatch" aspects of their behavior in which they naturally match their infants. The infants noticed these mismatches, which disrupted the infants' play. These findings further support the hypothesis that infants develop an expectation of being matched.

We suggest that as the infant makes progress toward a symbolic level of representation, the expectation of being matched, as well as the expectation of matching and participating in the state of the other, is one aspect of the infant's representation of self and object. The representation includes some prototype of the experience of what it is like to match and be matched, or not, on a moment-to-moment basis. That is, the representation includes the dynamic interactive process itself.

Once symbol formation develops, these experiences in matching affect and interpersonal timing may contribute to an expectation in the older child or adult of being "attuned," "known," or "on the same wavelength," in all the ways previously defined. We infer an experience not only of "I reflect you," but also of "I change with you; we are going in the same direction. I experience myself as tracking you and being tracked by you."

It is also possible that a dearth of experiences of matching creates important alterations in the capacity to represent the self symbolically as affectively well attuned or well related to the object. On the basis of Stern's (1985) data of experimental mismatch and the vocal data showing correlations between pause matching and infant positive affect, matching experiences can be said to constitute a positive state, certainly more positive than mismatch. Matching of interpersonal timing and affective direction, and matching interactions in general, may contribute to the positive coloration of self and object as representations increasingly become symbolic.

DERAILMENT AND EARLY COPING

The infant has a broad range of activities with which to cope with nonoptimal maternal stimulation. Part of this range is illustrated in the following vignette of a mother–infant pair at four months. It reveals the exquisite sensitivity and mutual responsivity that exist in interactions of infant aversion and withdrawal as well as in affectively more positive interactions. In between the obvious extremes of sustained mutual gaze and complete disruption of the play encounter, we find complex and subtle compromises between "engagement" and "disengagement." (See Beebe and Stern, 1977, for the original report of this study.)

Looking at a six-minute sample at the beginning of a videotape play session of this mother–infant pair at 4 months, we found that the usual long mutual gazes with positive affect were strikingly absent. Instead, we observed complex and rapid sequences in which the mother "chased" and the infant "dodged." The mother "chased" by following the infant's head and body movements with her own head and body, pulling his arm, picking him up to readjust his orientation, or attempting to force his head in her direction. The infant dodged by moving back, ducking his head down, turning away, pulling his hand from her grasp, or becoming limp and unresponsive. The infant exercised a virtual "veto power" over her attempts to engage him in a face-to-face encounter.

Statistical analysis revealed predictable sequences of mutual influence. The mother's rapid head-loom close in toward the infant's face was predictably followed by the infant's moving his head back and away from her. The mother's loom presumably elicited "defensive" reflexes to looming stimulation; these are identifiable as early as two weeks (see Bower, Broughton, and Moore, 1970). The infant's head movement away however, functioned as a stimulus for the mother to "chase" further. She followed with her head and body in the infant's direction of movement, pulled the infant's arm toward her or repositioned him. These maternal movements led, in turn, to further infant "dodges." The most striking dodges were extreme 90° head aversions, which have been described by Stern (1971). The infant also moved his head from one side to the other, "through" the center, directly face-to-face with mother, with eyes squeezed shut. Thus, the infant's withdrawal behaviors influenced the mother to chase, and the mother's chase behaviors influenced the infant to withdraw further.

The mother's reactions to these "dodges" were to become sober, grimace, bite her lip, jut out her jaw, or roughly thrust the infant away from her. Toward the end of the interaction, the infant increasingly lapsed into a limp, motionless headhang, which we term "inhibition of responsitivity" (which looks like "playing possum"; see Fraiberg's, 1982, description of "freezing"). No matter how vigorously the mother bounced, poked, or pulled, the infant remained motionless, giving an impression of a profound refusal to engage. At several points, the mother joined the infant in a limp headhang of her own. These gaze aversions, increasing head aversions, bodily aversions (pulling hand out of mother's grasp), and limp, motionless states can be seen as a series of increasing visual-spatial boundaries in relation to the mother.

In the sensitive interaction of "chase and dodge," each partner's adjustment to the other frequently occurred coactively; that is, one partner's "response" began before the other's behavior had been completed, with latencies under one half sec. The infant was thus sensitive to each maternal movement from moment to moment, although in the withdrawal direction, thus constructing a complex compromise between engagement and disengagement. Rather than "tuning out," this interaction points to a model of early coping capacity as continued responsivity and vigilance.

Implications of Mutually Regulated Aversive Patterns for the Organization of Infant Experience

We have suggested elsewhere (Beebe and Lachmann, 1988) that a mutual regulation structure may remain intact, and yet the pair may be "misattuned" in various ways: affect, arousal, timing, and so on. The "chase and dodge" interaction illustrates such a misattunement. Mother and infant continue a sensitive responsivity to each other. "Relatedness" per se, that is, the mutual influence structure, is not disrupted, because mother's "chase" behavior increases the probability of infant "dodges" and vice versa. Rather, it is the attunement of the relatedness that is compromised. Infant attention, affect, and arousal are not optimally regulated.

One form of misattunement can be conceptualized as the loss of contingent responsivity in either partner or as the loss of mutuality of influence. However, neither partner loses responsivity to the other in the "derailed" interaction just described. What makes this interaction atypical is that, although the infant's head aversion still influences the mother's behavior, it is in the direction of increasing the intensity of maternal stimulation. In the normative pattern, when the infant looks and turns away the mother temporarily decreases her stimulation (Brazelton et al., 1974; Donovan and Leavitt, 1978; Langhorst and Fogel, 1982; Hirschfeld, 1985; Hirschfeld and Beebe, 1987). The infant uses gaze aversion to reregulate his arousal. The infant's heart rate during play accelerates just before and decelerates just after a gaze aversion (Field, 1981). However, in this interaction, although the infant's own state of arousal decreased when he looked and turned away, the mother did not participate in the deescalation of arousal, in other words, in the infant's attainment of a calmer state. It appears that this mother had difficulty tolerating the infant's disengagement.

One could make various inferences about the infant's subjective experience in the "chase and dodge" interaction if this interaction proved to be typical of this particular pair. Normally, an infant experiences "efficacy": when events in the environment are contingent on his behavior, he experiences himself as the "producer" of these events (see DeCasper and Carstens, 1980). Because this mother's behavior was still contingent on the infant's behavior, this infant's experience of efficacy was to some degree intact. However, what this infant could "produce" in his mother's behavior was not typical, because he "produced" escalating intensity of maternal stimulation. Thus, he may have experienced having to calm himself "by himself." We speculate that the experience of efficacy itself was to some degree compromised because, although the infant's actions continued to "produce" effects, these effects are associated with negative affects and escalating arousal. The nature of the mutual regulation did not facilitate and may have actively interfered with this infant's optimal regulation of his own arousal.

Typically, as mutual regulation proceeds, infant affect and arousal remain within an optimal range, and mutual gaze with positive affect is readily available (Stern, 1977). In an atypical interaction such as this one, predictability and mutual influence remain, but, nevertheless, some aspect of the infant's behavior is not optimally regulated. Positive affect is dramatically interfered with, and the infant shows extreme postural aversion and withdrawal. Expectancies of misregulation organize such an infant's experience. That is, the aversive stimulation is contingent on his behavior, and the infant will come to expect this kind of negative interaction or "misattunement." If this interaction structure is characteristic of the pair, the infant chronically experiences extremes in certain affect and arousal states; these states have a greater or lesser tendency to dominate his experience; and the infant experiences less than optimal success in his extreme attempts to regulate these states. The mutual regulation structure thus retains interrelatedness but does not succeed in the optimal regulation of infant attention, affect, and arousal.

We suggest that expectancies of such misregulation or "misattunement" are stored as presymbolic representations. If they remain characteristic of the interaction, by the end of the first year they will be abstracted as prototypic. This composite prototype forms the basis for an emerging symbolic representation of self and object as misattuned.

DISCUSSION

We propose that interaction structures are represented over the early months of life and play a major role in the emerging symbolic forms of self- and object representations. The characteristic mutual influence patterns in purely social exchanges define interaction structures. An early presymbolic representational ability is used to store those interaction patterns that are recurrent, expectable, and characteristic. In the early months, the infant perceives, orders, and stores information about regularities and features of the environment. These capacities are used to store information about his social interactions as well. The infant is capable of comparing the nature of the interaction pattern at the moment with a stored model or representation of how the interaction typically goes and of evaluating whether the two are similar or different. The infant is organizing a "representational world" in the first half of the first year, prior to the emergence of symbolic capacity.

Although many issues are relevant to the origins of self- and object representations (see, e.g., Sandler and Rosenblatt, 1962; Fraiberg,

1969; Schimek, 1975; McDevitt, 1975; Blatt and Wild, 1976; Hadley, 1983; Main et al., 1985), we have described the dimension of self- and object representations having to do with the nature of the interrelatedness being represented. Several patterns of mutual regulation have been described, which can provide an empirical basis for conceptualizing this dimension. The dynamic interplay between the actions (including perceptions, affects, and proprioceptions) of infant and caretaker, as each influences the other, creates a great variety of mutual regulatory patterns. Not only are numerous matching experiences mutually regulated, but derailed interactions are mutually regulated as well. We suggest that the pattern of mutual regulation, when characteristic, is stored in the early presymbolic representations. Under conditions of matching, expectancies of matching are represented. The matching pattern and the shared states associated with matching are represented. Under conditions of "derailment" or misattunement, expectancies of misregulation of attention, affect, and arousal are represented. We suggest that not only is the derailed pattern represented, but also an associated disjunction or mismatch of states.

Not simply the infant's action nor the caretaker's responses, but rather the very process of reciprocal adjustments, as these create expected patterns, is the substance of these earliest "interactive representations" (Beebe, 1986; Beebe and Stern, 1977; see also Fast, 1988). Early representations of purely social exchanges should be conceptualized as interactive, that is, actions-of-self-in-relation-to-actions-of-objects (Beebe and Stern, 1977; Stern, 1977; Beebe, 1985). "Actions" include perceptions, affects, and proprioceptions. What is represented is an emergent dyadic phenomenon, interaction structures, which cannot be described on the basis of either partner alone. This interactive "process model" of early representations implies that in the social domain the experience of self and object are structured simultaneously. (See Sullivan, 1953; Sander, 1977, 983a,b; Stern, 1983; Atwood and Stolorow, 1984; Beebe and Lachmann, 1988, who have expressed similar views.)

The Prediction of Later Developmental Outcomes from Early Interaction Patterns

There is a large literature documenting that variations in early social interactions do make a difference in cognitive development and patterns of attachment during the first two years. For example, measures of mutual gazing, mutual smiling, and social play in the first 4 months predict cognitive measures at one and two years

(Cohen and Beckwith, 1979; Alper, 1982; Crockenberg, 1983). Studies of attachment show that infants identified as securely attached at one year show more looking, smiling, and excitement in social play at two to four months, whereas infants identified as anxiously attached at one year show more looking away, fussing, and unresponsiveness at four months (Blehar et al., 1977). Furthermore, maternal capacity to respond contingently to infant signals in the first six months has been shown to predict later cognitive (Cohen and Beckwith, 1979; Nelson, 1979; Alper, 1982; Crockenberg, 1983) and social (Ainsworth and Bell, 1974; Blehar et al., 1977; Langhorst and Fogel, 1982) outcomes. Maternal capacity to reserve stimulation for periods when the infant is attentive during social play predicts infant attachment and cognition in the second year (Donovan and Leavitt, 1978; Langhorst and Fogel, 1982). Maternal sensitivity during feeding at four weeks (rhythmic holding and facilitation of infant activity) predicts secure attachment at one year (Price, 1982).

A recent longitudinal study of 12 dyads has provided suggestive evidence that interaction structures at four months predict interaction structures at 24 months (Reich, 1988). The study showed that indices of the infant's capacity to track and be influenced by mother's engagement changes at four months (as measured by time series regression) predicted a measure of mutual influence to track the partner's engagement changes at 24 months. In addition, a measure of matching temporal patterns of vocalization at four months and a clinical evaluation of maternal sensitivity at four months also predicted mutual influence to track engagement changes at 24 months.

In proposing that interaction structures organize early representations, we cited various studies showing that early interaction structures predict cognition, attachment, and interaction structures in the second year. Cognition is a substrate of representation; attachment is an affective and relational dimension of representation; and interaction structures may both influence and be influenced by representations in the second year. From early interaction structures we can predict aspects of later representations and infer that early interaction structures are relevant to emerging self- and object representations.

VARIATIONS IN THE ORGANIZATION OF INFANT EXPERIENCE

In proposing interaction structures as central organizers of the infant's experience, we limit our discussion to the normal range of purely social interactions. In this range, mutual influence itself can be considered to define "relatedness," that is, an experience of affecting and being affected by the partner (see also Ruesch and Bateson, 1951; Sullivan, 1953). The stipulation that the mutual influence structures be characteristic in order to be candidates for organizing the infant's experience invokes the infant's capacity to expect predictable patterns, which eventually become generalized.

These criteria, however, still do not go far enough to allow us to infer the specific quality of the infant's subjective experience. Affective quality seems to be independent of mutual influence. For example, both the "chase and dodge" interaction and the mirroring exchanges are mutual influence structures, but they convey widely different affective tones. Mutual influence structures can encompass multiple patterns that convey a wide range of qualities or affective nuances. Within the mutual influence structures, it is necessary to define the specific nature of the mutual influence pattern in order to infer different qualities or affective nuances of interrelatedness and subjective experience being represented. We use the examples of mutual influence structures presented here, "misattuned" exchanges and "matching" exchanges, to speculate about specific qualities of the infant's subjective experience.

The kinds of withdrawal responses the infant shows and the interactive regulation of these withdrawal responses may affect later adaptations, defenses, representations, and subjective experiences. If the infant characteristically must resort to increasingly severe and prolonged withdrawal states in order to accomplish "time out" and a reregulation of arousal, his or her attention and information processing may be compromised (see, e.g., Brazelton et al., 1974; Donovan and Leavitt, 1978; Hirschfeld and Beebe, 1987). For example, an infant who typically uses inhibition of responsivity (playing possum) or seems to stare right through his partner ("glazing over") alters his capacity to stay alert and to be fully attentive and responsive to the environment. Later styles of adaptation and defense may be affected.

To translate from the chase-and-dodge interaction into the infant's subjective experience and into the language of adults, we take a step from the concrete action schemes of moving away to moving away in a metaphorical sense, that is, to psychological distance. We take the step from presymbolic representations to verbalized symbols. If infant withdrawal states are interactively regulated in a "chase-and-dodge" fashion, the symbolic representation of self and object may include experiences of "When I stay close to you, I feel overaroused and inundated. I feel you are moving in on me. No matter where I move in relation to you, I cannot find a way to feel comfortable. I can neither engage with you nor disengage from you." The easy balance between moments of engagement and disengagement is disturbed, and the interaction is dominated by the management of disengagement at the relative expense of engagement states. The later symbolic representation of the self as temporarily and partially "away from" the object may become more salient than the representation of states of engagement. In addition, the representation of the self as "away" is associated with the management of states of overarousal.

States of matching or similarity are key moments in the interaction. For example, Stern (1983) considered state sharing, such as vocal coaction or affect contagion, to be the basis of subjective intimacy. Demos (1984) accorded central importance to affective resonance, defined as the tendency to experience the same affect that is experienced by the other. The data presented here, documenting matching of temporal and affective patterns, go further in defining how the sharing of subjective states can occur. The findings of moment-to-moment mutual influence to match and track the other's behavior reveal particular forms of "resonance" or "state sharing." Ekman's (1983) and Zajonc's (1985) research indicate that reproducing the action patterns associated with the partner's emotional display evokes a psychophysiological state in the observer that corresponds to that of the partner. This correspondence, a mechanism of resonance or state-sharing, can be considered a precursor of empathy.

We suggest that the emerging symbolic representations are importantly different if matching is among the mutual influence structures that are easily available to the dyad. Matching the behavioral display of the partner provides more information about the partner than is available simply through the distance receptors, because one's own physiological state becomes an additional source of information. Thus, matching provides an approximation to the subjective state of the partner, which cannot be accessed directly. Regardless of whether the matching is of "positive" states (e.g., both mother and infant increasing the widening and opening of their smiles) or of "negative" states (e.g., mother sobering as infant frowns), the similarity provides a powerful link to the partner. The representation of self and object based on experiences of matching are proposed to be crucial to later symbolic experiences of feeling "known," "understood," or "involved."

To translate from the presymbolic matching interactions into a symbolic level of experience, we again make an inference to dimensions of affective experience, using such concrete sensorimotor spatial configurations as opening and closing the mouth and eyes or crescendos and decrescendos of smiles. Similarly, we infer from the concrete coordination of temporal patterns an experience of the coordination of feeling states. Again speaking from the subjective viewpoint of the infant, but in the language of adults, as symbolic capacities emerge, we suggest that the matching experiences may eventually be represented as the following self and object configurations: "I become similar to the way you look to me; I see you look like the way I feel; I feel similar to the way you feel. Our smiles and our heads move up and down together; it is both arousing and comfortable. I move at your pace; I feel you are matching my rhythm and balancing my tempo; we are on the same wavelength."

The derailment exchanges and the matching exchanges can be used to illustrate qualitative differences in the presymbolic organization of representations, which we assume continue to affect the emerging symbolic level of representations. These qualitative differences in the recurrent configurations of self- and object representations, based on the early interaction patterns, then continue to organize, alter, and potentially limit subsequent experience (see Atwood and Stolorow, 1984; Main et al., 1985). Main et al. argue that these representations form a set of conscious and unconscious "rules" that guide appraisals of experience and behavior, thus permitting or limiting access to the kinds of information and memories available regarding attachment figures. Many authors suggest that, once structured, these representations tend to resist restructuring because they operate largely outside conscious awareness and because they tend to be actively self-perpetuating (Freud, 1938; Sullivan, 1953; Bowlby, 1980; Main et al., 1985; Sroufe and Fleeson, 1986).

In summary, the characteristic patterns of mutual influence in purely social exchanges between mother and infant in the first six months of life provide an important basis for emerging self- and object representations. The dynamic, reciprocal interplay, as each partner influences the other, creates expected patterns of exchange that are represented in a presymbolic form during the first year. These early representations are abstracted toward the end of the first year and form the basis for emerging symbolic self- and object representations. Empirical studies have shown mutual influences in infant-caretaker matching of affect and timing. These matching experiences provide each partner with a behavioral basis for knowing and entering the other's perception, temporal world, and feeling state, and may contribute to later experiences of being attuned, known, tracked, or "on the same wavelength." An empirical study describing an interactive derailment illustrates that, even in aversive interactions, mutual influence prevails. These mutual influence patterns illustrate qualitative variations in the nature of the interrelatedness that will organize emerging self- and object representations.

REFERENCES

Ainsworth, M. & Bell, S. (1974), Mother–infant interaction and the development of competence. In: *The Growth of Competence*, ed. J. Connolly & J. Bruner. New York: Academic Press.
Allen, T., Walker, K., Symonds, L. & Marcell, M. (1977), Intrasensory and intersensory perception of temporal sequences during infancy. *Develop. Psychol.*, 13:225–229.
Alper, R. (1982), Mother–infant interaction and infant cognitive competence. Unpublished doctoral dissertation, Yeshiva University, New York.
Alson, D. (1982), Maternal empathy in relation to infant affective engagement at four months. Unpublished doctoral dissertation, Yeshiva University, New York.
American College Dictionary (1962), New York: Random House.
Atwood, G. & Stolorow, R. (1984), *Structures of Subjectivity*. Hillsdale, NJ: The Analytic Press.
Bahrick, L. & Watson, J. (1985), Detection of intermodal proprioceptive-visual contingency as a potential basis of self-perception in infancy. *Develop. Psychol.*, 21:963–973.
Beebe, B. (1973), Ontogeny of positive affect in the third and fourth months of the life of one infant. Doctoral dissertation, Columbia University. *Dissertation Abstracts International*, 35(2), 1014B.
———— (1982), Micro-timing in mother–infant communication. In: *Nonverbal Communication Today*, ed. M. Key. New York: Mouton, pp. 169–195.
———— (1986), Mother–infant mutual influence and precursors of self- and object representations. In: *Empirical Studies of Psychoanalytic Theories, Vol. 2*, ed. J. Masling. Hillsdale, NJ: The Analytic Press, pp. 27–48.
———— Alson, D., Jaffe, J., Feldstein, S. & Crown, C. (1988), Mother–infant vocal congruence. *J. Psycholing. Res.*, 17:245–259.
———— & Crown, C. (1988), Mutual regulation of engagement in mother–infant face-to-face play. Unpublished manuscript.
———— & Gerstman, L. (1980), The "packaging" of maternal stimulation in relation to infant facial-visual engagement. A case study at four months. *Merrill-Palmer Quart.*, 26:321–339.
———— Jaffe, J., Feldstein, S., Mays, K. & Alson, D. (1985), Interpersonal timings: The application of an adult dialogue model to mother–infant vocal and kinesic interactions. In: *Social Perception in Infants*, ed. T. Field & N. Fox. Norwood, NJ: Ablex, pp. 217–247.
———— & Kronen, J. (1988), Mutual regulation of affective matching in mother–infant face-to-face play. Unpublished manuscript.
———— & Lachmann, F. (1988), Mother–infant mutual influence and precursors of psychic structure. In: *Frontiers in Self Psychology: Progress in Self Psychology, Vol. 3*, ed. A. Goldberg. Hillsdale, NJ: The Analytic Press, pp. 3–26.
———— & Stern, D. (1977), Engagement-disengagement and early object experiences. In: *Communicative Structures and Psychic Structures*, ed. N. Freedman & S. Grand. New York: Plenum, pp. 35–55.
———— ———— & Jaffe, J. (1979), The kinesic rhythm of mother–infant interactions. In: *Of Speech and Time*, ed. A. W. Siegman & S. Feldstein. Hillsdale, NJ: Lawrence Erlbaum Associates, pp. 23–34.

Bertalanffy, L. von (1952), *Problems of Life*. New York: Wiley.

Blatt, S. & Wild, C. (1976), *Schizophrenia*. New York: Academic Press.

Blehar, M., Lieberman, A. F. & Ainsworth, M. (1977), Early face-to-face interaction and its relation to later mother–infant attachment. *Child Devel.*, 48:182–194.

Bornstein, M. (1979), Perceptual development: Stability and change in feature perception. In: *Psychological Development from Infancy*, ed. M. Bornstein & W. Kessen. Hillsdale, NJ: Lawrence Erlbaum Associates, pp. 37–81.

_____ (1985), Infant into adult: Unity to diversity in the development of visual categorization. In: *Neonate Cognition*, ed. J. Mehler & R. Fox. Hillsdale, NJ: Lawrence Erlbaum Associates, pp. 115–138.

Bower, T., Broughton, R. J. & Moore, M. (1970), Infant responses to approaching objects. *Percept. & Psychophysics*, 9:193–196.

Bowlby, J. (1980), *Attachment and Loss*, Vol. 3. New York: Basic Books.

Brazelton, T. B., Kozlowski, B. & Main, M. (1974), The origins of reciprocity. In: *The Effect of the Infant on Its Caregiver*, ed. M. Lewis & L. Rosenblum. New York: Wiley-Interscience, pp. 49–76.

_____ Tronick, E., Adamson, L., Als, H. & Wise, S. (1975), Early mother–infant reciprocity. In: *The Parent-Infant Relationship*, ed. M. A. Hofer. New York: Elsevier, pp. 137–154.

Byers, P. (1975), Biological rhythms as information channels in interpersonal communication behavior. In: *Perspectives in Ethology*, ed. P. Klopfer & G. Bateson. New York: Plenum.

Cappella, J. N. (1981), Mutual influence inexpressive behavior: Adult and infant-adult dyadic interaction. *Psychol. Bull.*, 89:101–132.

Church, J. (1961), *Language and the Discovery of Reality*. New York: Vintage.

Cohen, L. (1973), A two process model of infant visual attention. *Merrill-Palmer Quart.*, 19:157–180.

_____ DeLoache, J. & Strauss, M. (1979), Infant visual perception. In: *Handbook of Infant Development*, ed. J. Osofsky. New York: Wiley, pp. 393–438.

_____ & Gelber, E. (1975), Infant visual memory. In: *Infant Perception*, Vol. 1, ed. L. Cohen & P. Salapatck. New York: Academic Press, pp. 347–403.

Cohen, S. & Beckwith, L. (1979), Preterm infant interaction with the caregiver in the first year of life and competence at age two. *Child Devel.*, 50:767–776.

Cohn, J. & Tronick, E. (1988), Mother–infant face-to-face interaction: Influence is bidirectional and unrelated to periodic cycles in either partner's behavior. *Devel. Psychol.*, 24:386–392.

Crockenberg, S. (1983), Early mother and infant antecedents of Bayley skill performance at 21 months. *Devel. Psychol.*, 19:27–730.

Crown, C., Feldstein, S., Jasnow, M., Beebe, B., Wagman, I., Gordon, S., Fox H. & Jaffe, J. (1988), The cross-modal coordination of interpersonal timing: Infant gaze with adult vocal behavior. Presented at International Conference of Infant Studies, Washington, DC.

DeCasper, A. & Carstens, A. (1980), Contingencies of stimulation: Effects on learning and emotion in neonates. *Infant Beh. & Devel.*, 4:19–36.

_____ A. & Fifer, W. (1980), Of human bonding: Newborns prefer their mothers' voices. *Science*, 208:1174.

_____ & Spence, M. (1986), Prenatal maternal speech influences newborns' perceptions of speech sounds. *Infant Beh. & Devel.*, 9:133–150.

Demos, V. (1984), Empathy and affect: Reflections on infant experience. In: *Empathy*, Vol. 2. ed. J. Lichtenberg, M. Bornstein & D. Silver. Hillsdale, NJ: The Analytic Press, pp. 9–34.

Donovan, W. & Leavitt, L. (1978), Early cognitive development and its relation to maternal physiologic and behavioral responsiveness. *Child Devel.*, 49:1251–1254.

Eimas, P. D. (1985), Constraints on a model of infant speech perception. In: *Neonate Cognition*, ed. J. Mehler & R. Fox. Hillsdale, NJ: Lawrence Erlbaum Associates, pp. 185–197.

————— & Miller, J. L. (1980), Contextual effects in infant speech perception. *Science*, 209:1140–1141.

Ekman, P. (1983), Autonomic nervous system activity distinguishes among emotions. *Science*, 221:1208–1210.

Emde, R. (1981), The prerepresentational self and its affective core. *The Psychoanalytic Study of the Child*, 36:165–192. New Haven, CT: Yale University Press.

Erikson, E. (1950), *Childhood and Society*. New York: Norton.

Fagan, J. F. (1974), Infant recognition memory: The effects of length of familiarization and type of discrimination task. *Child Devel.*, 45:351–356.

Fagen, J. W., Morrongiello, B. A., Rovee-Collier, C. & Gekoski, M. J. (1984), Expectancies and memory retrieval in three-month-old infants. *Child Devel.*, 55:936–943.

Fairbairn, W. R. D. (1954), *An Object Relations Theory of the Personality*. New York: Basic Books.

Fantz, R., Fagan, J. & Miranda, S. (1975), Early visual selectivity. In: *Infant Perception, Vol. 1*, ed. I. Cohen & P. Salapatek. New York: Academic Press, pp. 249–346.

Fast, I. (1988), Body image: An alternative perspective. Unpublished manuscript, University of Michigan, Ann Arbor.

Feldstein, S. & Welkowitz, J. (1978), A chronography of conversation: In defense of an objective approach. In: *Nonverbal Behavior and Communication*, ed. A. W. Siegman & S. Feldstein. Hillsdale, NJ: Lawrence Erlbaum Associates, pp. 329–377.

Field, T. (1981), Infant gaze aversion and heart rate during face-to face interactions. *Infant Beh. & Devel.*, 4:307–315.

————— Woodson, R., Greenberg, R. & Cohen, D. (1982), Discrimination and imitation of facial expressions by neonates. *Science*, 218:179–181.

Finkelstein, N. W. & Ramey, C. T. (1977), Learning to control the environment in infancy. *Child Devel.*, 48:806–819.

Fraiberg, S. (1969), Libidinal object constancy and mental representation. *The Psychoanalytic Study of the Child*, 24:9–47. New York: International Universities Press.

Fraiberg, S. (1982), Pathological defense in infancy. *Psychoanal. Quart.*, 51:612–635.

Freud, S. (1938), An outline of psychoanalysis. *Standard Edition* 23:139–207. London: Hogarth Press, 1964.

Gianino, A. & Tronick, E. (1988), The mutual regulation model: The infant's self and interactive regulation and coping and defensive capacities. In: *Stress and Coping*, ed. T. Field, P. McCabe & N. Schneiderman. Hillsdale, NJ: Lawrence Erlbaum Associates, pp. 47–60.

Gottman, J. (1981), *Time Series Analysis*. Cambridge: Cambridge University Press.

Greco, C., Rovee-Collier, C., Hayne, H., Griesler, P. & Early, L. (1986), Ontogeny of early event memory: I. Forgetting and retrieval by 2- and 3-month olds. *Infant Beh. & Devel.*, 9:441–460.

Hadley, J. (1983), The representational system: A bridging concept for psychoanalysis and neurophysiology. *Internat. Rev. Psycho-Anal.*, 10:13–30.

Hayne, H., Greco, C., Earley, L., Griesler, P. & Rovee-Collier, C. (1986), Ontogeny of early event memory: II. Encoding and retrieval and 2- and 3-month olds. *Infant Beh. & Devel.*, 9:461–472.

Hirschfeld, N. (1985), Maternal intensity and infant disengagement in face to face play. Unpublished doctoral dissertation, Yeshiva University, New York.

————— & Beebe, B. (1987), Maternal intensity and infant disengagement in face-to-face play. Presented at the Society for Research in Child Development, Baltimore, MD.

Horner, T. (1985), The psychic life of the young infant: Review and critique of the psychoanalytic concepts of symbiosis and infantile omnipotence. *Amer. J. Orthopsychiat.*, 55:324–344.

Horowitz, M. J. (1972), Modes of representation of thought. *J. Amer. Psychoanal. Assn.*, 20:793–819.

Jacobson, E. (1964), *The Self and the Object World*. New York: International Universities Press.

Jaffe, J. & Feldstein, S. (1970), *Rhythms of Dialogue*. New York: Academic Press.

_____ Anderson, S. & Stern, D. (1979), Conversational rhythms. In: *Psycholinguistic Research*, ed. D. Aronson & R. Rieber. Hillsdale, NJ: Lawrence Erlbaum Associates, pp. 393–431.

Jasnow, M. (1983), Temporal accommodation in vocal behavior in mother–infant dyads. Unpublished doctoral dissertation, George Washington University, Washington, DC.

Kagan, J. (1978), The enhancement of memory in infancy. *Newsletter of the Institute for Comparative Human Development*, pp. 58–60.

_____ (1979), Structure and process in the human infant: The ontogeny of mental representation. In: *Psychological Development in Infancy*, ed. M. Bornstein & W. Kessen. Hillsdale, NJ: Lawrence Erlbaum Associates, pp. 159–182.

Kaye, K. (1982), *The Mental and Social Life of Babies*. Chicago: University of Chicago Press.

Kohut, H. (1971), *The Analysis of the Self*. New York: International Universities Press.

_____ (1977), *The Restoration of the Self*. New York: International Universities Press.

Kronen, J. (1982), Maternal facial mirroring at four months. Unpublished doctoral dissertation, Yeshiva University, New York.

Kuhl, P. (1985), Categorization of speech by infants. In: *Neonate Cognition*, ed. J. Mehler & R. Fox. Hillsdale, NJ: Lawrence Erlbaum Associates, pp. 231–262.

_____ & Meltzoff, A. (1984), The intermodal representation of speech in infants. *Infant Beh. & Devel.*, 7:361–380.

Lamb, M. (1981), The development of social expectations in the first year of life. In: *Infant Social Cognition*, ed. M. Lamb & L. Sherrod. Hillsdale, NJ: Lawrence Erlbaum Associates, pp. 155–176.

Langhorst, B. & Fogel, A. (1982, April), Cross-validation of micro-analytic approaches to face-to-face interaction. Presented at International Conference on Infant Studies Austin, TX.

Lewis, M. & Brooks, J. (1975), Infant's social perception: A constructivist view. In: *Infant Perception. Vol. 2*, ed. L. Cohen & P. Salapatek. New York: Academic Press, pp. 102–148.

_____ & Goldberg, S. (1969), Perceptual-cognitive development in infancy: A generalized expectancy model as a function of the mother–infant interaction. *Merrill-Palmer Quart.*, 15:81–100.

Lewkowicz, D. & Turkewitz, G. (1980), Cross-modal equivalence in early infancy: Audio-visual intensity matching. *Devel. Psychol.*, 16:597–607.

Lichtenberg, J. D. (1983), *Psychoanalysis and Infant Research*. Hillsdale, NJ: The Analytic Press.

Mahler, M., Pine, F. & Bergman, A. (1975), *The Psychological Birth of the Human Infant*. New York: Basic Books.

Main, M., Kaplan, N. & Cassidy, J. (1985), Security in infancy, childhood, and adulthood: A move to the level of representation. *Monogr. Society for Research in Child Development*, 50 (1–2, Serial No. 209):66–104.

Marler, P. (1965), Communication in monkeys and apes. In: *Primate Behavior*, ed. I. Devore. New York: Holt, Rinehart & Winston, pp. 544–584.

Mast, V., Fagen, J., Rovee-Collier, C. & Sullivan, M. (1980), Immediate and long-term memory for reinforcement context: The development of learned expectancies in early infancy. *Child Devel.*, 51:700–707.

Mayer, N. & Tronick, E. (1985), Mother's turn-giving signals and infant turn-taking in mother–infant interaction. In: *Social Perception in Infants*, ed. T. Field & N. Fox. Norwood, NJ: Ablex, pp. 199–216.

Mays, K. (1984), Temporal accommodation in mother–infant and stranger–infant kinesic interactions at four months. Unpublished doctoral dissertation, Yeshiva University, New York.

McCall, R. (1979), Qualitative transitions in behavioral development in the first two years of life. In: *Psychological Development in Infancy*, ed. M. Bornstein & W. Kessen. Hillsdale, NJ: Lawrence Erlbaum Associates, pp. 183–224.

McDevitt, J. (1975), Separation-individuation and object constancy. *J. Amer. Psychoanal. Assn.*, 23:713–742.

Mehler, J. (1985), Language-related dispositions in early infancy. In: *Neonate Cognition*, ed. J. Mehler & R. Fox. Hillsdale, NJ: Lawrence Erlbaum Associates, pp. 7–28.

Meltzoff, A. (1985), The roots of social and cognitive development: Models of man's original nature. In: *Social Perception in Infants*, ed. T. Field & N. Fox. Norwood, NJ: Ablex, pp. 1–30.

———— & Moore, M. (1977), Imitation of facial and manual gestures by human neonates. *Science*, 198:75–78.

Millar, W. S. & Watson, J. S. (1979), The effects of delayed feedback on infancy learning reexamined. *Child Devel.*, 50:747–751.

Natale, M., Dahlberg, C. & Jaffe, J. (1979), The effect of LSD and dextroamphetamine on therapist-patient matching of speech "rhythms." *J. Comm. Dis.*, 12:45–52.

Nelson, K. (1979), The role of language in infant development. In: *Psychological Development in Infancy*, ed. M. Bornstein & W. Kessen. Hillsdale, NJ: Lawrence Erlbaum Associates, pp. 307–337.

Papousek, H. & Papousek, M. (1977), Mother and the cognitive head start. In: *Studies in Mother-Infant Interaction*, ed. H. R. Schaffer. New York: Academic Press, pp. 63–85.

———— & ———— (1979), Early ontogeny of human social interaction. In: *Human Ethology*, ed. M. Von Cranach, K. Koppa, W. Lepenies & P. Ploog. Cambridge: Cambridge University Press, pp. 63–85.

Piaget, J. (1937), *The Construction of reality in the child* (M. Cook, Trans.), New York: Basic Books, 1954.

Pine, F. (1985). *Developmental Theory and Clinical Process*. New Haven, CT: Yale University Press.

Price, G. (1982, July), Maternal sensitivity at four weeks and attachment status at one year as manifestations of maternal empathy. Presented at Tenth International congress of the International Association for Child and Adolescent Psychiatry, Dublin, Ireland.

Reich, M. (1988), The prediction of social interaction at two years from mother–infant interaction at four months. Unpublished doctoral dissertation, Yeshiva University, New York.

Robson, K. (1967), The role of eye-to-eye contact in maternal-infant attachment. *J. Child Psychol. Psychiat.*, 8:13–25.

Rose, S. (1979), Cross-modal transfer in infant: Relationship to prematurity and socioeconomic background. *Devel. Psychol.*, 14:643–682.

Ruesch, J. & Bateson, J. (1951), *Communication*. New York: Norton.

Sander, L. (1977), The regulation of exchange in the infant-caretaker system and some aspects of the context-content relationship. In: *Interaction, Conversation, and the Development of Language*, ed. M. Lewis & L. Rosenblum. New York: Wiley, pp. 133–156.

Sander, L. (1978, May), New knowledge about the infant from current research: Implications for psychoanalysis. Presented at Annual Meeting of American Psychoanalytic Association, Atlanta, GA.

_____ (1983a), Polarity paradox, and the organizing process in development. In: *Frontiers of Infant Psychiatry*, ed. J. D. Call, E. Galenson & R. Tyson. New York: Basic Books, pp. 315–327.

_____ (1983b), To begin with: Reflections on ontogeny. In: *Reflections on Self Psychology*, ed. J. Lichtenberg & S. Kaplan. Hillsdale, NJ: The Analytic Press, pp. 85–104.

Sandler, J. & Rosenblatt, B. (1962), The concept of the representational world. *The Psychoanalytic Study of the Child*. 17:128–145. New York: International Universities Press.

Schaffer, H. R., (1977), *Studies in Mother–Infant Interaction*. London: Academic Press.

Schilder, P. (1964), *Contributions to Developmental Neuropsychiatry*. New York: International Universities Press.

Schimek, J. (1975), A critical re-examination of Freud's concept of unconscious mental representation. *Internat. Rev. Psycho-Anal.*, 2:171–187.

Seligman, N. (1975), *Helplessness*. San Francisco: Freeman.

Spelke, E. S. & Cortelyou, A. (1981), Perceptual aspects of social knowing. In: *Infant Social Cognition*, ed. M. Lamb & L. Sherrod. Hillsdale, NJ: Lawrence Erlbaum Associates, pp. 61–84.

Spitz, R. (1959), *A Genetic Field Theory of Ego Formation*. New York: International Universities Press.

Sroufe, A. & Fleeson, J. (1986), Attachment and the construction of relationships. In: *Relationships and Development*, ed. W. Hartup & Z. Rubin. New York: Cambridge University Press, pp. 51–71.

Sroufe, L. A. (1979), The ontogenesis of emotion. In: *Handbook of Infant Development*, ed. J. Osofsky. New York: Wiley, pp. 462–516.

Stechler, G. & Kaplan, S. (1980), The development of the self. *The Psychoanalytic Study of the Child*, 35:85–105. New Haven, CT: Yale University Press.

Stern, D. (1971), A microanalysis of the mother–infant interaction. *J. Amer. Acad. Child Psychiat.*, 10:501–507.

_____ (1977), *The First Relationship*. Cambridge, MA: Harvard University Press.

_____ (1981), Early transmission of affect. Presented at First International Congress on Infant Psychiatry, Cascais, Portugal.

_____ (1983), The early development of schemas of self, of other, and of "self with other." In: *Reflections on Self Psychology*, ed. J. Lichtenberg & S. Kaplan. Hillsdale, NJ: The Analytic Press, pp. 49–84.

_____ (1985), *The Interpersonal World of the Infant*. New York: Basic books.

Strauss, M. S. (1979), Abstractions of proto-typical information by adults and 10 month old infants. *J. Exper. Psychol.*, 5:618–632.

Sullivan, H. S. (1953), *The Interpersonal Theory of Psychiatry*. New York: Norton.

Tobach, E. (1970), Some guidelines to the study of the evolution and development of emotion. In: *Development and Evolution of Behavior*, ed. L. Aronson, E. Tobach, D. Lehrman & J. Rosenblatt. San Francisco: Freeman, pp. 238–253.

Trevarthen, C. (1979), Communication and cooperation in early infancy. In: *Before Speech*, ed. M. Bullowa. New York: Cambridge University Press, pp. 321–347.

Tronick, E. (1982), Affectivity and sharing. In: *Social Interchange in Infancy*, ed. E. Tronick. Baltimore, MD: University Park Press, pp. 1–8.

Waddington, C. H. (1940), *Organizers and Genes*. Cambridge: Cambridge University Press.

Watson, J. (1985), Contingency perception in early social development. In: *Social Perception in Infants*, ed. T. Field & N. Fox. Norwood, NJ: Ablex, pp. 157-176.

Weiss, P. (1973), *The Science of Life*. Mt. Kisco, NY: Futura.

Werner, H. (1948), *Comparative Psychology of Mental Development*. New York: International Universities Press.

Werner, H. & Kaplan, B. (1963), *Symbol Formation*. New York: Wiley.

Winnicott, D. W. (1974), The mirror role of the mother and family in child development. *Playing and Reality*. Middlesex, England: Penguin.

Zajonc, R. B. (1985), Emotion and facial efference: A theory reclaimed. *Science*, 228:15-22.

Zelner, S. (1983), The organization of vocalization and gaze in early mother-infant interactive regulation. Unpublished doctoral dissertation, Yeshiva University, New York.

6

Dialogues as Transitional Space

A Rapprochement of Psychoanalysis and Developmental Psycholinguistics

ADRIENNE HARRIS

Many contemporary academic disciplines seem haunted by schizoid phenomena. Mainstream psychology, for example, is deeply fissured, its boundaries often marked by alienation, misunderstanding, and contempt. Developmental psychology produced many internal splits, separating the study of the child from that of the adult, and most crucially, isolating the study of the speaking and thinking child from that of the feeling and loving child. A child's brain, mind, emotions, and relationships are each taken as the province of methodologically incompatible intellectual and research enterprises.

Curiously, one practice seems to unify these subdisciplines. It is the disavowal of psychoanalysis. The repudiation of such a dominant and seminal body of intellectual and clinical thought by the academic practice of psychology is striking. This repudiation is organized primarily through appeals to method and scientific rigor. And these debates about explanation, verification, and proof rage within psychoanalysis as well (Holt, 1989).

My project here is to argue for rapprochement. I want to explore the possibilities of an engaged encounter between two matured and maturing systems of thought—psychoanalysis and the study of cognitive and linguistic development. There is, of course, a wonderful precedent. Initiated by the empirical and theoretical work of Daniel Stern (1975; 1983) and developed through a generation of infancy research, there is now a substantial body of writing and research that focuses on the early relational history of the infant and parent and its impact on representation and psychic structure[1].

The elaboration of infant life and interactive mother-child experience has been one of the great developments of modern mid-century developmental psychology. In the 1960s the work on infancy focused on the sensory, perceptual, and processing capacities of infants. We are now so accustomed to thinking of the intricacy and nuance of infant responsiveness that it is stunning to remember how undeveloped the psychology and psychiatry of the 1940s and 1950s actually was. "Until cortical development occurs (at almost a year) the motor behavior of the infant resembles that of the precordate animal" (Stone, Smith, and Murphy, 1973), hardly a suitable partner for attunement and mutual regulation. The first wave of modern infancy research in the 1960s focused on what has been termed "the competent infant." This work had a somewhat mechanistic orientation, colored by the information processing models of adult cognition (Stone et al., 1973). I have seen this as a "rationalizing" tendency in child study, antithetical to the whole project of psychoanalysis (Harris, 1987). I use the term "rationalizing" both to highlight and critique the view of the infant as a simply adaptive reactor, whose cognition is privileged over and split off from affect. There was no space within that model of infant mind for any unconscious phenomena or more inchoate experience.

In the 1970s this split between infant cognition, sociability, and affect was addressed through the work of Stern (1983) and his colleagues. In Stern's work and in the psychoanalyst/infancy researchers who have built on his ideas, what has been privileged is the power and persistence of early, pre-verbal, action-based patterns. Stern's claim was that the mood, quality, style, and rhythm of parent-infant interaction found stable but evolving representation in infant experience. These representations—RIGS, or Representations of Interactions that have been Generalized—become the bedrock of the self. The dyad of a mother and her infant provided a rich site in which to observe the capacities of the infant developing in response to and in the service of an evolving self structure. The development

---

[1]Analysts and clinicians are among the primary consumers of this empirical tradition and several theoreticians in psychoanalysis draw on infancy studies explicitly in model building (Lichtenberg, 1983; Beebe, 1988; Beebe and Lachmann, 1991). Fast's (1984) work on event theory constitutes a bridging activity between cognitive developmental psychology and psychoanalysis. Most recently, Furth (1987) has begun to work out a rapprochement between Freud and Piaget. These very exciting interdisciplinary projects are probably best thought of as a form of paradigm shift, to use Kuhn's (1962) model for scientific transformation.

of elaborated patterns of mutual interaction of mother and child are represented in the child's mental life as early forms of identity (Lachman and Beebe, 1989). Identity and self arose initially in the context of shared experience central to which is the infant's experience of regulation of both feeling levels and activity levels. An attuning mother is one who matches and manages the emotional and physical decibel level of her child, mapping the contours of excitement. The quality of attunement (i.e., its adequacy, distortion, or disruption) has implications for the character of the child's developing self. Stern's (1983) work claimed to marry academic and empirical traditions to ideas drawn from psychoanalysis, particularly psychoanalytic theory focusing on the role of the mother and early experience.

Yet if this was a marriage, it has been an embattled one. Infancy studies offered significant challenges to Freudian metapsychology and to the neoFreudian psychoanalytic theories of early development, in particular Mahler's (Mahler, Pine, and Bergman, 1975) model of a primary symbiotic phase preceeding the process of separation and rapprochement. Several debates have ensued. Are the representations stable and permanent features of self-structure? What are the parameters of these representational structures? These questions have been guiding the work of Beebe and Lachmann (Beebe, 1988; Beebe and Lachmann, 1991), who stress the simultaneous development both of experiences of attunement and experiences of difference.

For my purposes, the question to pursue is: What is the relationship of representation in the preverbal period to symbol use and symbol development? Less fully explored are the role and impact of human language and developing symbolization upon this interactive process and upon the child's developing identity. Yet the symbolization of experience, its meaning, the organization of primary process, anxiety, or emotion through linguistic expression, has always been the paramount focus of psychoanalysis.

In this paper, I want to show how the process of language development is implicated in the evolution of the self and of subjectivity. I am interested in looking at toddlers using the same synthesizing agenda as the work on infancy. Drawing on the core contributions of work in language development, I want to explore ways in which symbolic representation is layered onto but also embedded within the preverbal representational patterns. The child who is held, cuddled, nursed, and gazed at is also crooned and spoken to, by a grownup person who even as she modulates her speech to her baby does speak "as if" the baby were an already comprehending, rational little communicator. Mothers bring to their speech to babies all the rich fantasy elaborated around and on behalf of the child. The child is already an object of desire, a symbolically meaningful other. As Benjamin (1988) has suggested, the baby is both known and new.

My aim here is to build on the study of language acquisition and on developmental psychoanalytic theory (primarily object relations theory) to demonstrate the power of an integrative and relational approach in looking at the impact of *symbol use* upon the development of both self and object relations and upon their representation.

Language, as it is constituted in any human group we know of, is a profoundly intricate system of meaning and structure. Any person entering or being entered by language is profoundly transformed in thought, feeling and experience. Entry into the speech system is one of the great watersheds of human growth and experience. Yet paradoxically, at the same time, any child, from the moment he or she is *imagined* by a parent, is coming into being as an *already interpreted* social subject.

The dialogues of mothers and toddlers are sites for self construction and the evolution of the child's identity, just as the earlier representations of mother-infant interaction form the bedrock of self structure. This idea builds on Stern's (1983) model of the evolving structures of self, here focusing on one of the later stages—the verbal self. Beebe and Lachmann (1991) have recently elaborated this model to describe three principles of representation: ongoing regulations, disruption and repair, and heightened affective experience. The question would be: Can we find in the verbal exchanges *interactive schema* parallel to earlier pre-verbal patterns?

Children's language skill develops out of their shared linguistic and social experience with a parent, usually the mother. But these dialogues can never be only experiences of cognitive development or language learning. Instead the child is brought into an experience of self and social consciousness. In the transactions conducted through speech to and with a parent, the child is drawn into a world of words that establishes as the anthropologist Geertz (1983) notes, "the way the world is talked about—depicted, charted, represented—rather than the way it intrinsically is" (p. 12).

I am assigning to mother–toddler dialogues features of language and speech which derive from what has been termed "the language turn" in philosophy; that is, a tradition in philosophy that has provided a well grounded, critical alternative to positivism[2]. These

---

[2]Rorty (1980), in describing this shift in philosophy speaks of a shift in the kinds of questions one asks. This is a shift away from the question how do you know something to be true? Such a question pushes off in a fruitless search for first principles and fixed, objectively determined meanings. The interesting question becomes, how is it that you

debates have radiated from philosophy into many other disciplines and scholarly practices and enter our own field through the spirited discussions over whether to ground psychoanalysis as a natural science-based research enterprise or as a hermeneutic activity based on the constructive role of interpretation (Spence, 1982; Holt, 1989).

The dominant intellectual influence in this philosophical tradition is the American pragmatist Charles Sanders Peirce whose theories of meaning have influenced much of contemporary semiotics. Drawing on Peirce (1955) and on the latter work of Wittgenstein (1965), contemporary thinkers such as Giddens (1976), Bateson (1970), Geertz (1983), Taylor (1989), and others have worked to dismantle any firm conviction in fixed, pre-suppositionless truths. Meaning is established contextually, not objectively. In William James's fresh phrase, the real is "anything we are obliged to take into account" (James, 1950, p. 186).

From this perspective a crucial function of all social discourse is the making and adjudicating of meaning and it is through these speech activities that the self and the self-in-relation-to-other is constructed and played out. The dialogues of mothers and toddlers, the setting for language acquisition, would be one important setting for self structure.

> There is no way we could be inducted into personhood except by being initiated into a language. . . . This is the sense in which one cannot be a self on one's own. I am a self only in relation to certain interlocutors. . . . A self exists only within what I call a "web of interlocution" [Taylor, 1989, p. 36].

DEVELOPMENTAL PSYCHOLINGUISTICS

In reviewing child language studies I want to react to the rationalizing tradition and instead draw on work in child language that views the process of language acquisition as a constructive, collaborative

---

find what you say persuasive? With this shift in focus, language and interpretive practices, rather than objective scientific method, arbitrate meaning. This perspective has implications for the study of dialogues between an adult and a developing child. Giddens (1976) describes dialogues as "skilled performances" (p. 29) enabling people to produce and maintain themselves by the production and working out of what they mean when they talk. All family- and couple-therapy systems based on the communication models of Bateson (1976) draw on this idea, finding the pathology in any human system in the distortions and constructions worked out in language and communication.

meaning-making experience[3]. This makes mother–child dialogue an exceedingly complex, often paradoxical process. Concerning this complexity, I want to briefly note two points. First, although in this paper I am focusing on the construction and elaboration of the child's sense of self in a shared collaborative process, these ongoing dialogues are part of a process through which the mother evolves a *maternal* self. Second, these complex activities of self construction and identity making are set in dialogues between unequally powerful participants. This idea drives much theory in family systems and family therapy. Mother–toddler dialogues may be the site for profound distortion and projective identification as well as collaboration. Quite probably the process of collaborative meaning making (in mother–child discourse and in psychoanalytic dialogues) always combines distortion and recognition.

Studies of children's acquisition of language took a quantum leap in sophistication and power when Chomskian linguistics replaced behaviorist-dominated learning principles as the explanatory engine of comprehending and producing speech (see Brown, 1973, for an extended account of this work). There were many insights from the large empirical data based analyzed through Chomsky's (1965) generative grammar. The language that children produce was not solely imitative. Children used words in their own particular syntactic structures, building models of how the speech system worked. Over the first four years of life these structural models are fine-tuned and altered by the child in order to conform more and more closely to the adult forms of speech.

This was a view of language mastery that made the child a creative actor and constructor, not a reactive, passive learner. The power and pace of children's entry into the communicative system has been well documented. Children, on average, begin to work with single-word sentences at the beginning of the second year and by three-and-a-half or four have elaborated syntactic, pragmatic, and semantic structures of quite astonishing range.

This dramatic developmental process was made unnecessarily mysterious in the early work on child language by the claim that such skill was unlearned, hence innate. It was argued that the appearance of control over syntax and semantics in three- and four-year-olds was

---

[3]There has been some fascinating, provocative work pointing in the direction of integration of psychoanalytic theory and developmental psychology. Edgcumbe (1976) has been mapping stages of language development to unfolding self-structure. Horton and Sharp (1985), in their study of solacing in children and in adults, points to the use of language as a soothing device and as a transitional object. Urwin (1984) has done a critical analysis of Winnicott's conception of self and subjectivity in transitional space.

not based on prior experience or the social surrounding. This view, essentially a non-developmental, nonsocial perspective on the child's growth, seems most indebted to the heavily Cartesian features of Chomsky's (1975) theories.

Another problem with that early Chomsky-dominated period of child language studies was the exclusive focus on the rational and cognitive properties and functions of language. A child mastering language *is* expanding her cognitive and representational possibilities. But language learning is not simply the isolated mastery of the world of words and the world of objects. This, in a rather crude summary, is the child of Chomsky and the child of Piaget. There is also a tradition in child development of seeing the mastery of language as the mastery over the body and its activities. The study of verbal regulation or verbal control in the work of Luria and American interpreters of that tradition (see review in Zivin, 1979) stresses the power of speech to manage impulse, and to organize and plan sequences of action and reaction.

It has taken several decades to put in place a more interactive, relational model of the child's language development[4]. I want to draw out six distinct themes and concepts from the developmental psycholinguistic literature. Together they create a picture of early language development as a dialogical and interactional event. The attention to communicative interaction, the analysis of discourse and dialogue, allows us to see language development in the context of a social relationship. Mastery over the sounds and symbols of human language arises in a profoundly social and interpersonal sphere. Language is not some maverick, isolated skill erupting without apparent cause in two-year-olds, but a slowly evolving process rooted in children's play, their needs, their actions, their relationships.

First, there is the centrality of *meaning* and *semantics*, rather than syntax. Children have something to say and construe ways to say it. Halliday's (1975) insight was to see language acquisition as the outcome of a more general project; "learning how to mean." Meaning making arose first in activity. A child "meant" through doing,

---

[4]Bates's (1976) work connecting language acquisition to cognition drew on Piaget's theory of sensory motor and preoperational thought and its correlation with unfolding semantic schemes. The linguist who has developed the most subtle account of this interdependence of social, cognitive, and linguistic process is Halliday (1975), who has influenced a group of British psycholinguists working on child language. The work of Wells (1986), Shotter (1978), and Trevarthan (1980) places the growth of a child's mastery over symbols in a very complex interactional network. This model is quite compatible both with Piaget's idea of the transformation of internal schemes from sensorimotor to preoperational structures and with Fast's (1984) event theory.

gestures, looking, touching, etc. Later vocalizing could be brought into the service of meaning making. Halliday's (1975) account of the development of his own child, Nigel, charts a stage in which Nigel had highly idiosyncratic but predictable sound patterns, each tailored to a need, an action or a referred-to object. Finally the formal language system (culturally derived sets of symbols and their rules of use and combination) is used by the child to extend and elaborate his or her intentions.

Second, we know that children's mastery over language includes the appreciation and skillful use of *pragmatics*, the rules of how language is used in particular context. For example, it is a well-documented observation that mothers of young children use a high percentage (20%–35%) of interrogatives in their speech to children. Dore (1974) and others have shown that by the age of three or four children understand that certain questions are not innocent probes for information but unequivocal demands for action.

A nursery school teacher at the end of snack time sees an empty juice glass in front of a child. The query, "Whose juice glass is this?" prompts the child to action as well as to acknowledgment. The routines and rules of nursery snack-time—throwing the paper cup out, or taking the glass to the sink for washing—are immediately put in play. Silence or inaction would clearly be understood as transgression. These rules of speech usage, *pragmatic* rules, are conveyed in tone, intonation, and probably with lots of nonverbal cues as well. Children process them accurately and easily. So we add to our view of children's mastery over language that this fast-forming skill will include grammar, word meaning, pronunciation rules (phonology), and pragmatics.

Third, dialogue is the site for *intersubjectivity*. Trevarthan (1980) detailed the evolution of what he has called primary and secondary intersubjectivity. Displays, turn-taking patterns, intrinsic patterns of interaction become coordinated under the management and orchestration of the mother. He described a process at the end of the first year in which the mother helps the infant triangulate with her and an object through the joint gazing at an object that may also be touched and spoken about. At the same time, much of maternal speech to children draws another triangle of mother-child-context by commenting on and describing the ongoing situation, in this way setting an interpretive context for what is happening.

By way of illustration is a brief vignette, a conversation between a mother and her two-year-old daughter. They are seated at a table, both looking at a doll house. The child identifies the house and the mother in her answer and starts to weave a story about the dollhouse.

Child: Barbie's new house.

Mother: She lives in Barbie's new house. That's right. That's where she is going to live sometimes, right?

Then the child shifts the topic, pointing to a bandaid on her mother's finger.

Child: Lemme see your boo-boo.

Mother: You wanna see my boo-boo? OK Are you gonna kiss it for me. (Child nods, looking at the cut on her mother's finger.) OK, it's much better today. Much better. Don't forget, once I take off this bandaid, I can't put it back on. (Mother removes bandaid and child kisses her finger.) Oh thank you, thank you. See, it's getting better; isn't it? It's getting all better. Pretty soon it's gonna be all right, right?

In this way gestures, sounds, words, and sentences all enter a system of social exchange. In this communicative interchange the mother's speech is used for social connection and for commentary. This capitalizes on one of the paramount features of human language: its capacity for reflective and self-reflective use. The mother's speech to her child can thus carry and expand the triangulating function Trevarthan (1980) describes, shaping the child's focus on the world of objects and the conventional meanings and experiences in the social world surrounding the child.

Triangulation, in a subtle way, offers the simultaneous experience of connection (mother and child are sharing a moment) and novelty (jointly they focus on a new third item). Gazing, gesturing, and speaking alternate between a dyadic interplay and a triangulated system. The dialogues of mothers and children bear both functions of connection and support and the uniquely symbolic function of creating new structures to stand in for and communicate experience. Dialogues are, in this way, experiences in which both the practicing subphase and later rapprochement can be enacted.

Fourth, in dialogue the speech of adults and older children is subtly and skillfully *attuned* to the level and capacity of the young interlocuter. Snow and Ferguson (1977) analyzed a form of speech they came to call "motherese" or the "baby register." Speech by mothers to children turns out to have its own unique forms and styles. Slower, higher pitched, with more intonational contours and simpler structure, the baby register (with variants used for pets, sick people, and lovers) provides children with an accessible model of speech and one which is attention grabbing and promotes interaction. Code switching—the move into the baby register—occurs almost intuitively in the presence of a small child and can be seen even in the speech of siblings to a smaller brother or sister. We have thus in the verbal sphere something analogous to the attuning and matching of the mother and her preverbal infant.

Fifth, the parent-child dialogues reveal the complex interplay of *interpretation* and *social construction*. Symbols like language are not simply neutral tools to be adapted to any child's particular needs, wishes, and intentions. Speech is imbued with culture and social significance. So harnessing language to a child's intention is an essentially paradoxical move in which aspects of the child's intent are lost to the social meaning in words themselves.

This is what Halliday (1975) meant in considering the "social semiotic" of speech (p. 43). Any sign produced by a child has intentional value for a receptive adult. Thus there is always a social level to any act of symbol use. In the term "signs" one must include sounds, words, facial expressiveness, gazing, gestures, the surrounding context, the background to the symbol, the appearance of the sign at certain times of day or in certain contexts. Any child-produced or socially mediated activity can and probably will become endowed with symbolic meaning for the mother.

One of the principles outlined by Beebe and Lachmann (1991) is "ongoing regulation." Regulation takes a new and expanded form in the realm of language and dialogue. Hence the sixth theme from the psycholinguistic research is the creation and maintenance of *narratives* in parent–child dialogue. Bruner (1990) has described and analyzed children's developing capacity and passion for making a coherent narrative of their experience. He has drawn on movements in philosophy and linguistics that privilege the *ordering* or *knowledge constituting* properties of language. Language with its structure, its linear movement, its associations of meaning, is an ideal format for the drawing together of disparate experiences in order to make some coherent sense of things. This idea will be very familiar to psychoanalysts. One strong trend within psychoanalytic theory recently has been to see the project of an analysis as the making of a narrative and the establishing of coherent narrative truth (Spence, 1982).

VYGOTSKY AND THE EVOLUTION OF INTERSUBJECTIVITY

All these features of mother–child dialogue and the complex activity of meaning construction map well to the work of Vygostky (1963;

1975). For Vygotsky, any process, any mental representation and experience was played out first in the social domain and only then internalized as an individually based conscious experience. Consciousness and thinking originate in dialogue, in social interaction. This idea parallels insights from infancy research, that mental structures of self arise in patterned experience shared between mother and infant.

Vygotsky outlined a process of development arising in what he termed "the zone of proximal development." Social interaction has potential as a site for growth. He was also speaking against the practice of measuring individual performance solely on the basis of what a child could do unaided. He defined the zone of proximal development as "the distance between the actual developmental level as determined by independent problem solving and the level of potential development as determined through problem solving under adult guidance or in collaboration with more capable peers" (Vygotsky, 1975, p. 86).

Bruner (1983, 1990) has been investigating parent-child dialogues as potential sites for this zone of proximal development, or transitional space. Linguists make a distinction in speech between subject and predicate, topic and comment, the "given" and the "new." In the dialogue between child and parent, Bruner noted the way that speech establishes what is common between the dyad (the topic; the subject) and then embellishes it, adds something new (the comment). In this way, more complex and nuanced forms of thought are produced. Initially, this synthesis of the known and the new cannot be managed by the child alone. It is first built and maintained through dialogue.

The regulating and connecting aspect of dialogue is simultaneous with another property of dialogues, their use in establishing difference, in expanding autonomy for the child. In the context of dialogues, meaning will sometimes be shared and sometimes mismatched. There is agreement and misunderstanding, distortion and repair.

Looking at dialogue in this way we might be able to see, almost diagnostically, how difference and merger are managed. Toddler dialogues, then, would be the site for subtle, fine-grained experiences of sameness and difference between mother and child. Simultaneously these dialogues are the site for self creation. Narratives, scripts, routines of social life are practiced and played out in discourse. Aspects of such dialogues are then material for internalization as the child both plays in the world and creates and elaborates an internal world with its actors and dialogues and scripts.

Bringing psychoanalytic theory to bear on this experience, we might say that dialogue holds the paradox of same/different. Dialogue allows the child both the safety of a holding environment and the possibility of a new experience. In a micro-moment of dialogue this would be an experience of refueling, or practicing. Mother–child speech, then, could be seen as a site for separation/reunion sequences, just as in early infancy face-to-face play permits match, mismatch, and repair (Lachmann and Beebe, 1989).

Finally, Vygostky embedded language use in culture and social formations. Signs, the term he used for symbols or words, were a kind of tool and all tools derived from the social space in which they developed. Individual consciousness, developed out of social interaction with socially mediated tools, would inevitably come to have a profoundly social or cultural marking. Although Vygotsky does not explicitly speak of the *un*-conscious, perhaps that too develops on the basis of the child's encounters with tools and signs and social others.

LANGUAGE AS TRANSITIONAL OBJECT

I now want to integrate these concepts from Vygotsky with Winnicott's (1971) developmental theory, in particular his work on transitional objects. Vygostky's term "zone of proximal development" has a somewhat abstract quality. Analysts, I think, will find a ready translation for this concept by thinking of Winnicott's concepts of "transitional space" as an intersubjective space and "auxiliary maternal ego." Winnicott places central importance on the relationship as a holding environment in which symbol and creativity arise in the psychic terrain between a mother and her child. In this context, the mother provides an auxiliary ego function to enable her child to evolve an experience of self and self mastery. This auxiliary ego function must take many different forms, appropriate to the particular developmental level of the child. A mother's *discourse* to her child constitutes one such format. As in Vygotsky's concept of the zone of proximal development, there is a dialectical process in Winnicott's thinking about transitional objects and the evolution of the self. Only in a transitional space – an experience of rupture or absence – can symbolic activity arise. But only with the appearance and play with *symbolic* objects that both stand for and are aspects of the mother, can the absence or loss of the mother be assimilated and integrated.

Transitional objects are transitional in two distinct senses. They are transitional as symbolic forms, embodying both symbolic and what I will call *protosymbolic* properties. The preverbal and verbal levels of representation are always inextricably intertwined. It is an attribute of symbols that they are exchangeable, that something stands for something else. Word meaning and symbolic meaning arise in a system of differences and a system of exchange. Metaphors and synonyms call on this property of substitution. In psychoanalytic terms symbols entail a sublimation or displacement. But transitional objects are also characteristically not fully exchangeable. Winnicott pointed out the tenacity of a child's requirement that the object retain its smell, its shape, its qualities. The protean character of this object, offered by the mother but created by the child, are simultaneously symbolic and presymbolic.

This duality is captured by Kristeva's (1980) work on semiotics and in particular her analysis of the semiotic function of maternal speech. She makes a distinction between the "semiotic" and the "symbolic" The semiotic features of speech are its sounds, its rhythms, its prosody, its material forms, its sinewy presence as an extension of the maternal body. These features are likely to hold quite private meanings and translations. The term "symbolic" captures the more abstractable exchangeable aspect of any word, its meaning within a system of meaning within the public form of language. Transitional objects carry both the semiotic and the symbolic. The material quality in these objects is not substitutable but profoundly cathected as an extension of the parent. Yet through the evolving play of the child, the object is moved beyond being a concrete extension of the mother into the realm of the symbolic. The child's creativity arises when the object comes to be symbolic, having as "as if" character.

The mother's speech to her child, the babbling interactive language play of mother and child, the evolving dialogues and protoconversations of mothers and toddlers expand our understanding of transitional objects and transitional space. The dialogue constitutes a space in which both an experience of self and other and self-in-relation-to-other are developed. Dialogue is precisely that which Winnicott (1971) conceptualized as potential space. There is in dialogue both safety and creative potential because the child is held in an imaginative conversation through the mother's mature dialogic capacities, and because the mother's speech to her child (at least ideally) retains the material and sensuous aspects of her nonverbal forms of maternal holding.

This treatment of language is markedly different from the more provocative Lacanian account of the process and power of symbolization. Lacan's (1970) stage theory marks discrete characterizations of an early preverbal mirror stage (dominated by the child's relation to the Imaginary) interrupted by a necessary but humbling encounter with the Symbolic. Symbols, particularly in their paramount form in human speech, break the hold of the Imaginary. The Symbolic does yeoman service, as it is through entry into the Symbolic that any child establishes a relation to desire, a subjectivity, a gender, and an unconscious.

Winnicott, in a certain way, is more surrealist than Lacan. If language and the Symbolic order are sites for both rules and the play of meaning, Lacan's tropism is for rules and Winnicott's for playfulness. Acquiescence to the Symbolic order (in development and in analysis) is one form of the resolution of the Oedipus complex, acknowledging loss and deferral of satisfactions[5]. For Winnicott, absence is one crucial press toward the use of symbols in a creative act of self construction. But symbols have elasticity and infinite playfulness. The maternal experience is both empathic holding and creative space. In this sense, the mother simultaneously maintains both an Imaginary and a Symbolically mediated connection to her child.

There is a strong affinity between Winnicott's use of symbol as the site of self development and the linguistic theories of Bakhtin (1981). First, they have in common a sense of language as the site for laughter and subversion. Secondly, they both connect the experience of loss and absence in symbols with *expansions* in consciousness.

For Bakhtin, human speech has the capability of holding and expressing all the varieties and shifts in social life. it is "impregnated by the practical situations" (p. 240). Moreover speech has what

---

[5]In Lacan's (1970) concept of the mirror stage, mother and child are initially bound in a mirroring and quasi-delusional system. The child experiences self reflected in the mirroring mother. But this reflection gives back a more coherent and whole image than the child is able to generate, ego being more fragmentary and unintegrated in the child's early experience of self. I believe this idea of the realm of the Imaginary as the early site of child ego owes more to Winnicott's idea of the mirroring mother and to Klein's work on part-objects integrating into whole-objects than Lacan ever acknowledged. Officially, Winnicott's notion of a supportive environment as a characterization both of child growth and analytic work was anathema to Lacan. An analytic process that imitated the maternal holding environment would only perpetuate the Imaginary.

Lacan's theory of language and the role of the Symbolic, drawn from Saussure (1959) and strongly influenced by semiotic theory, treats language as a system of fluid and displaceable meanings. The heart of the symbolic function is the capacity of one sign to stand in for something else. Meaning is displaced into other systems and signs. Yet foremost in a Lacanian account of the Symbolic is its connection to loss and to castration. Entry into the speech system comes at a price. Only a lost object can be symbolized. Only in absence can a symbolic representation arise. A word arises in the system of human speech, laden with culture and with already assigned meanings. When a child maps his own needs and wishes to these public meaning systems, in Lacan's view, need is reworked as desire but a desire coded as the desire of the Other. We lose the illusion of a whole subjectivity in our entry into the expanding and expansive world of symbols.

Bakhtin termed a *horizon*. What he means by this is that symbols, drawn from human language, are sites where different subjectivities encounter each other. This is so because of an "irreducible duality of speaker and listener" (p. 201). For any person speech has a public character; it draws on a public code but also on an unalienable private character, rooted in the person's own consciousness and unique individuality.

When two people, a child and a parent, for example, join in conversation, there is a potential for an encounter of two subjectivities which, when the conversers use the same words, could have sometimes overlapping and sometimes quite distinct meanings. Shared meanings and misunderstandings then are crucial sites for *expansions* of consciousness of self and of consciousness of the other. The discovery that someone using the same word as you means something different is a chance to explore ways in which you and someone else are both alike and different. Self-consciousness, an expanded reflection of the object relation and a dawning appreciation of the other's subjectivity, may thus arise within the transitional space, the parent–child dialogues in which symbol use develops.

This process underlies Winnicott's (1958) account of the importance of aggression for emotional development. An act of aggression, carefully contained by a parent, creates for the child an experience of externality, of something outside, of a limit. It brings relief from the terrors of omnipotence (i.e., the omnipotent fantasy: I can kill you in my fantasy and you will really be destroyed). In using speech to establish differences, a child and parent have the possibility to go beyond the establishment of self–other distinctions. Dialogues have the potential for the development of a position, described by Benjamin (1988). This is the discovery of an object (the mother) who is at the same time also a subject. It may be true that there is no full understanding of another's meaning. Unlike Lacan, for Winnicott and Bakhtin this is a cause for hope, not defeat. Winnicott's strong feeling for analytic interpretation as an act of inquiry rather than an act of knowing is allied to this position.

There is a second sense in which transitional objects, including language, are transitional. They are transitional in an interpersonal sense. These objects constitute a bridge between the parental imaginative holding environment and the developing child ego.

For Winnicott, maternal environment has always played a crucial role in the evolution of the child's psychic life. Two familiar terms, "primary maternal preoccupation" and "holding environment," contain the heart of this idea. I want to extend the use of these terms to include the mother or parent's holding the child in *imagination*. This means that the child exists as, and in a symbolic representation of, the mother. These representations are expressed and elaborated in the mother–infant and, later, mother–child dialogues. I include in this concept both the intense imaginative reverie of the primary maternal preoccupation at the earliest stage of life and the more elaborated verbalized communications, containing both the conscious and the unconscious formations that parents evolve in imagining and speaking to their growing children.

Maternal speech and mother–child dialogue can also be considered as a skin or a container. The narratives, vocal play, and streams of discourse through which parent and child build and maintain contact can be thought of as a kind of membrane in the auditory mode, with a complex feedback capability in which speech simultaneously serves as contact for another and transformation of the self. We might map the way Bruner (1983, 1985, 1990) and others have thought of child narratives to Bion's (1962) concept of container and contents. Speech to the child can frame and format experience, providing a container for the child's developing experience in the world of objects and the world of people. But speech also fills in the details elaborating the child's experience. In this way the contents of experience are consti-tuted for the child.

McDougall (1980, 1989) and Green (1986), among others, have writ-ten of the disastrous consequences of a failure in maternal psychic holding. Margaret Little's (1985, 1989) account of her analysis with Winnicott elaborates the power of this psychic holding in the analytic setting. We might note also that for Little this psychic holding some-times had to be grounded in actual skin contact, in Winnicott's con-taining touch. Coltart's (1991) work with silent patients must also draw on this experience. The analyst, while silent with the patient, is deep in reflective thought about the patient; the patient is held in mind.

Green's (1986) elaboration of this idea is perhaps the most provoc-ative and relevant here. He speaks of the impact on a child when the mother is taken up with concerns and bereavements outside her relation to the child. An empty mirror, reflecting absence, is consid-erably more dire for the child than a depressive or angry tie between parent and child. Even with a negative tie, there is at least an attachment to some object. Green asks us to imagine a mother devoid of fantasy about her child, a mother profoundly preoccupied else-where, again both at the conscious and unconscious level. Such a parent leaves traces of a kind of absent presence – a deadly emptiness. This highly abnormal situation, that of the child with a "dead" mother, allows us to see the potency of maternal fantasy in the more normal parent-child dyad where the parent's elaborated imaginings of the child create one element of the holding environment.

If mother–child dialogues constitute one important site in which to observe the maternal fantasy in play, given the asymmetry in social, cognitive, and linguistic power, we might imagine these maternal fantasies and projections as extremely powerful vectors in the shared construction of the child's self.

Evidence of this power can be seen in a fascinating collaborative study of the dialogues and monologues of a two-year-old girl named Emily. Led by Katherine Nelson, a group that included Jerome Bruner, John Dore, Daniel Stern, and Carol Feldman, speculated on and analyzed Emily's cognitive and emotional and linguistic processes (Nelson, 1990). They studied two different types of Emily's language play. There were transcripts from Emily's crib talk—time spent alone in her crib before nap-time, a rather key moment for the use of transitional objects. They also recorded and analyzed actual dialogues between Emily and her father.

Feldman noted that Emily's dialogues were "much duller" than her monologues. Emily's speech when she was alone in her crib trying to fall asleep has longer, more complex utterances, more pragmatic markers, and a much richer narrative structure and emotional texture. Feldman describes the difference this way: "It is her world that constitutes the domain of monologue, her father's that provides the basis for dialogic discourse" (cited in Nelson, 1990, p. 119). But the difference here may also take into account the powerful impact of the social constructive activity of the adult in these dialogues. Emily's monologues may constitute a transitional space relatively free from parental projection, more like the situation Winnicott (1965) points to in considering the "capacity to be alone in the presence of another" (p. 30). These two situations, social discourse with a parent and private monologue (which, following Bahktin, I argue, is actually a special kind of dialogue) develop in tandem as sites for self-structuring. Emily, in monologue at two-and-a-half to three years, uses speech both as her own holding environment and as transitional space perhaps less dominated by the parental projective fantasies. In dialogue, Emily must struggle with an infinitely more powerful interlocutor and a more articulated interpretation of who she is and what she means. While the origins of self may arise in shared pattern interchanges, there are important and substantial elaborations of self that arise in conditions of solitary play.

BLANKIE'S BIRTHDAY: FANTASY PLAY AND TRANSITIONAL OBJECTS

In this excerpt from an extended conversation recorded between a mother and her two-year-old daughter, I want to offer some preliminary illustrations of how mother–toddler dialogues may be studied as the site of self- and self-and-object structure. In this particular episode, there is also ample evidence of the powerful parental constructions that can arise in fantasy play.

The content, subject matter, and forms of the dialogue give insight into the dynamics of the dyad. I am suggesting that the format and experience of conversation, like the pattern of mother infant play, become part of the child's self-structure. In this study, done in home visits in which the mother chose what to play out and do with her child, her choices illuminate something of her expectations and fantasies of herself and her child. In this example, the mother, Miranda, is an artist who has stopped working to be at home with Mary. Fantasy and "let's pretend" games were a feature of all the taping made of this mother and child. Both parents in this family are involved in creative work, and both explicitly place a premium on games and activities involving creativity, imaginative use of language, and dramatic play. A different mother–child pair in the same study produced no episodes of fantasy play. In the tapings of the second pair, games of reading and naming objects, all enacted in a rather tutorial style of discourse, predominated.

Mother–child discourse can be studied as one site for the making of family meaning and social context. Almost every one of the interactions of Mary and Miranda filmed featured long narrative accounts and evocations by Miranda of what she and her daughter were doing, and many reminders to her child of the events and people of the previous year. Miranda had spent that year living geographically close to her parents with her husband close at hand, working on a project conducted at home. She spoke of the year as an idyllic time. It was quite striking, for example, how frequently Miranda's parents were brought up in conversation. There are many references to events and people no longer in the child's daily life and many accounts of past activities and future plans for shared activities with husband and friends. This focus on what is absent or in the past is in marked contrast to most mother–child dialogues, in which the conversation is based on immediate and concrete references (see Snow and Ferguson, 1977, for extended treatment on the features of "motherese").

Perhaps we might think of this mother's talk to her child, part conversation and part reverie, as Miranda's creation of a holding environment both for herself and for her child in a context of considerable isolation. Another factor contributing to the sense of aloneness was her own developmental history. Prior to having children, she had an active professional career. The arrival of her first child had radically altered her conversational and interpersonal world. Although she experienced this change as a choice and also experienced great pride and pleasure in her mothering, like many women in similar circumstances, parenting a small child had, nonetheless, inevitable features of solitude and separation from adult company.

Her stories, narratives, and ongoing conversation with her child, which evoked the past so consistently, created an ongoing experience of social and familial reality that seemed deeply comforting to her. She also offered this narrative reverie as a soothing and enlivening experience for her daughter. In a subtle and nondidactic way, this conversational style communicated steadily and reliably to the child, "This is who we are as a family, this is what matters, these people and events are what we care about."

Another striking feature of this parent–child communication is the mother's highly elaborated and extensive speech to her child. Looking at the pragmatic features, we can also note the asymmetry, the degree to which Miranda controlled and shaped the flow of discourse just as she often controlled the topic and direction of dialogue. Such discourse features as sentence ratio, turntaking, and average utterance length bear out the impression of asymmetry in this dialogue.

A discourse with long maternal sentences and long sequences of sentences but short, infrequent child responses is really more of an extended monologue, a pseudodialogue where one partner dominates. At the time of this first taping, when the child was 20 months old, the ratio sentences of mother to child was 2.1:1; later it rose to 2.8:1. Even at the end, when Mary was two-and-a-half and had a MLU of 3.35, the ratio was still 1.8:1. Miranda seemed to create a broad framework of talk, a river of words in which her daughter's briefer, single-word or short-phrase utterances bobbed like small boats.

The sequence I examine here and analyze in some detail occurred just after Mary's second birthday. It is typical of their conversations. The mother initiates a fantasy game, sets the stage for a narrative sequence, and uses household objects to operate symbolically for elements in the game. This game, a birthday party for Mary's blanket, uses a symbolic object in whose creation Mary has collaborated.

Her blanket, named Blankie, was a transitional object. It was carried about, taken to bed, and often held close to her ear while she also sucked her thumb. A small tassel that had apparently fallen off the blanket was reconnected to it with a safety pin. This object had also been given a name ("Tassel") and an identity, which both Mary and Miranda used in their play. The blanket, then, was a transitional object with its own transitional object—the tassel—and both these symbolic and emotionally laden objects occupied a psychic and interpersonal space in Miranda and Mary's discourse.

Transitional objects are both material objects and linguistic objects, part symbol, part fetish. Work with these objects is part of the process of self-construction in the collaborative presence of another person. The term self construction can be something of an abstraction. But the concept can be given particularity if we can trace it through the intricacy of parent–child dialogue. In the sequence I examine in some detail, we can watch for the movement of these symbolic objects, the way in which mother and child alternately speak *as* and *on behalf of* the transitional object, that is, for its benefit and as its representative. It is possible to see that identity moves fluidly through speech and that mother, child, and symbolic objects alternate in representing experience and interaction.

In the staged birthday party scene that follows, Miranda, the mother, initiates many of the elements and rituals of the event. Over a 20-minute sequence, 19 new narrative elements were added to the game, all initiated by Miranda. In this dyad, the child is much less able to control or shift the direction and form of the play. She responds to requests and probes and seems genuinely caught up in an activity her mother is shaping and promoting.

	M: What does Blankie want, Mary?
C: Wan cake	M: And what does Blankie want to drink for his party?
C: Appa juice.	M: Ok, we'll do that.

The two go through several turns arranging who is to drink the little glasses of juice, thus establishing which is Mary's glass and which Blankie's. Then the mother directs Mary to set out plates for the cake and introduces the conventional birthday ritual of candles. All Mary's contributions are elicited by Miranda, who uses questions both as tutorial and action prods.

	M: What are you going to sing for Blankie when we cut the cake?
C: Happy birthday dea' blankie.	M: (laughs) Ok, here we go. Ready to sing?

After the singing, the mother persuades Mary to blow out the candle saying that Blankie needs help. Then she instructs Mary in pulling out the candle from the cake, taking paper off the cup cake and cutting the cake. In this segment, the mother produces 28 utterances; Mary, 3. Each of Mary's comments is some lexical variation on "I want" (I wa', I wan, . .) as she tries to hold the knife and cut the cake under her mother's supervision. Then there is a sequence of eating the cake in which the mother tries to establish that Mary gets a piece and Blankie a piece while Mary determinedly eats both pieces.

C: I get . . dat piece.   M: Why don't you give a
   Piece. I get two piece.   piece to Blankie and then
                                     maybe you could eat it
                                     for him later.

Mary is seen and talked to as herself but also is encouraged to act *as if* she were Blankie. Then Miranda continues the scene by bringing up a new aspect of the birthday routine: giving Blankie his present. There is then a small bout of misunderstanding where Miranda tries to elicit Blankie's age from Mary while Mary continues to talk about which pieces of cake are hers.

                                 M: Don't forget, we're gonna
                                    give Blankie his present
                                    too. How old is Blankie,
                                    Mary?

C: Eh mine.   M: He's one, only one year
                                    old.

C: Eat that, dollie.

The mother comments on Blankie's nice present, but the child continues eating;

C: Ah got to ha' a little piece of ca'.

Miranda responds in an interesting way. She picks up on Mary's cue and talks to Mary *as though* Mary were Blankie.

M: Ooh, bet Blankie likes that, eh. I think Blankie likes his
   cake.

Miranda, moving the sequence on to a new element in birthday rituals, probes Mary for suggested activities to take place after the party meal.

Mary responds "Pa games" and then "Dance" but returns to the immediate circumstances of the birthday meal and continues to ask for more cake. Miranda distracts her with an account of an upcoming party where Mary will have cake. Then the mother introduces two other dolls into the game as guests and seats them at the table. The child continues to focus on the cake and eats each of the dolls' portions, which Miranda has put on plates. Several times when Mary eats or drinks, Miranda speaks as though Mary were Blankie or one of the other dolls, sometimes making little nibbling sounds as Mary eats.

	M: We better get your special Tassel up here. Yes. Now, Tassel, eat your cake. Teh. teh teh. . . . teh teh teh. Gonna eat that too?
C: Last piece.	M: That's the last piece. Well, you eat it. Teh, teh Blankie. You ate all your cake.

Miranda then introduces a final element in the event, telling Blankie a story but is unable to enlist Mary, who says instead:

C: Blankie wants some milk.	M: Oh, Blankie wants more milk.
C: W wan . . . tum mo milk.	M: You and Blankie both.

Milk is poured into two little cups, and Mary drinks hers. Miranda starts to initiate a game with the Blankie, but notices the second cup of milk and says:

	M: Oh, Blankie never drank his milk. It's gonna get all spilled. You drink it for him.
C: Can	M: Which hand? OK.
C: I dink em for Blankie.	

Miranda has created, with her daughter as an occasionally willing, occasionally resistant junior partner, a web of meaningful social actions, linked to future events and to the past. Miranda reproduces the formal rituals, what Nelson (1986) would call "scripts" of birthday parties (the routines involving cake, candles, songs, games, and presents). Winnicott (1965) has noted the importance of establishing the experience of "going on being" (p. 40). There must be many modalities of experience, nonverbal but sensual and palpable, through which a parent gives an infant a feeling of "going on being." This encompassing narrative with which parents surround their children, these commentaries through which parents verbally communicate their sense of the child's past, present, and future, of patterns of action, scripts (to revive Nelson's term), routines of life, may on the symbolic and verbal level contribute to the child's experience of "going on being." Parental narratives thus seem an important continuation of the parental holding function and the mirroring function arising in the early patterns of parent–infant interaction described earlier in this paper.

Yet this mother–child discourse is markedly asymmetrical. Other dyads show a more equal give-and-take, with mothers producing shorter and briefer communications that permit the children gradually to initiate and shape the conversation with their own input. This power differential in mother–child dialogue raises the question of a true- or false-self-construction. Might toddler dialogues be a setting in which to examine the power of parental constructions to impose a false self-structure upon the child? Parents hold social and linguistic power in these discourses, and thus their dialogues with their child contain evidence both for the sustaining holding environment that provides security and structure and also for the overwhelming and subtle *reproduction* of the adult's construction as the child's experience and social reality.

Miranda also works out several levels of symbolic activity that Mary plays with but perhaps cannot quite elaborate for herself. Blankie is made into an actor at the birthday. Sometimes Mary acts as herself and sometimes is seen and treated by her mother as though she *were* Blankie. Some rudimentary ideas of sharing and taking turns are also introduced. In examining Mary's contribution, mostly reiterating comments of Miranda's and sometimes supplying a term or word Miranda elicits, Mary participates or is rehearsed in this fantasy narrative game orchestrated and managed by her mother. The symbolic and named object, "Blankie," is both self and symbol, used by the mother and accepted by the child. Throughout the activity there is a kind of slippage between Mary, mother, and Blankie with both participants speaking sometimes *as* and sometimes *about* the object. This interchange might be seen as a microgenetic moment of intersubjectivity in which discourse is a field available for playing out identity and meaning. The fantasy figure and fantasy game present a setting in which the adult, offering the routines of social and family life, shapes an identity for the child through enactments with the transitional object.

TRANSFERENCE COUNTERTRANSFERENCE

Winnicott (1965) saw the empathic and receptive maternal holding environment as a model for analytic listening. It seems also that he saw play in the transitional space as a model for analytic interpretation. Interventions were not made for the purpose of reality testing but rather to put into play—in a transitional, probabilistic, "what if," *imaginative* space—the projections, internal ambivalence, and conflictual fantasies of internal life.

To conclude, I want to use the integrative work on early symbol use developed in this chapter to speculate on transference and countertransference interactions. I will make three points.

First, the view of speech I have been proposing breaks with any idea that speech is ever monologic. Speech is always addressed to some other, whether that listener is real or imaginary. Analytic dialogues carry and reproduce each speaker's history of these dialogues hidden inside monologues. An "object relation," then, is what is carried and represented in the discourse. Transference phenomena simply concentrate and promote what is a feature inherent in any conversation, the presence of an imaginary, internally represented other (part or whole) as the intended listener and interlocutor.

Second, I expand the meaning of the term "holding environment" to include the mother's holding the child in thought, both consciously and unconsciously. This form of holding is manifest in the style and content of her speech to her child. Her dialogues, the construction of fantasy and play and narrative through discourse, elaborate the mother's deep construction of her child. In this holding environment, the child can come into consciousness and relationship as an already imagined being. Winnicott identifies a fulcrum moment when the mother turns from holding to reacting to her infant's signals. In the realm of speech and discourse we would see the same developmental growth at the point where the mother makes space in her fantasy play for the child's own production.

Social construction may be distorted if the parent refuses her child's contribution and requires instead that the child be the container of projection and projective identifications. In an extreme case, of, say, deadness or depression in the mother, the child may, psychologically speaking, be erased. Extrapolating to analytic discourse, we might watch for the properties of the dialogue, the capacity to enter, share, and shape meaning. The dialogic features in analytic conversations might illuminate the potential for collaboration or for distortion and loss of self the patient may have experienced in early parent–child dialogues.

Third, we can explore the similarities between the transitional space in mother–child dialogue and the transitional space in the analytic setting as sites for self-*construction*. Analytic dialogues would be seen as creative spaces for the making of meaning. This perspective is aligned to hermeneutic models of interpretation as collaborative conversations in which meaning and understanding is adjudicated, and also to Vygotsky's (1963) idea that internal representation, particularly verbalized thought, arises first in the social plane and then is internalized in the individual mind. In the analytic setting, transference/ countertransference play would provide, in dialogic format, representations of self-in-relation, which would become aspects of the internal object world. Psychic changes in the internal world, then, involve changes in the dialogic audience and the internal conversations.

A final word from Vygotsky. Words, "signs," are tools, and tool use transformed ways of thinking and being. If we think of words as socially derived tools and as transformative features of mental and emotional life, we have to give up comfortable, sharp distinctions between public and private, as well as between self and other. One of the extraordinary services psychoanalysis has made to gender studies has been to see the potency of cultural construction in intrapsychic life. Language is both the medium for this social installation and its liberation. But gender is only one social structure among many. To return to mother child conversation, the meaning of speech in that small, two-person society affects the self-construction in the child. A commitment to intersubjectivity and a relational self is a commitment to a complex subjectivity, contaminated by cultural meaning but also elusive, split, as language is, between the private and the public, between longing and expression.

REFERENCES

Bakhtin, M. (1981), *The Dialogic Imagination*, ed. M. Holquist. Austin: University of Texas Press.

Bates, E. (1976), *Language in Context*. New York: Academic Press.

Bateson, G. (1970), *Steps to an Ecology of Mind*. Boston: Beacon Press.

Beebe, B. (1988), The contribution of mother–infant mutual influence to the origins of self- and object representations. *Psychoanal. Psychol.*, 5:305–337.

_____ & Lachmann, F. (1991), Representational and selfobject transferences: A developmental perspective. *Progress in Self Psychology, Vol. 8*. Hillsdale, NJ: The Analytic Press, pp. 3–15.

Benjamin, J. (1988), *The Bonds of Love*. New York: Pantheon Press.

Bion, W. R. (1962), *Learning from Experience*, London: Heinemann. (Reprinted in: *Seven Servants*, New York: Aronson, 1977.)

Brown, R. (1973), *A First Language*. Cambridge, MA: Harvard University Press.

Bruner, J. (1983), *Child's Talk*. New York: Norton.

_____ (1985), Historical and conceptual perspectives on Vygotsky. In *Culture Communication and Cognition*, ed. J. Wertsch. Cambridge, MA: Cambridge University Press, pp. 39–53.

_____ (1990), *Acts of Meaning*. Cambridge, MA: Harvard University Press.

Chomsky, N. (1965), *Aspects of a Theory of Syntax*. Cambridge, MA: M.I.T. Press.

_____ (1975), *Reflections on Language*. New York: Random House.

Coltart, N. (1991), The silent patient. *Psychoanal. Dial.*, 1:439–453.

Dore, J. (1974), A pragmatic description of early language development. *J. Psycholing. Res.*, 4:343–351.

Edgcumbe, R. (1976), Towards a developmental line in language acquisition. *The Psychoanalytic Study of the Child*, 30:159–176. New Haven, CT: Yale University Press.

Fast, I. (1984), *Event Theory*. Hillsdale, NJ: Lawrence Erlbaum Associates.

Furth, H. (1987), *Desire in Knowledge*. New York: Columbia University Press.

Geertz, C. (1983), *Local Knowledge*. New York: Norton.

Giddens, A. (1976), *New Rules of Sociological Method*. New York: Basic Books.

Green, A. (1986), *On Private Madness*. London: Hogarth Press.

Halliday, M.A.K. (1975), *Learning How to Mean*. London: Edward Arnold Press.

Harris, A. (1987), The rationalization of infancy. In: *Critical Developmental Theory*, ed. J. Broughton. New York: Plenum Press.

Holt, R.R. (1989), *Freud Reappraised*. New York: Guilford Press.

Horton, P. & Sharp, S. (1985), Language, solace and transitional relatedness. *The Psychoanalytic Study of the Child*, 38:167–195. New Haven, CT: Yale University Press.

James, W. (1950), *Principles of Psychology*, Vol. 1. New York: Dover Press.

Kuhn, T. (1962), *The Structure of Scientific Revolution*. Chicago: University of Chicago Press.

Kristeva, J. (1980), *Desire in Language*. New York: Columbia University Press.

Lacan, J. (1970), *Ecrits*. Paris: Seiul.

Lachmann, F. & Beebe, B. (1989), Oneness fantasies revisited. *Psychoanal. Psychology*, 6:137–149.

Lichtenberg, J. (1983), *Psychoanalysis and Infant Research*. Hillsdale, NJ: The Analytic Press.

Little, M. (1985), Winnicott working in areas whereof psychotic anxieties predominate. *Free Associations*, 6:9–42.

Mahler, M., Pine, F. & Bergman, A. (1975), *The Psychological Birth of the Human Infant*. New York: Basic Books.

McDougall, J. (1980), *Plea for a Measure of Abnormality*. New York: International Universities Press.

_____ (1989), *Theatres of the Body*. New York: Norton.

Nelson, K. (1986), *Event Knowledge*. Hillsdale, NJ: Lawrence Erlbaum Associates.

_____ (1990), *Narratives from the Crib*. Cambridge, MA: Harvard University Press.

Peirce, C. S. (1955), *The Philosophical Writings of Peirce*, ed. J. Buchler. New York: Dover.

Rorty, R. (1980), *Philosophy and the Mirror of Nature*. Princeton, NJ: Princeton University Press.

Saussure, F. de (1959), *Course in General Linguistic*. New York: Philosophical Library.

Shotter, J. (1978), The cultural context of communication studies: Theoretical and methodological issues. In: *Action, Gesture and Symbol*, ed. A. Lock. New York: Academic Press.

Snow, C. & Ferguson, C. (1977), *Talking to Children*. Cambridge: Cambridge University Press.

Spence, D. (1982), *Narrative Truth and Historical Truth*. New York: Norton.

Stern, D. (1973), *The Primary Relationship*. Cambridge, MA: Harvard University Press.

_____ (1985), *The Interpersonal World of the Infant*. New York: Basic Books.

Stone, J., Smith, H. & Murphy, L. (1973), *The Competent Infant*. New York: Basic Books.

Taylor, C. (1989), *Sources of the Self*. Cambridge, MA: Harvard University Press.

Trevarthan, C. (1980), The foundations of intersubjectivity: Development of interpersonal and cooperative understanding in infants. In: *The Social Foundations of Language and Thought*, ed. D. R. Olson. New York: Norton, pp. 183–230.

Urwin, C. (1984), Power and the acquisition of language. In: *Changing the Subject*, ed. J. Henriques. London: Methuen Press, pp. 79–110.

Vygotsky, L. (1963), *Language and Thought*. Cambridge, MA: MIT Press.

_____ (1975), *Mind in Society*. Cambridge, MA: Harvard University Press.

Wells, G. (1986), *The Meaning Makers*. London: Heineman.

Winnicott, D.W. (1958), *Through Paediatrics to Psychoanalysis*. London: Hogarth Press.

_____ (1971), *Playing and Reality*. London: Tavistock.

Wittgenstein, L. (1965), *The Blue and Brown Books*. New York: Harper Torchbooks.

Zivin, G. (1979), *The Development of Regulation through Private Speech*. New York: Wiley.

7

Mutative Factors in Child Psychoanalysis

A Comparison of Diverse Relational Perspectives

SUSAN C. WARSHAW

The work of such child psychoanalysts as Melanie Klein, Winnicott, and Mahler, and of infant researchers such as Stern and Bowlby has figured prominently in the thinking of many analysts of adults who consider themselves to be working within a broadly defined relational perspective. The observations of these child researchers/practitioners have contributed significantly to developmental theory and frequently have been used to support relational model theories of the mind and corresponding evolving theories of adult psychoanalytic treatment. The various contemporary relational-model theories, while differing from one another in major ways, share a belief that personality is essentially forged in the context of relatedness to others (Greenberg and Mitchell, 1983). While not negating the importance of the body and its requirements in the development of personality, Greenberg and Mitchell suggest that the relational-model theories have shifted emphasis from the primacy of the drives in the shaping of personality development to the primacy of relatedness. With the shifts to relational conceptualizations of mind have come shifts in the conceptualizations of the nature of the unconscious along with widespread debate about the mutative factors in treatment, for example, the balance and significance of interpretive and relationship factors as those most essential for change to occur.

As has been well documented elsewhere, all the just mentioned child analysts/observers have made individual contributions to an evolving relational perspective (Greenberg and Mitchell, 1983, Mitchell, 1988). Their thinking, however, varies significantly from one to another with respect to their conceptualization of the developmental process, their beliefs about the nature of the core conflicts in pathology, and the role they ascribe to experiences with the real parents in the development and perpetuation of internal relational configurations, including the experience of self. To some extent, child psychoanalysts whose work evolved out of these different traditions have also developed different perspectives about the factors in child treatment that are mutative. To date, the major discussions of the implications of the shift to relational models of mind have been with respect to adult psychoanalysis. My focus here is to consider some of the contributions of the foremost child analysts and developmental researchers to the process of child psychoanalysis. I will thus include a discussion of the work of Anna Freud in this context. I shall look at the place of relational concepts in the work of each and particularly emphasize the implications of each point of view for our conceptions of the mutative factors in child treatment.

The major contemporary schools of psychoanalytic child treatment—ego psychological (British as well as American), British middle school (essentially Winnicottian), and Kleinian—developed their treatment approaches from models of the mind that integrate relational concepts in significantly different ways. While having their roots in drive theory, they varied in their emphasis and differed in the extent to which they incorporated the concept of drives into their perspectives. Each of the theories wrestles with different conceptions of the mutative factors in child treatment. They seem to be in different places at different times with respect to the primacy of interpretation, insight and analysis of transference, and the beliefs regarding the mutative aspects of the relationship with the analyst. Despite the contributions that observations of child analysts have made to relational-model theories of mind, it is interesting to note that within the voluminous literature on child psychoanalysis proportionately little has been written about child treatment from what Greenberg and Mitchell (1983) describe as a "purely" relational perspective, such as that developed by the Fairbairnian object relations theorists or American interpersonalists, perspectives that disavow drive theory.

Thus until the relatively recent work of such researchers as Bowlby (1988) and Stern (1985), the primary support for the focus on the development of the internal world of self and object relations, and the concern with the significance of the facilitating environment in the development of that world, came from child analysts with significant ties to instinct theory. Alfred Adler developed an approach to child treatment utilizing a nondrive perspective, but his ideas with respect to child therapy are not widely referred to by current practitioners who consider themselves to be psychoanalytic. Bryt (1972) reviewing non-Freudian perspectives on child analysis, presented treatment approaches all of which were rooted in models of development that were entirely retrospective. Most striking in this review was the relative lack of contribution of *child observers or child practitioners* to the *developmental theories* from which the theories of mind and of child treatment evolved. For reasons that are not particularly clear, the entire field of child treatment from an interpersonal perspective seemed to take a back seat to those perspectives being developed by the British and American child analysts (Anna Freud, Mahler, Winnicott, and the Kleinians). At the very least, interpersonal approaches to child analysis have not been widely described in the literature.

With the support derived from contemporary infant research, and the research derived from attachment theory, there has been a renewal of interest in conceptualizing the child-treatment process from a nonclassical/nondrive psychoanalytic perspective. (To some this might appear to be an oxymoron.) Tentative steps in this direction have begun to be taken within recent years. Speigel (1989) has adapted a basically Sullivanian approach to work with children. Some articles have begun to appear in psychoanalytic journals exploring the implications of contemporary infant research for issues of psychotherapeutic technique with children (see, e.g., Lombardi and Lapidos, 1990). The work of Bowlby and his followers (Bowlby, 1988; Belsky and Isabella, 1988) and of Stern (1985) provides empirical support for the conceptualization of a model of mind rooted in a purely relational matrix. In the final portion of this chapter, I will explore the possibilities and some implications for child treatment of the use of a nondrive relational model of mind. First, however, I shall describe some of the issues with which child analysts have grappled when attempting to develop their treatment approaches.

In its formative years, child psychoanalysis was a *derivative* of adult analysis. The model of the mind and concepts of development used by practitioners were derived primarily from reconstructive work with adults. The adult-treatment technique was the yardstick against which the emerging approaches to child analysis were measured. Thus, in the literature of child analysis much was written about the ways in which the child-treatment process deviated technically from the adult process, the sorts of parameters that were necessary for work with children were elaborated upon, and the priority goals were debated. But always in the background was the yardstick of classical adult psychoanalysis, the sine qua non of technique.

Through the process of direct observation of children, psychoanalytic developmental theory has been altered significantly; and through the astute observations of generations of child analysts, bodies of clinical knowledge and technique have emerged that can be considered to constitute the primary approaches to child psychoanalytic treatment: contemporary Freudian, which in child work is largely ego psychological, British middle school, and Kleinian (including contemporary Kleinian). (This is not to suggest that most contemporary clinicians do not integrate insights derived from all perspectives in daily work but, rather, to note that, in fact, the models of the mind from which these treatment approaches operate are different and these differences influence technique as well as beliefs regarding what is mutative in child treatment.)

Despite the fact that child psychoanalysis has become a distinct and separate field, it is still affected by its historical roots in adult psychoanalysis and its contemporary association with adult psychoanalysis. We still come to know about it through comparison with its adult counterparts. We struggle to integrate the observations of those who work with children into the model of mind originally developed as a result of work with adults; it is hard to alter our metapsychology. We evaluate the ways in which the process with children is like or unlike the process with adults, perhaps because most practitioners who work psychoanalytically with children also have been trained as analysts of adults, often prior to coming to child work. In addition, even if trained primarily as child clinicians, all child psychoanalysts have had their own adult psychoanalysis, which is generally acknowledged to be a most significant aspect of one's training. Thus one's reconstructive perspective of one's own development, as well as the theoretical models and experiential aspects of the adult model, is always at the scene of psychoanalytically informed child treatment. Any attempt to understand and develop a child-treatment model must be informed by an awareness of the important issues raised in the still extant struggle to emerge from under the dominance of the adult perspective and develop a truly child-oriented psychoanalytic treatment. This is as true for any attempt to develop a child-treatment model from a purely relational perspective as it was for models emerging out of the drive model.

All psychoanalytic treatment perspectives employ some model of the mind, as well as developmental theory, in order to assess pathology and hypothesize its genesis. In varying degrees these models and theories influence technique and at the very least provide hypotheses that shape the interventions and interpretations analysts provide their patients. With respect to adult psychoanalysis, there are variations in the extent to which alterations in developmental theories as well as shifts in models of the mind are reflected in technique. With respect to work with children, perhaps the same can be said, although shifts in technique predated shifts in the model of the mind, developmental theory, changes in conceptualization of cause of pathology, and shifts in the basic treatment goals. From the beginning, practitioners working analytically with children had to alter their technique to accommodate the different developmental statuses of children. Thus, flexibility of approach, or deviation from the basic treatment model, was taken as a given in child treatment almost from its inception. The realities of the child's immature level of cognitive and emotional development along with dependence on the primary caretakers, led to the early debates about the process and goals of child analysis. The questions raised in these debates still have their relevance today.

The first and most obvious modification in technique is related to the child's inability to lie on the couch and utilize the method of free association. Both Hug-Hellmuth (1921) and Klein (1946) are credited with the development of the technique of play therapy, which they believed to be a substitute for free association in providing access to the unconscious. Klein suggested that the material thus produced by the child be interpreted in the manner of a dream. In her early work, she perceived of the goal of treatment with children as the same as the goal with adults, and the main principle of treatment as identical.

> Consistent interpretation, gradual resolution of the resistances, steady reference back of the transference, whether positive or negative, to earlier situations—these maintain a correct analytic situation with the child not less than with the adult [Klein, 1975, p. 12].

She sought to facilitate the rapid emergence of unconscious sexual and aggressive material related to a very early development of the Oedipus complex. Klein believed that rapid and deep interpretation was the surest way to reduce the painful anxiety that youngsters experience: "Taking the shortest cut across the ego, we apply ourselves in the first instance to the child's unconscious and from there gradually get into touch with its ego as well" (p. 12).

Anna Freud (1945) was a leading critic of the assumption that play could be considered a substitute for free association. Offering several criticisms of Klein's approach, she stated that one could not accept the child's play activities as equivalents of the free associations of adults for at least two reasons. First, she disagreed with Klein's technique of deep interpretation, which did not involve defense analysis. She criticized it for "aiming to lay bare the deeper layers of the child's mind without working through the resistances and distortions of the preconscious and consciousness" (p. 70). She did not believe that one could interpret the play material that emerged in this context as though it were a symbolic equivalent of the unconscious. Second, she did not believe that children engaged in play with the same intention or therapeutic aims that motivated adults when engaging in free association with the analyst. Inasmuch as the free associations of the adult are produced within the analytic transference, she raised the question as to whether the relationship of the child to the analyst could be considered parallel to the transference.

Thus, by raising issues regarding the equivalence of free play with free association, Anna Freud also raised issues with respect to the child's motivation for treatment, as well as the type of transference relationship in which the child engaged. These questions became the basis of debate for decades (A. Freud, 1945, p. 70). She did not disagree that play is a useful medium for engaging a child in treatment, but in later discussions she clarified her perception of play as but one medium among many for becoming familiar with children and their conflicts (Sandler, Kennedy, and Tyson, 1980).

Thus, in early approaches to child treatment, for both Melanie Klein and Anna Freud play was conceived of as a technical tool, as a means to an end, the end being to facilitate the child's capacity to engage in an analytic process modeled after the adult process. One central disagreement had to do with the literal equivalence of play with free association and the degree of its interpretability as an equivalent of unconscious communication. It was left to others (Winnicott, 1971a, for one) to elaborate the therapeutic importance of the process of playing as a growth-facilitating experience particularly in the development of the self.

As noted earlier, a second central area of disagreement had to do with the nature of the transference developed by the child, the extent to which it could be considered equivalent to that developed by adults, and whether it could be worked with in the same manner. Anna Freud and others noted that the child's failure to use the couch and the constancy of direct interaction with the analyst had a major impact on the child's relationship with the analyst by interfering with the desired anonymity and making her "real" presence unavoidable. Thus it became more difficult to attribute feelings and behaviors directed toward the analyst as emanating solely from the fantasy life of the child. This forced a reconsideration of the phenomenological role of the analyst in the child-treatment situation. In addition (as noted earlier) Anna Freud focused on the issue of the child's capacity to develop an analyzable transference neurosis in the light of the continuing presence of the original love objects (the parents). This would then bring into question the goal of treatment, that is, the resolution of the transference neurosis through analysis. Here the divergence between Miss Freud and Melanie Klein occurred with respect to the nature of the transference in child treatment. (For an elaboration see Altman, this issue).

Klein had little problem with viewing the child as being able to engage in an analyzable transference. Early in her work, she described her belief that children develop a spontaneous transference immediately. In fact, her observations of children in treatment had led her to begin to make significant shifts in developmental theory that further supported her belief in the capacity of young children to produce an analyzable transference neurosis that was rooted in their primitive relations to their objects. Very early in her work, Klein began to observe that the origins of the Oedipus complex lay in the second half of the first year of life, a much earlier period than Anna Freud believed. The failure adequately to resolve anxieties and guilt in relation to the early oedipal complex led to the persistent use of very primitive defenses and resulted in pathological functioning.

For Klein, the internal object world developed primarily out of the child's inherited instinctual world, projected onto parental objects, part and whole, and reintrojected. The external object was primarily the recipient and processor of the child's projections, either confirming or negating the best and the worst. With her emphasis on an inherited knowledge of objects and her concept of projective identification as a normative defensive process in earliest infancy and one that is central to the development of the internal object world, she had little difficulty perceiving the development of a transference of very early object relations. Because of her primary emphasis on the child's contribution to the development of object relations, as well as her belief in the formative influence of the earliest relations to the primitive part- and whole-objects, she was less concerned with the presence of the currently existing parents, though she did mention her awareness that their "complexes" could pose an obstacle to treatment. She took the stance, however, that except in extreme circumstances it was best to avoid too much involvement of the parents in the treatment (Klein, 1975).

With the child as creator of the object world, the analyst became a recipient of the child's projections of primitive transferences. The projections apparently were not seen as being reserved for those currently nearest and dearest to the child, the contemporary parents, but rather as having been shaped in the historical past of infancy, still lacking resolution with respect to the internal objects of the past, and transferable to the analyst in much the same manner (perhaps even more readily) as the adult transfers relationships with old objects. In Klein's work, the analyst's prime role was as *interpretor* of the transference.

Anna Freud was acutely aware of the child's dependence on the primary caretakers and of the child's loyalty to the parents as being of major significance to the treatment. She emphasized the presence of the real parent as a shaping force in the child's development to a much greater degree than did Klein. She was also much more acutely concerned with the continuing presence of the parents as the primary love objects in the life of the child. Hence she was cautious about the extent to which the child could develop an analyzable transference neurosis or in essence transfer the passionate conflicts originating in relation to the still-present parents to a figure of significantly less real importance in the child's life.

Several issues, then, were presented by Anna Freud in her dis-agreements with Melanie Klein that have continuing relevance to our work with children. Among those issues were the nature of the transference and the impact that the continuing dependence of the child on the still-present parents had on the treatment. Many years after she began her work with children, Sandler et al. (1980), in their discussions with Anna Freud, elaborated upon the types of relation-ships they believed a child develops with the analyst. From their perspective, the child makes many uses of the analyst, only some of which are transferential. They described four different types of transference (though not as rigid categories): transference of predom-inately habitual ways of relating, transference of current relation-ships, transference of past experiences, and transference neurosis (p. 78). The child also may use the analyst as an object for externalization of internalized conflicts by transferring one aspect of a conflict onto the analyst. They also described the child as being capable of developing a relationship to the analyst as a "real" object. Not only is the child capable of perceiving the analyst as a "real" object, but there are ways in which the relationship to that object are important to the development of that child's personality. The child may use the analyst as an object for identification, as an auxiliary ego, or as a new love object serving as an alternative to parents insufficiently available. Thus the relationship to the analyst is perceived as mutative in a variety of ways in addition to the traditional role as interpretor of transference and internal conflict.

From the perspective of Anna Freud and her followers, these other uses of the analytic relationship, while therapeutic and while occur-ring in all analyses to some extent or another, are not the main elements in a psychoanalytic treatment of a child. They vary in importance, depending, in part, on the diagnosis of the child. The greater the pathology of the child, the more likely the nontransferential relational components will be of significance as therapeutic factors. Sandler et al. (1980) wrote: "Analytic therapies are distinguished from play therapies in that interpretation, insight and the self-awareness consequent on interpretation are the major therapeutic agents" (p. 70). In that same volume Anna Freud is quoted as stating:

> Analysis is neither abreaction which would be associated with play therapy, nor "corrective emotional experience" as Franz Alexander called it. It is rather the changing of the inner balance or focus to bring about that widening of consciousness which is insight into motivation [p. 70].

She and her followers go a long way toward introducing the significance of the relationship to the "real" analyst and the "real" parents into the work of the analytic treatment. Yet they do not utilize a relational model of the mind as described by Greenberg and Mitchell (1983), that is, a mind composed of relational configurations. Rather they utilize the Freudian structural theory of mind. They conceive of the analytic process as one whose aim is to effect the balance of forces within the personality structure, to widen the areas of consciousness, which means to expand the power of the ego in relation to the id and the superego. The chief tool employed in the service of that goal is interpretation of transference and resistance.

Both Anna Freud and Melanie Klein maintained a belief in the centrality of interpretation and, in particular, interpretation in the transference. Neither altered these views, which were central to the process of child analysis. However, as noted earlier, they engaged in the process of interpretation in significantly different ways, with Miss Freud emphasizing defense analysis and support for the development of ego functions and Mrs. Klein emphasizing direct and rapid id interpretation.

Anna Freud (1965) noted that *while the aim of analysis for both children and adults* is the widening of consciousness, the type of material to be interpreted differs.

> With adults, analysis deals for long stretches of time with material under secondary repression, that is with the undoing of defenses against id derivatives which have been rejected from consciousness at one time or another. Only from there does it proceed to elements under primary repression, which are preverbal, have never formed part of the

organized ego, and cannot be "remembered" only relived within the
transference. Although this procedure is the same with older children,
it is different with the youngest where the proportion between elements of the first and second kind and also the order of their
appearance in analysis are reversed [p. 32].

She believed that for young children the process of interpretation
goes hand in hand with the process of verbalization of numerous
strivings that are not incapable of consciousness, but that have in
essence never been put into words. Thus she ascribed a major
developmentally facilitating role to analysis, support for the development of verbalization, which is a prerequisite for secondary-process
thinking. At the same time, however, she maintained the primacy of
the interpretative role by including this verbalization process as part
of the interpretive process.

It was Bion (1962) who ascribed a developmentally facilitating role
to Kleinian analysts. Pick and Segal (1978), discussing Bion's elaborations of Klein's ideas, noted that

the setting and the analyst's interpretive role within that setting can
provide the patient with the experience of a containing object (Bion,
1962) or the equivalent of what Winnicott has called the good enough
mother [p. 440].

Pick and Segal stress, however, that there are differences between
Winnicott's concept of the holding experience and the Bionian
concept:

The Kleinian child analyst might differ from Winnicott in technique
because of the conviction that an essential part of the holding experience resides in the analyst's function of observing the transference and
putting the child's feelings and experiences into words for him. This
enables the child to internalize an object that helps him hold experiences in his mind. Kleinian analysts take the view that verbalizing,
actually interpreting, is an essential part of child analytic technique [p.
440].

It should be apparent by now that Melanie Klein and Anna Freud
integrated their concerns with relational factors in significantly different ways. Klein proposed an elaborate theory of the development
of the child's relation to his or her internal objects; she believed that
infants were born with an instinctual and innate knowledge of these
objects. Rather than focusing on the contributions of the real environment to the development of the internal world of object relations,

Klein's theory emphasized the contributions of the infant that emanated from his or her instinctual endowment. Her developmental perspective significantly affected the focus of her interpretations, but she did not reconceptualize the treatment process as a result of her developmental theory.

Anna Freud, on the other hand, was acutely aware of the environmental influences on the development of the young child. Development occurred in an interaction with real external objects, and pathology could occur as a result of environmental failure, shaping, or inducement. The role of the environment was important in facilitating ego functioning, as well as in contributing to the development of fixations and regressions in drive development. Despite her awareness of, and emphasis on, the role of the parents in development, however, Anna Freud's theory views the development of object relations as occurring within the context of drive theory. Relations to the objects are an outgrowth of gratification or frustration of the instincts. Relatedness does not achieve independent motivational status within the drive/structural theory. The child's dependence on the parent was of concern to the analyst both because of the parent's continuing impact on the child's development and the need for the parent to be the facilitator of the child's treatment.

Anna Freud (1965) cautioned, however, that

> in spite of accumulated evidence that adverse environmental circumstances have pathological results, nothing should convince the child analyst that alterations in external reality can work cures, except perhaps in earliest infancy. . . . Such an assumption runs counter to the experience of the analyst. Every psychoanalytic investigation shows that pathogenic factors are operative on both sides, and once they are intertwined, pathology becomes ingrained in the structure of the personality and is removed only by therapeutic measures which affect the structure: . . . The child analysts have to remember that the detrimental external factors which crowd their view achieve their pathological significance by way of internalization with innate disposition and acquired, internalized libidinal and ego attitudes [pp. 51–52].

Anna Freud, in her later works (1965) and in Sandler et al. (1980), sounds increasingly like a contemporary relational theorist. However, she at no point disavowed drive theory or elevated relatedness to central motivational status. She also maintained that in the process of a child analysis, the goal of treatment is the widening of consciousness (the expansion of the ego's dominance over the id), and that goal is achieved through interpretation, the primary mutative factor.

Winnicott and Mahler each have made significant contributions to contemporary relational thinking. Each paid exquisite attention to the role of the parent in the development of the child's mind. The primary focus of each was with the elaboration of an understanding of the development of the self and the self in relation to the object. Each was concerned with the implications of failures in the parent child relationship for the pathological development of the self and its object relations. Neither explicitly disavowed drive theory, and Mahler explicitly stated that her concentration on the development of object relations was supplemental to the structural theory (Mahler, Pine, and Bergman, 1975). Nevertheless her contributions to developmental theory, which have shaped our contemporary beliefs about the origins of a broad range of problems in living, are most notable in the area of object relations.

While Mahler's major interest in the development of object relations stemmed from her concern with the treatment of severe pathology, the findings of her research had a significant impact on her conceptualization of the roots of less severe pathology and normal developmental struggles as well. One need only compare psychological reports written within the past 10 years with those written 20 years ago to note the extent to which the clinician's focus has shifted from a concern with the child's level of psychosexual development to the development of the child's object relations. Mahler's work in no small measure contributed to that shift in focus. She emphasized relational conflicts: the eternal struggle against fusion on one hand, and isolation on the other; the expression of individuality and autonomy occurring in the context of, and sometimes in conflict with, the development of a capacity for intimacy. Mahler's major contributions were in the area of psychoanalytic developmental theory, shaping our understanding of dynamics and thereby affecting our conception of the data of treatment as well as the content of our interpretations. Mahler's (1968) work has influenced treatment technique in relation to treatment of severely disturbed youngsters. In addition, her work has affected technique insofar as others have reconceptualized interventions as a result of the new developmental understandings she and her coworkers provided. Pine (1985), for example, coinvestigator with Mahler, utilized developmental theory to enhance our understanding of the noninterpretive, developmentally facilitating aspects of the analyst's role.

Winnicott's work also has had a major impact on our understanding of the development of the self within a relational matrix. He made major contributions to developmental theory through his explication of the environmental role in facilitating the development of the self and the self in relation to its objects. He contributed to our theory of technique through his emphasis on the mutative function of the noninterpretive aspects of the analytic situation. Though he worked extensively with children in psychoanalysis and consultation, Winnicott published relatively little about the process of psychoanalysis with children. Rather, most of his writing about interventions with children focused on brief consultation (e.g., Winnicott, 1971b) or the application of a psychoanalytic understanding of early development to the nonanalytic setting.

Believing as he did in the central role of the caretakers in the child's development, Winnicott was significantly concerned with helping caregivers learn to provide a facilitating environment, an environment in which the individual self could develop, along with the capacity to relate to objects that are "of the environment" (Winnicott, 1961, p. 105). Thus he emphasized working with parents, as well as nurses, teachers, physicians, and social workers, in order to ensure appropriate environmental provision.

He also emphasized the importance of detailed history taking (Phillips, 1988) in understanding the development of pathological symptoms. Phillips notes that Winnicott saw "symptoms as communications to the environment," as a sign that to some extent the child's individuality has been threatened. The healthy child has a "flexible repertoire of symptoms" (p. 50), and in health the symptoms do their job. In pathology however, "symptoms become rigidified, habitual and part of an illness pattern" (p. 50). Winnicott emphasized the importance of gathering detailed data around the formation of the child's symptoms. "What is repressed in the symptom is the context that makes it intelligible" (p. 51). The analyst helps gather the details together for the parent as well as the child: "Obtaining basic data from the interviews with the parent is in itself a psychotherapy if it be well done" (Winnicott, 1961, p. 102). The work need not always go beyond the consultation with the parent, for when the symptoms become understandable in the context of the pattern of the child's life in the family, the parent may feel able to manage. Similarly, when the analyst is consulting with the child, the job is to facilitate the emergence of whatever in the person is waiting for acknowledgment, not what is remotely unconscious, but what is there and unnoticed, unattended, the result perhaps of dissociation, perhaps of parental anxieties.

It is difficult to discern from any one of his papers the way that Winnicott worked in the actual process of a child analysis. One must piece together his ideas from various writings and take into account the evolution in his thinking over time and the vacillation in his allegiances to Anna Freud and Melanie Klein. One must also rely to some extent on the elaboration of his position by contemporary analysts who were trained in the Winnicottian tradition (Phillips, 1988, for example).

In his earlier writings, while one can discern his emphasis in the treatment on the mutative aspects of the analyst's behavior, Winnicott stated a position similar to that taken by Sandler, Kennedy, and Tyson in their discussions with Anna Freud. That is, he suggested that psychoanalysis as a treatment cannot be described without reference to diagnosis (Winnicott, 1958):

> The classical psychoanalytic situation is related to the diagnosis of psycho-neurosis, and it might be convenient to speak only of psycho-neurosis. . . . It must be emphasized . . . that in the technique of psycho-analysis there are very big differences according to whether the child is neurotic or psychotic or antisocial. . . . It should be added for completeness, that the difference between the child and the adult is that the child often plays rather than talks. This difference however, is almost without significance, and indeed some adults draw or play [p. 117].

In that same paper he endorsed the importance of interpretation, particularly when appropriately timed: "the earliest moment that the material makes it clear what to interpret" (p. 122).

Elsewhere, Winnicott (1961) expanded further the idea of the differences in the treatment process related to the diagnosis of the patient (pp. 101–111). He made clear that for those cases in which the cause of illness is a failure in early nurture, what must be provided is an appropriate holding environment in which the innate growth tendencies are given a chance to flourish:

> These growth tendencies are present all the time in every individual, except where hopelessness (because of repeated environmental failure) has led to an organized withdrawal. The tendencies have been described in terms of integration, of the psyche coming to terms with the body, the one becoming linked with the other, and of the development of the capacity for relating to objects. These processes go ahead unless blocked by failures of holding and of the meeting of the individual's creative impulses [p. 107].

I will not elaborate on his beliefs regarding the treatment of the antisocial tendency except to state that he believed it could be treated psychotherapeutically only at an early stage.

Speaking of psychoneurosis, Winnicott (1961) stated:

If illness in this category needs treatment, we would like to provide psychoanalysis, a professional setting of general reliability in which the repressed unconscious may become conscious. This is brought about as a result of the appearance in the "transference" of innumerable samples of the patient's personal conflicts. In a favourable case the defenses against anxiety that arise out of the instinctual life and its imaginative elaboration become less and less rigid, and more and more under the patient's deliberate control system [p. 106].

Phillips (1988) writes:

From a psychoanalytic perspective the patient is always suffering from the self knowledge he has had to refuse himself. Winnicott emphasizes in his first analytic papers that it is an attitude . . . relatively free from anxiety, not exclusively the interpretive process which can be a part of that attitude, that enables the child to become intelligible to herself. He does not so much as interpret the child's defenses as allow for them. He assumes that the child has a wish to make sense to herself, but that she cannot be directly informed of what she already knows. The invitation in the analyst's attitude facilitates her self representation [p. 53].

Thus the analyst is depicted as benign, one who minimizes anxiety by being an *unanxious observer* of the child's distress. Early on Winnicott described the observational stance as having considerable mutative value. This is not to suggest that he did not clarify, or question, verbalize or formulate. He did, however, emphasize the development of an environment in which the patient would creatively discover his own self as well as his objects. Cautioning against too much interpretation, he likened the overinterpretive analyst to the intrusive mother (Winnicott, 1963).

The Piggle (Winnicott, 1977) written toward the end of his analytic career and published posthumously, presents the flavor of the psychoanalytic work in which he engaged with a prelatency child. Though this was an intermittent analysis, not unusual for Winnicott, an analysis conducted in part "on demand" by the patient, it is possible to get a sense of the process in which he engaged. The use of the psychoanalytic setting as a playground for the elaboration of the inner life of the patient is beautifully depicted. In *The Piggle* Winnicott exposes the reader to the power of play as a medium through which the child becomes able to express her inner worries and experience the deep understanding of another. The child is free within the analysis to "make up" the analyst, to "create him," and in so doing to make herself "known." Striking to the reader of *The Piggle* is the extent to which Winnicott does interpret to the child in the context of the play relationship. Thus, despite his emphasis on the mutative aspects of the analyst's relationship to the child, it is clear that Winnicott did see interpretation as of importance, particularly when appropriately timed.

In *Playing and Reality* Winnicott (1971a) presented his clearest statement on the roles of play and interpretation in psychotherapy:

> Psychotherapy takes place in the overlap of two areas of playing, that of the patient and that of the therapist. Psychotherapy has to do with two people playing together. The corollary of this is that where playing is not possible then the work done by the therapist is directed towards bringing the patient from a state of not being able to play into a state of being able to play [p. 38].

Winnicott noted that playing can be a form of communication in psychotherapy. With respect to psychoanalysis, he stated that it is a very specialized form of playing in the service of communication with oneself and others.

Winnicott did not eliminate interpretation from his repertoire of mutative factors in analysis, although he believed that psychotherapy of a very deep kind could be done without interpretive work. He made several significant statements about interpretation, among them the following: "Interpretation when the patient has no capacity to play is simply not useful, or causes confusion. When there is mutual playing, then interpretation according to accepted psychoanalytic principles can carry the therapeutic work forward" (Winnicott, 1971, p. 51). In addition, he cautioned against interpreting too early, before the material suggests readiness. He stated that premature interpretation might produce compliance and is akin to indoctrination. Is this perhaps a reaction to Melanie Klein's heavily interpretive approach to the work?

Clearly, Winnicott was a child analyst who made major contributions both to the developmental theory of self and object relations and to psychoanalytic technique. He articulated a theoretical position that delineated what a child needs from the environment, particularly with respect to its facilitating role in the development of the sense of the self and the capacity to relate to objects. His focus on the contributions of the primary caretakers in development were then integrated into his perspective on the role of the analyst as a facilitator of development. His theory of the role of play in development and its function in psychotherapy and psychoanalysis is particularly useful for work with children, as play is the prime communicative mode in child analysis and therapy.

As noted at the beginning of this chapter, there is as yet no single approach to psychoanalytic treatment that can be considered to be relational. Within the field of child psychoanalysis, various individuals have contributed on both theoretical and technical levels to an emerging relational perspective. One can discern a shift over time in the degree to which the impact of a child's relationships with the real parent are granted importance as significant for development, pathogenesis, and treatment. In addition, one can discern a significant shift over time in the degree to which the noninterpretive functions of the analyst and the analytic setting are granted significance as mutative factors in treatment. Anna Freud, Winnicott, and Mahler (to name but a few) have all emphasized the highly important parental function in development, and their work certainly contributes to our perspective on the child's development within a relational matrix. They have all also attempted to delineate the developmentally facilitating aspects of the treatment, particularly in the light of the immature cognitive and affective state of the children with whom they worked. Each in his or her own way credits the environment as a significant force in the child's development and considers the relationship with the analyst as mutative in ways that are not solely interpretive. What, then, is added to an already vital and growing child psychoanalytic discipline by considering alternative and purely relational perspectives from which to conceptualize the work?

Greenberg and Mitchell (1983) suggested that the fundamentally different understandings of human development that underlie the drive/structure and relational/structure models lead to different conceptions of the psychoanalytic situation as well as to different beliefs as to what is mutative. Greenberg and Mitchell present strong arguments for their position that the treatment goals that emerge from approaches within the relational/structure model are quite different from those which evolved out of theories emanating from the drive/structure model.

> Within the drive/structure model, development is conceptualized in terms of the integration of infantile impulses (the component drives) into structured unitary aims. These aims are then brought under the control of the ego, which can exert a decisive role in organizing, channeling, delaying or gratifying particular needs. Pathogenic conflicts arise because for one reason or another the drives have not been brought adequately under the ego's domination [p. 390].

Within the treatment situation these conflicts become projected onto the "abstinent" analyst and are thus recreated in the transference.

The goal of psychoanalytic treatment within this model is the strengthening of the dominance of the ego over the id. The psychoanalyst strives to bring into the patient's awareness unconscious, drive-derived infantile conflicts so that resolution can occur under the aegis of the more mature ego; the chief technical tool for the psychoanalyst is interpretation of transference and resistance. Thus we see that within the work of Anna Freud and her followers, the central concern is with the variety of ways in which the ego can be strengthened with respect to the id. Within the purely relational models, not positing the libidinal and aggressive drives as of central motivational significance leads to different goals as well as to different beliefs as to what is mutative.

The diverse relational theories conceptualize the psychoanalytic situation and the treatment process using significantly different models of mind. These different models lead inevitably to different understandings of the clinical data. For example, a contemporary Kleinian analyst such as Segal (1985) will formulate the data of treatment differently than will a Sullivanian analyst such as Spiegel (1989). These different formulations will have an impact on the treatment goals and will lead to different technical emphases. Greenberg and Mitchell (1983), however, suggest that within the broad relational model there are some commonalities of focus that are worthy of note. For example, they suggest that just as mind is essentially a dyadically constructed structure, for relational model analysts the psychoanalytic situation is inherently dyadic. Events within the analysis are created in the interaction between the patient and the analyst. Thus, there is a significant focus within the analysis on the behaviors of the analyst as a coparticipant in the process.

Some theorists who are viewed as *relational,* such as Winnicott, view the participation of the analyst as a rather quiet one, the analyst's role being as a facilitator of the emergence of the self in a relational matrix. Within the analytic setting, the Winnicottian analyst, while a background participant, still assumes a neutral stance. The patient "makes up" the analyst, in essence projects his or her internal relational world onto the analyst.

Within other relational theories, however, particularly the interpersonal theories evolving out of Sullivan's (1953) work, there is an emphasis on the patient's, as well as the analyst's, awareness of the analyst's participation in the creation of the transference. Thus, while the transference is evolved from the patient's historically significant relationships, the analyst's participation is believed to shape the transference as well. The analyst can never be perceived of as anonymous, in the manner sought after by analysts working within the drive/structure model. The analyst is inevitably a coparticipant in the patient's world. Through the use of the countertransference, the analyst comes to develop an understanding of the patient's relational patterns:

> The task of the analyst is not to remain outside of a process which is unfolding from within the mind of the patient, because this is theoretically impossible in terms of the model's basic premises, but to engage the patient, to intervene, to participate in, and to transform pathogenic patterns of relationship [Greenberg and Mitchell, 1983, p. 390].

A theoretical perspective that can conceptualize the ideal analyst–patient relationship as other than anonymous is particularly appealing to the child analyst. As has already been noted by A. Freud in Sandler et al. (1980), children relate to their analysts in many different ways, only some of which are considered to be transferential. To this extent, the recognition of those authors of the other aspects of the relationship to the analyst suggests that they have incorporated into their work aspects of a relational orientation. Maintaining a stance of analytic anonymity is obviously difficult in child analysis in part because of the child's inability to participate in the standard procedure, which includes analytic abstinence, the use of the couch for the free-associative process, and the like. The child analytic literature is replete with discussions about the necessity for the analyst of children to deviate from the basic adult treatment stance at times. There appears to be a good deal of debate, however, about the specifics of such deviation. Should the analyst answer the child's questions? Celebrate birthdays? In innumerable ways, the child analyst is brought into direct interaction with the child, who has an extremely difficult time grasping the concept of anonymity. The analyst breaks anonymity to assure the continuation of the process and also as a result of having to manage the realistic issues that must be dealt with between an action-oriented child and a caretaking adult. Within the drive/structure model, however, these breaks are to some extent still viewed as necessary inconveniences for the analytic aspect of the work. As anonymous a stance as possible is sought, so that the child's transference projections will become clearly delineated (Scharfman, 1978, pp. 285–288).

Within the interpersonally oriented relational models, anonymity is neither possible nor something to strive for. The child will always have some degree of awareness of the analyst's subjectivity and will be working to interact with, connect with, or avoid the analyst on the basis of the child's personal processing of this real experience, albeit an experience shaped by and understood in the light of the child's internal models derived from prior experience. The entire focus of the analysis will be on *understanding* and *transforming* the pathological aspects of this relatedness.

There are certainly many other ways in which the adoption of a purely relational perspective will affect the analyst's understanding of the psychoanalytic situation and beliefs about the mutative factors in treatment. It is beyond the scope of this chapter to review all of them. I also will not offer a revised metapsychology, nor a totally new child-treatment model. I do believe that the findings of contemporary infant research are leading us in such directions. Though we are on the road, however, we have not yet reached our destination. Because I believe that all our interventions develop out of our understanding of the clinical data and that that understanding is shaped by the models of mind that we use, in what follows I will briefly describe the emerging relational model of mind and present some relational perspectives on the conceptualization of pathology. I will then describe some treatment implications.

Beginning in earliest infancy, our relationships with others and our experiences of ourselves in interactions with these others set processes in motion that will shape subsequent relatedness; the child is an active coconstructor of his interactional and internal worlds. Within purely relational model theories, mind is composed of relational configurations that are developed in the context of interaction with others.

Bowlby (1988) believed that children develop "working models" of the parents, the self, and the self in interaction with the parents on the basis of real experiences with the caretakers during the first years of life. These "working models" also reflect images that parents have of the child and that are communicated verbally (and, some believe, nonverbally) as well as behaviorally. "Once built, evidence suggests, these models of a self, and a parent and self in interaction, tend to persist and are so taken for granted that they come to operate at an unconscious level" (p. 180). The child's working models of self and other, tending to reinforce basic continuity but at the same time being open to elaboration, modification and change (Sroufe, 1988) will have a shaping influence on new experiences.

Stern (1985), in an extensive discussion of research and methodology, put forth his hypotheses about the manner in which preverbal infants come to encode their interactive experiences and consequently become able to create experiences of self. In his innovative exploration of the evolution of the infant's interpersonal world, Stern described the development of the self within an interpersonal environment. He designated the building blocks of that self as internal representations, which he called *Representations of Interactions that have been Generalized*, or RIGS.

Others, too, have explored the development of psychic structure within the interactional parent–child matrix. The recent infant research of Beebe, Jaffe, and Lachmann (this volume), and Beebe and Lachmann (this volume) presents additional data that supports the hypothesis that structure is built as a result of the internalization of parent–infant interaction patterns. Subsequent patterns of relatedness emerge out of, and are colored by, earlier patterns developed through the *mutual regulation of parent and infant*.

It is particularly important for child practitioners to realize that the role of the body and its maturational unfolding is not ignored within relational perspectives. Some, such as Mitchell (1988) suggest, rather, that relationships assume primary motivational status and sexuality and aggression are understood as powerful physiological responses "generated *within* a biologically mandated relational field and therefore deriving their meaning from that deeper relational matrix" (p. 20). Others may not feel the need to attribute sole motivational primacy to the relational connection but propose that individual development, including physiological responsivity, cannot be considered outside of the relational context in which it occurs. Within relational model theories, the *need for social relations*, and the tools that enable the infant to engage in them, are *biologically rooted*, genetically encoded.

Within these models of mind, how does one understand pathology, its emergence and continuance? Again there are alternative possibilities, and no fully developed new metapsychology. Rather the work is in process. Mitchell (1988), in presenting his integrated relational perspective, suggested:

> All important human relationships are necessarily conflictual, since all relationships have complex, simultaneous meanings in terms of self-definition and connection to others, self-regulation and field regulation [p. 276].

He also noted, "The prolonged condition of childhood dependency makes the discovery and forging of reliable points of connection not just a necessity, but an apparent condition for physical survival" (p. 275). Like drive theorists, Mitchell suggested that conflicts within the personality are inevitable. Neurotic symptoms, however, are not rooted in conflicts between wishes and defenses but, rather, are perceived of as manifestations of conflictual relational configurations.

Conflicts revolve around and between various points of connection and identification with early significant others. Like drive theorists, relational theorists view symptoms as reflecting attempts at adaptation. Unlike the adaptations of the individual as understood within drive theory, however, the adaptation achieved is not concerned with instinctual gratification. Rather the adaptations reflect the individual's best attempts at integrating the senses and needs of the self (including regulation of physiological needs) within an interpersonal matrix in which the striving for and maintenance of connectedness to others is central.

Within relational perspectives, the development of the self and the self in relation to the primary environmental figures are the focus of the work. Pathology reflects a limited range of experience of self, or problems in the development of aspects of the experience of self. Some aspects of pathology may be the result of an excessive need to deny what one knows and feels and a consequent lack of freedom to perceive new experience. A fixity to a rigid pattern of relatedness, loyalty to archaic objects, anxiety about entertaining new experiences, difficulties in revising working models of self and other, all are indicative of pathology. These problems in living are understood to be outgrowths of our relationships with the significant people in our lives.

For Bowlby (1988), the potential for psychological health was bound up with security of attachment to primary caretakers. There appears, in fact, to be a growing body of literature suggesting that the research-defined construct of security of attachment in infancy (12–18 months) has considerable predictive value for competent functioning in a variety of nonfamilial situations through the early elementary school years. (For a review of the research in this area see Belsky and Nezworski, 1988.) However, Sroufe (1988) cautioned that we remember that "anxious attachment classifications are not equivalent to psychiatric diagnoses of infants" (p. 28). He suggested that, instead, anxious attachment may be conceived of as a risk variable. "Anxious attachment does not cause later pathology, for many anxious infants are not clinically disturbed as children, but it may place individuals at greater risk for pathology" (p. 29). Sroufe suggested that there may be an interaction between anxious attachment and stress, the combination of which may lead to pathology.

Bowlby (1988) believed that security of attachment is related to maternal sensitivity and attunement to the signals and needs of the infant, as well as the degree of loving responsivity to the child's comfort and protection-seeking behaviors. Here, too, there is a fair amount of data to support Bowlby's beliefs, but there is also competing data that does not support his hypotheses. Belsky and Isabella (1988) conclude that there is sufficient evidence to suggest that the "sensitivity-security linkage" is at the very least a viable working hypothesis (p. 45). However, rather than simplistically "blaming" the mother for the interactional difficulties that seem to relate to anxious attachment, there is a need to understand the full range of possible antecedents. The factors that contribute to the mother's capacity for sensitive attunement to her infant are the subject of extensive research (Belsky and Isabella, 1988, pp. 3–17) and include such possibilities as infant temperament; environmental support, including the absence or extent of external stress factors; and the mother's maternal experiences with her mother.

Mitchell (1988) noted that different relational theories use different explanations for our tendency to maintain pathological self-structures and recreate maladaptive patterns of relatedness.

> From the point of view of self organization, psychopathology is repeated because it provides the organizational glue that holds the self together. . . . From the point of view of object ties, psychopathology is repeated because it functions to preserve early connections to significant others. . . . From the point of view of transactions, psychopathology is repeated because it works interpersonally; it functions to minimize anxiety [p. 291].

From the perspective of the self, what is new is frightening because the person's basic sense of continuity is disrupted and she becomes unfamiliar to herself. From an object relations perspective, new experiences threaten old object ties and basic loyalties. From an interpersonal perspective, what is new is frightening because it is associated with past parental anxieties. These ways of understanding are all integrated by Mitchell into his way of looking at clinical data.

Bowlby (1988) presented an interesting hypothesis that adds yet another dimension to our understanding of the difficulties people have in modifying pathological patterns. In essence, he suggested that openness to new emotional experiences of self and other is itself learned in the context of particular styles of parent–child communication. Citing the research of Bretherton, Bowlby noted that parents and their securely attached children had demonstrably more open patterns of communication than did parents and anxiously attached children. He suggested that this learned pattern of open communication provides securely attached children with a greater ability to revise working models of the self and the other than are available to anxiously attached children (p. 130). The ability to be aware of the point of view of the other, to respond sensitively, to negotiate and adjust, are all behaviors learned in an interactional matrix.

Bowlby further used this communication model to postulate the basis for the splitting off of major aspects of the child's personality, thereby rendering them inaccessible both to consciousness and further modifiability. He believed that the child's self-model is so profoundly influenced by the way the mother sees and treats him, that whatever she fails to recognize in him he will fail to recognize in himself (p. 132). This perspective seems to be entirely congruent with an interpersonal relational perspective.

The use of a relational model of mind alters our perception of the clinical data. Although most relational treatment approaches emphasize mutative aspects of the relationship to the analyst as of great significance, the adoption of a relational point of view does not necessarily lead to a highly interactive stance. It does not mean that the analyst never interprets, nor does it mean that the analyst does not wish to assist the patient in developing a greater awareness of motivations, some of which may be outside of awareness, or, as in the case of many children, never formulated. What we notice, however, what we choose to interpret, what we believe is motivating, is intimately bound up with our understanding of mind and conflict. Thus, by adopting a model of development in which, for example, the finding and maintaining of connectedness is of prime importance, we articulate the dynamics of the case in terms that bring conflicts with respect to these issues to the forefront. By understanding resistance as related to anxiety about loss of connection to significant others, or anxiety about the possibility of engendering anxiety in a primary caretaker, we may tailor our interventions accordingly.

Classical child analysts have tended to separate the processes of child analysis and child therapy. Analysis has historically been perceived as a treatment approach whose goal is the restructuring of personality. Through the use of interpretation of the transference and resistance, the patient gains insight into hitherto unconscious conflicts between the agencies of the mind, and structure is altered in the direction of greater ego control. While a variety of aspects of the analytic relationship are considered to facilitate personality growth, Interpretation is the primary analytic tool. The other mutative factors in analytic treatment, such as the use of the analyst as a figure for identification, as a new object, as an educator, are granted importance as "therapeutic" elements but are distinguished from the analytic elements. The more nonanalytic or psychotherapeutic treatments have tended to rely more heavily on the noninterpretive aspects of the patient–analyst relationship. Thus any treatment that emphasizes the mutative aspects of the relationship with the analyst tends to be considered a "psychotherapy," not a psychoanalysis.

The nature of interpretation in child analysis and the explication of its developmentally facilitating function have been topics of discussion in all psychoanalytic circles. As stated earlier, Anna Freud (1965) noted that for young children a significant aspect of the interpretive function was the verbalization of hitherto unverbalized experience. It was not so much that repressed material was lifted into consciousness through interpretation, but that preverbal material, never before part of the organized ego, was formulated, put into words, and thus brought within the ego's purview. Thus, the idea of an additional perspective on the mutative aspect of interpretation was introduced into child analytic treatment by Anna Freud.

Within many of the relational perspectives, the distinctions between psychoanalysis and psychotherapy are not drawn with the degree of specificity noted in the Freudian orientation. Particularly with respect to child treatment, the mutative elements are not perceived as belonging more to one type of treatment than to another. Employing different perspectives on the nature of mind, conflict, and pathology leads to a consideration of mutative factors as those which expand the child's awareness of the self and open the child up to the possibility of new forms of relatedness. Within this context, the verbalizing function of the analyst may be understood to be mutative in a variety of ways. For the contemporary Kleinian analyst, interpretation is mutative in part because it creates for the child the experience of being profoundly understood. The analyst can know and speak about things that have previously been conceived of as unthinkable. Through internalization of the experience of being with such an analyst, the child will come to be able to bear and think about aspects of experience that were previously intolerable (De Folch, 1988). From Bowlby's (1988) communication perspective, one can think of the interpretative function of the analyst as having some similar qualities. That is, the analyst creates for the patient the experience of being responded to sensitively, of being known and heard, of being attuned to. In this context, the analyst dares to say the unsayable, notice the unnoticeable. Within this model, the analyst will also validate awful realities that were previously not validated by the central people in the child's life. Within Bowlby's model, as in most interpersonal perspectives, real experience (albeit processed at the child's level of cognitive and affective development) is a central pathogenic factor.

REFERENCES

Beebe, B. & Lachmann, F. (1988), The contributions of mother–infant mutual influence to the origins of self- and object representation. *Psychoanal. Psychol.*, 5:305–337.

Belsky, J. & Isabella, R. (1988), Maternal, infant and social-contextual determinants of attachement security. In: *Clinical Implications of Attachment,* ed. J. Belsky & T. Nezworski. Hillsdale, NJ: Lawrence Erlbaum Associates, pp. 41–94.

Bion, W. R. (1962), *Learning From Experience.* London: Heinemann. (Reprinted in: *Seven Servants.* New York: Aronson, 1977.)

Bowlby, J. (1988), *A Secure Base.* New York: Basic Books.

Bryt, A. (1972), Non-Freudian methods of psychoanalysis with children and adolescents. In: *Manual of Child Psychopathology,* B. Wolman. New York: McGraw-Hill, pp. 865–899.

De Folch, T. (1988), Communication and containing in child analysis: Towards terminability. In: *Melanie Klein Today,* ed. E. Bott-Spillius. New York: Routledge, pp. 206–217.

Freud, A. (1945), Indications for child analysis. In: *The Psycho-Analytical Treatment of Children.* New York: International Universities Press, 1946, pp. 65–93.

_____ (1946), *The Psycho-Analytical Treatment of Children.* New York: International Universities Press.

_____ (1965), *Normality and Pathology in Childhood.* New York: International Universities Press.

Greenberg, J. & Mitchell, S. (1983), *Object Relations in Psychoanalytic Theory.* Cambridge, MA: Harvard University Press.

Hug-Hellmuth, H. (1921), On the technique of child-analysis. *Internat. J. Psycho-Anal.,* 2:287–305.

Klein, M. (1946), The psychoanalytic play technique: Its history and significance. In: *New Directions in Psychoanalysis,* ed. M. Klein, P. Heimann & R. Money-Kyrle. New York: Basic Books, 1955, pp. 3–22.

_____ (1975), *The Psycho-Analysis of Children,* Vol. 2. New York: Free Press.

Lombardi, K. & Lapidos, E. (1990), Therapeutic engagements with children: Integrating infant research and clinical practice. *Psychoanal. Psychol.,* 7:91–103.

Mahler, M. (1968), *On Human Symbiosis and the Vicissitudes of Individuation,* Vol. 1. New York: International Universities Press.

_____ Pine, F. & Bergman, A. (1975), *The Psychological Birth of the Human Infant.* New York: Basic Books.

Mitchell, S. (1988), *Relational Concepts in Psychoanalysis.* Cambridge, MA: Harvard University Press.

Phillips, A. (1988), *Winnicott.* Cambridge, MA: Harvard University Press.

Pick, I. & Segal, H. (1978), Melanie Klein's contribution to child analysis: Theory and technique. In: *Child Analysis and Therapy,* ed. J. Glenn. New York: Aronson, pp. 427–449.

Pine, F. (1985), *Developmental Theory and Clinical Process.* New Haven, CT: Yale University Press.

Sandler, J., Kennedy, H. & Tyson, P. (1980), *The Technique of Child Psychoanalysis.* Cambridge, MA: Harvard University Press.

Scharfman, M. (1978), Transference and the transference neurosis in child analysis. In: *Child Analysis and Therapy,* ed. J. Glenn New York: Aronson, pp. 275–307.

Segal, H. (1985), The Klein-Bion model. In: *Models of the Mind,* ed. A. Rothstein. Madison, CT: International Universities Press, pp. 35–47.

Spiegel, S. (1989), *An Interpersonal Approach to Child Therapy.* New York: Columbia University Press.

Sroufe, L. A. (1988), The role of infant–caregiver attachment in development. In: *Clinical Implications of Attachment,* ed. J. Belsky & T. Nezworski, Hillsdale, NJ: Lawrence Erlbaum Associates, pp. 18–38.

Stern, D. (1985), *The Interpersonal World of the Infant.* New York: Basic Books.

Sullivan, H. S. (1953), *The Interpersonal Theory of Psychiatry.* New York: Norton.

Winnicott, D. W. (1958). Child analysis in the latency period. In: *The Maturational Processes and the Facilitating Environment.* New York: International Universities Press, 1965, pp. 115–123.

_____ (1961), Varieties of psychotherapy. In: *Home Is Where We Start From.* New York: Norton, 1986, pp. 101–111.

_____ (1963), Communicating and not communicating leading to a study of certain opposites. In: *The Maturational Processes and the Facilitating Environment.* New York: International Universities Press, 1965, pp. 179–192.

_____ (1965), *The Family and Individual Development.* London: Tavistock.

_____ (1971a), *Playing and Reality.* London: Tavistock.

_____ (1971b), *Therapeutic Consultations in Child Psycho-Analysis.* London: Hogarth Press.

_____ (1977), *The Piggle.* London: Hogarth Press.

_____ (1986), *Home Is Where We Start From.* New York: Norton.

8

Relational Perspectives on Child Psychoanalytic Psychotherapy

NEIL ALTMAN

JULIA

An 11-year-old girl in the termination phase of a year-long, once-a-week psychotherapy wrote the following letter to her therapist:

> Dear ___
>
> I love you very much.
> I allways love you you know that.
> I know you are leaving me.
> I hope you forgive me
> for calling you name I'm sorry
> I love you I wish you wasing leaving
> I will miss you very much. I hope your
> marriage is well. I love you
> Come back to me. I do not want you
> to leave me I won't let you leave me
> You hear me. I hope you hear me well.
> and you are sorry. You want me to clean your ears.
> If I have to make you clean your ears

I wish to express my gratitude to Stephen Mitchell for his careful reading of an earlier draft of this chapter and his comments, which guided me in its revision. I also want to thank Marsha Levy-Warren, who read my paper with care and offered me comments from a different theoretical perspective. Finally, I acknowledge the editorial support of Neil Skolnick, who worked with me on this chapter, and the support of Susan Warshaw, who, in a variety of ways, helped this chapter come into being.

175

I will come down to your house I will do it for you.
You hear me miss ___

In another session, during the last month of the treatment, the following exchange occurred:

Julia: I don't want to talk to you anymore. I hate you for leaving. I want to eat you.

Therapist: So you could keep me forever.

Julia: Yes.

Therapist: Who else is in there?

Julia: My mother, so she won't leave me. And my father, he's been in there for a long time.

Julia's father, to whom she had been close, was murdered when she was four years old. Her mother had been in psychiatric care since a suicide attempt shortly after her husband was killed. When Julia was eight, her mother attempted to smother her with a pillow, then made a second suicide attempt with pills. Julia was removed from her mother's care and placed with her maternal grandparents, who found her behavior extremely provocative and unmanageable. Her teacher described her as obstinate and demanding, occasionally and for no apparent reason screaming as if she were being killed.

Julia was placed in a residential treatment center where she stayed for two years. Her gains in almost all areas of her functioning there were described as considerable. She was described as manipulative of the staff, but she was also said to be amenable to discipline. During her stay she was informed of her mother's rape in her own apartment, and the murder of an uncle. She was discharged from the residential treatment center back to her maternal grandparents, who shortly thereafter were burned out of their apartment and forced to live with one of their sons and his family in overcrowded conditions. Julia was referred to a community mental health center for psychotherapy because she fought in school shortly after being returned to her grandparents.

During the course of her psychotherapy, Julia's behavior in school ceased to be a problem. Her reactions to the multiple losses she experienced seemed to find expression in her interaction with her therapist. In sessions she would say to her therapist, "I am going to cut you with a knife. I'm going to cut you up like a piece of meat. I'm going to hunt you down with a gun. I'm going to eat all the food in the clinic." On occasion she would grab a handful of crackers, take them back to the therapy room, stuff her mouth with them, and pretend to choke. The therapist was to revive her. At other times, she would become a harsh teacher, forcing the therapist-student to stand at the blackboard and endlessly write the alphabet. At the end of sessions, Julia would usually refuse to leave; she would lie on the floor and pretend to be dead. One day, the security guard in the clinic had to be called to get Julia out of the office at the end of a session.

Julia's behavior outside of the sessions was not problematic. She would enter the clinic, immediately regress, then reconstitute on leaving the session. A powerful transferential process was clearly at work. Julia's sense of loss and the rage associated with the losses she had experienced found expression in partially symbolic form, in her relationship to her therapist.

The concept of transference has its roots in Sigmund Freud's basic concepts of drive and defense. Theoretical difficulties arise, however, in accounting for transference phenomena in children within this model. In what follows I outline the nature of these difficulties; then I consider the concept of transference in children from the perspective of an alternative theoretical model based on the object relations theories of Klein, Winnicott, Fairbairn, and Bion. Along the way I offer some thoughts on an integration of the contributions of these thinkers. I then return to the case of Julia and some other clinical material with consideration from the point of view of these various theoretical models.

THE CONCEPT OF TRANSFERENCE IN FREUDIAN CHILD PSYCHOANALYSIS

Freudian concepts of transference applied to analytic work with children derive from the concept of transference in adult work. The classical position is that psychological symptoms arise from intrapsychic conflicts between drives and defenses. These conflicts originate in childhood, typically in the oedipal period, when sexual drives are directed toward the parent of the opposite sex. The entire conflict is unconscious, thus unalterable. When a person enters psychoanalysis, the neutrality and anonymity of the analyst evoke a regression. Derivatives of the repressed drives, as well as the associated defenses, are transferred onto the analyst. The analyst's task, through interpretation, is to make the repressed conflict conscious, subject to a new resolution by the mature ego of the adult. Interpretation, in this context, refers to the establishment of a linkage between the feelings the patient has toward the analyst and the original feelings the patient had toward the parents. Transference is valuable as a way of bringing the repressed pathogenic conflict into the here and now, and as a way of vividly and convincingly demonstrating to the patient the nature of that conflict in the service of making it conscious.

The difficulties in applying this adult-based model to work with children seem threefold. First, the parents are still very much part of the child's life. Insofar as the child's drive-defense conflicts are still focused on the parents, the analyst is less likely to become the object involved. If one adopts Freud's economic model, in which psychic energy is assumed to exist in finite quantity, then there is less drive energy available with which to invest the analyst. From another point of view, one could say that, when the parents are still so present, there is less need to repeat conflicts involving them with substitute objects such as an analyst.

A second difficulty arises from the classical assumption that the analyst's anonymous and neutral stance is necessary to induce the regression necessary for transference. Deviation from an abstinent stance results in drive gratification, which makes analysis difficult or impossible. But children are less able than adults to tolerate analytic abstinence, and no child analyst has advocated the kind of "blank screen" stance that is classically adopted with adults. Once the analyst begins to engage the child patient actively, can a transference reaction occur in an analyzable form?

The third difficulty appears to arise from the cognitive immaturity of the child. In the adult, the process of the development of insight through interpretation involves a highly complex form of abstract and analogical thinking. For example, drawing parallels between feelings and perceptions directed toward the analyst, and those which have the parents as object, requires analogical reasoning not commonly encountered until adolescence.

Anna Freud (Sandler, Kennedy, and Tyson, 1980), Scharfman (1978), and many other child analysts have attempted to adapt the classical analytic model to children in the light of these difficulties. With respect to the first—the current and ongoing presence of the parents as primary objects—Anna Freud (1926) stated that the transference neurosis as it occurs in adults could not occur in children. Without the transference neurosis, how are the child's conflicts to be brought into the here-and-now of the analysis? The analyst may interpret current conflicts involving the parents to a young child still in the midst of an oedipal situation. To the older, postoedipal child, the analyst may interpret distortions in the youngster's perceptions of his parents today, based in past conflicts which have been repressed. In either case, interpretation refers to a conflict involving a third person, not the analyst. Given the child's cognitive concreteness, presumably it is more important to talk about here and now events and feelings involving the analyst. Here child analysis seems to face a formidable problem.

Furman (1957) and others have proposed one solution: the treatment of young children via their parents, usually their mothers. The parents are guided toward a psychoanalytically-based understanding of their childrens' difficulties that allows them to make interpretations to their children, such as an analyst might otherwise make. Sigmund Freud (1909) used this approach with Little Hans, the first child psychoanalytic patient. While making sense in terms of helping the child deal with here and now conflicts, this puts a great demand on the parent. As analysts or therapists, we are in a better position to maintain our objectivity when we are involved in a transference struggle with a patient, when we see the patient at most for an hour per day in very structured circumstances. Imagine having to spend most of one's waking hours with a patient, with responsibilities such as getting him or her out of bed and off to school, or into the bath at the end of a long and tiring day at work. Nonetheless, psychoanalytic understanding can be very useful to a parent in gaining perspective on and managing a child's otherwise incomprehensible and difficult behavior.

Treatment via the parents, then, requires very special parents. The problem remains, in the great majority of cases, of dealing with the conventional, dyadic, analytic situation without the assistance of a here and now transference relationship to the analyst. Anna Freud's (1936) pioneering work in ego psychology gave her the means to deal with this problem in another way. Without renouncing her father's emphasis on the id, and conflict involving id impulses, she expanded her focus to include ego functions, such as defense mechanisms, reality testing, cognitive functions, and so on, allowing for an expansion of the nature of the analytic work as well. She discussed the analyst's educational function in relation to the child patient, clarifying reality for him or her. Or, with respect to the young child's limited capacity for verbalization and self-observation, the analyst may "lend" to the child his or her own skills in the session, for example by verbalizing feelings for the child who has not yet learned to do so. The vacuum created by the relative absence of transference is thus filled by ego-supportive activities on the part of the analyst; these activities are thought of as preparatory to the true work of analysis, which is interpretation of conflict over id impulses, none-theless. In this way, the nature of the analytic work is broadened without challenging the classical model.

Anna Freud later acknowledged the existence of transference phenomena in children. First she stated (A. Freud, 1946) that the current presence of the parents mitigated, but did not preclude, transference to the analyst. She spoke of this as a quantitative issue, that it was a matter of how much of the child's psychic energy was attached to the parents, and not to the analyst, at any given time.

Second, (Sandler, Kennedy, and Tyson, 1980) she broadened the definition of transference to include such phenomena as "transfer-ence of habitual modes of relationship," "transference of current relationships," and "transference of past experiences" (pp. 79–99). The child's view of and feelings about the analyst could be condi-tioned by the child's usual way of being with people, or by current or past events in the child's life at home or school. These transference phenomena were to be distinguished, however, from the transfer-ence neurosis per se, in which the child's infantile conflicts crystallized around the analyst. Here again Anna Freud enlarged the scope of psychoanalytic work without disturbing the basic model developed by Sigmund Freud. If a child locked in a power struggle with a parent at home, for example, engaged in a similar behavior with the analyst, there might be echoes of anal stage conflicts over toilet training; but they are only echoes from the primary infantile conflict being played out at home. These are matters for the analyst to clarify for the child patient, but the real drama is going on elsewhere. The way in which the analytic situation can promote deep and thorough-going change in the child remains a problematic issue.

I now turn to a brief consideration of how Anna Freud and her followers dealt with the issue of the analyst's neutrality and anonym-ity. Scharfman (1978) acknowledges that it is not possible for the analyst to assume the same kind of abstinent stance that classical analysts take with adults. More ready, perhaps, to acknowledge the phenomenon of transference neurosis in children than Anna Freud, he nevertheless says that the analyst's interaction with the child as a "real object" (p. 286) should be kept to a minimum because it impairs the development of the transference. Anna Freud (Sandler, Kennedy, and Tyson, 1980) defines the issue not in terms of hindering or facilitating the development of transference, but in terms of assessing how much frustration the child can tolerate. One gratifies the child, or interacts like a "real object," only to the extent necessary to avoid losing the child's cooperation in the work. Framed in this way, the issue again becomes an ego-psychological one: insofar as the child's frustration tolerance is insufficient to tolerate abstinence, the analyst accommodates and gratifies. This action is necessary because it prepares the way to true interpretive work later.

Anna Freud and Scharfman also acknowledge that children make use of their analysts in various ways as "real objects," as objects of identification or even, to some extent, as surrogate parents who can fulfill the child's current developmental needs. Freud (Sandler, Kennedy, and Tyson, 1980) cites children whose fathers are not at home and are often referred to male therapists. Scharfman (1978) gives the example of a boy who had had a very conflictual relationship with his mother's boyfriend, followed by the man's death. Scharfman felt that this boy had a second chance to achieve a masculine identity in the relationship with his male analyst. In Anna Freud's view, such experiences of the analyst may be therapeutic, in the sense of promoting positive change but they are not truly the stuff of analytic work. Yet Scharfman describes cases in which the analyst at first seems to become a true transference object; it is only when he or she has taken on this sort of significance for the child that the analyst can have an impact as a "new" object. Scharfman believed that, in the transference of the boy just mentioned, the analyst was first identified with the mother's boyfriend. Many conflicts originating in that relationship were played out in relationship to the analyst, who did not behave as the mother's boyfriend did; for instance, he did not die. In this example, the boundary between the analyst as transference object and as new object is blurred.

THE KLEINIAN REVISION

A radically different point of view about transference in child analysis was initiated by Melanie Klein (1952). Klein thought in terms of projection and reintrojection of internalized objects created from the child's own fantasy life. She adopted Freud's (1920) dual instinct theory in which he postulated a death instinct, a source of innate aggression, along with the life instinct, the source of libido. In Klein's view, derivatives of these two instincts, projected onto the parents and then reinternalized, create an inner world populated by aggressive and frightening, as well as idealized, objects. These internal objects are continually reprojected onto people, such as parents and analysts, and reintrojected. Klein viewed transference in terms of these processes, that is, the projection of the internalized objects onto the analyst. In this sense, one might say that parents can be transference objects in the same way as an analyst can be. There is no "economic" theory of psychic energy here. The presence of the parents in the child's life in no way precludes transference in relation to the analyst, or anyone else in the child's life for that matter. All significant people in the child's life will be viewed in terms of the hopes, fears, anxieties, expectations, and so on, derived from the child's inner world of good and bad objects.

In Klein's theory, instincts become structured in the form of good (invested with libido) and bad (invested with aggression) objects. Instincts are no longer seen, as they were by Freud, as a "seething cauldron" (Eagle, 1984, p. 116) of unstructured energy. For Klein, instinctual energy and structured object representations are inherently intertwined.

There are ways, however, in which Klein followed in the Freudian tradition. In both theoretical systems, mental life is seen as largely intrapsychically, or endogenously, determined. The child's perceptions, feelings, anxieties, and conflicts derive from innate instincts and their vicissitudes, not from the influence of events in external reality. For Klein, as for Sigmund Freud, it followed that the analyst should adopt a rigorously abstinent, anonymous, strictly interpretive stance in order to facilitate the emergence of endogenous mental phenomena. Klein did not follow Anna Freud in recommending technical alterations in work with children; she developed no ego-psychological theory to provide a rationale for ego-supportive activities by the analyst. Thus emerged a major point of controversy between Freudian and Kleinian child analysts. Anna Freud and her followers rejected not only the Kleinian tendency to make direct interpretations of unconscious material, bypassing defenses, but also the Kleinian postulation of complex mental processes in the earliest months of life.

Working during the latter part of Klein's career, Winnicott broke with the emphasis on the innate, the endogenous. Winnicott believed that children brought with them innate potential for growth and development, but that the behavior of the actual mother or parents was crucial to how these potentials unfolded. Correspondingly, the technical approach of Winnicott (1963a) and his followers emphasized the participation of the analyst as a "facilitating environment," (p. 223) like a "good-enough" parent (Winnicott, 1960, p. 145). In this theoretical context the role of interpretation underwent a change. For Winnicott, the emphasis was not on the informational content of an interpretation, or the degree to which a psychic phenomenon could be made conscious; he focused instead on the way in which the analyst's comments represented a participation with the patient in the analytic setting. An interpretation was often seen by Winnicott as an intrusion on the patient, although there were times when interpreting advanced the analyst's "holding" function (Winnicott, 1963b, p. 240).

At points throughout her writing, Klein took account of the impact of the actual mother on the child's development (Greenberg and Mitchell, 1983). For example, in explaining how the child became able to allow for the integration of loving and destructive feelings toward the mother in the depressive position, Klein acknowledged that good experiences with the mothering person could facilitate this development. Klein did not, however, develop in her technical approach a role for the analyst as participant. This development, within the context of Kleinian theory, was carried forward by Bion. In order to understand his contribution, we must briefly review the roots of his work in Klein's theory.

When Klein (1946, 1955) introduced the concept of projective identification, she saw it as a defensive, intrapsychic phenomenon, a process involving a defensive fantasy of expelling a "bad" psychic content into another person, in which form the projected content can be brought under control. The concept of projective identification was used by Klein's followers as a more interpersonal process with communicative as well as defensive purposes. Bion (1959) introduced the idea that a child's projections could have an actual recipient or an impact on the analyst. The analyst's awareness of the patient's impact on his or her state of mind becomes data concerning the mental contents that are being disowned and projected by the patient. Pick and Segal (1978) give as an example a child who comes into his session and reads comics. The analyst feels left out and annoyed, a reaction seen as evidence that the child may be projecting into the analyst his own feelings of being abandoned and angry consequent to feeling left out in some way.

Projective identification can lead to vicious circles of projection and reintrojection. In the above example, if the analyst reacts overtly with annoyance, the patient may feel rejected or further left out. The analyst's feelings of being left out and angry, and the same feelings in the patient, feed and reinforce each other. In this way the patient's world remains a "closed system" (Fairbairn, 1958, p. 380). Internalized objects remain unmodified insofar as people in the outside world are induced to play their assigned roles in the pre-written script.

How can such vicious circles be broken? Klein (1948) believed that they were broken by an increase in love, relative to aggression, as children grow and mature. She also introduced the idea that positive experiences with others in the outside world could have an impact on one's internal object world (Klein, 1932). But if projective identification tends to reproduce negative expectations of others, how are positive experiences generated?

Bion (1988) contributed an answer to this question with his concepts of "container" and "contained (p. 106)." He proposed that the vicious circle of projective identification could be broken if a mother or analyst could contain the child's projection. Bion (1983) said that the recipient of a projection could "detoxicate" (pp. 122, 125) the projection in such a way that the mental content would be reintrojected by the child in a less extreme less pathological form (see also Ogden's, 1986, Grotstein's, 1987, and Burke and Tansey's, 1985 discussions of this process). What constitutes the "detoxication" of a projection? For Bion, the analyst must be able to receive the projection and "know" it, in the sense of allowing it to have an impact, to think about it, to understand it. Failure to contain means that the recipient rejects the projection and reprojects it, thus maintaining the vicious circle. The analyst who asks the child to put down the comic, returning to Pick and Segal's (1978) example, or makes some other rejecting comment, is seen as rejecting the child's projected feelings of abandonment. The analyst who contains these projected feelings allows himself or herself to experience them, to know them, and then to view them as a communication from the child about his or her own disowned experience.

As container, the analyst emerges as a coparticipant with the patient in the analytic work, someone whose function involves more than simply being a blank screen for projections. Let us now reconsider the role of interpretation in the Kleinian analyst's repertoire. For the early Klein, the analyst interpreted from a position outside the patient's transference. The disowned impulses or feelings were called to the patient's attention with the goals of undermining splitting and fostering psychic integration. In Bion's emendation of Klein's theory, interpretation becomes the means by which psychic content is reprojected by the analyst, in more or less "detoxicated" form; it appears that silent "processing" (Ogden, 1986, p. 36) of experience takes an important place in the analytic process. The analyst contains the projection by using his or her own reaction as a source of information about the child's experience and then using the understanding gained thereby to formulate an interpretation (Folch, 1988; O'Shaughnessy, 1981). To return to Pick and Segal's (1978) example of the boy with the comic book, the analyst might say to the child that he or she believes that the child, by reading the comic, is showing the analyst how left out he feels in relation to the analyst or some other person. The interpreting analyst allows the child to reintroject him or her as a containing object; thus the child develops the capacity to contain his own feelings and reactions (de Folch, 1988). In this way, the child's need to disown or project his own feelings is reduced, and progress is made toward breaking out of the vicious circle. The mechanism of therapeutic change, from this vantage point, is no longer primarily through insight as it is for Freudian adult analysts, or through ego enhancement as the Freudian child analysts have added. Rather the relationship between the child and analyst promotes an alteration in the child's projective–introjective processes. The Kleinian analyst working in this way does not interpret from a position outside the patient's presumably self-contained inner world. The analyst's stance, rather, entails being powerfully engaged and affected by the patient, all the while serving a containing function. The inner worlds of patient and analyst are deeply connected, each affecting the other. This interconnectedness is the matrix of analytic change.

Bion's work allows for a Kleinian rapprochement with the Winni-cottians on the issue of the importance of parents, and analysts, in the external world. But important differences remain. The issue for Winnicott and his followers is not the alteration of internalized objects so much as the facilitation of the emergence of a "true self." For a more complete discussion of the relationship of Kleinian and Winni-cottian theories, see Phillips (1988).

FURTHER INTERPERSONAL AND OBJECT RELATIONS THEORIES

The British object relations theorists have made a significant departure from the classical position by presenting transference as an interactive process. American interpersonal analysts, following in the tradition of Sullivan, have moved in a similar direction. Sullivan's (1953) concept of participant-observation opened the way in America for an interactive view of the psychoanalytic process. Modern interpersonal analysts (Gill, 1982; Levenson, 1972, 1983), have elaborated on the nature of this process. Levenson's (1972) concept of the "transformation" (pp. 33–44) of the analyst describes how the analyst becomes a participant in the patient's interpersonal world. Collaborative inquiry into the analytic relationship on the part of patient and analyst allows the analyst to resist being transformed, while offering the patient a new and unexpected experience. Although the focus is on the interpersonal rather than the inner stage, this process seems analogous to that described by the British object relations theorists of being inducted into the patient's world through projective identification, then working one's way out through containing and interpretation.

Fairbairn (1958) described a similar process with different language. In his terms, patients "pressgang" (p. 385) people in the outside world, including analysts, into behaving in the ways which they expect, based on the nature of their internal objects. The patient who expects to be attacked provokes attack; or the comments of the therapist tend to be perceived as critical attacks. In either case, the patient's world remains what Fairbairn calls a "closed system" (p. 380). The internal object world determines how people in the outside world are experienced; there is no room for people to be experienced in new ways, or as new objects. Fairbairn defines the goal of psychoanalytic treatment as opening up this closed system so that people can be experienced by the patient in new, more flexible ways.

More recently Greenberg (1986) proposed some balance between the degree to which the patient perceives the analyst as a new object and an old object. The analyst needs to be seen as an old object, especially at first, in order for the patient's internal object world to become manifest in the treatment situation, and in order for the analyst to become significant to the patient. The analyst needs to be perceived as a new object, to some degree, for change to occur; if not, there is an unmanageable transference situation, one that is too "hot." The analyst finds that everything he or she does confirms the patient's preconceptions. If the analyst is not enough the old object, the relationship lacks significance: for instance, when the analyst forgets a session with the patient and the patient dismisses the significance of the incident ("Oh well, everyone makes mistakes.") When the analyst is not enough the new object, the patient may perceive abandonment whenever the analyst looks away momentarily. When there is a balance, the patient can experience the analyst as abandoning while still collaborating with the analyst in the exploration of these perceptions. One can translate this process into Bion's terms as follows: seen as old object, the analyst becomes the recipient of the patient's projections. As new object, the analyst is recognized as containing the projections and feeding them back to the patient in the form of an interpretive intervention which only minimally, if at all, feeds the vicious circle.

I further propose that, aside from specific perceptions of the analyst as, for instance, abandoning, transference or "old object" status involves a particular quality of relatedness. This status involves the analyst assuming an enhanced significance to the patient, such as that lovers or parents and small children have to one another. This was a prominent aspect of what Breuer and Freud (1895) encountered in their interaction with Anna O., which led to the initial conceptualization of transference. I propose that it is only because the analyst has this special status in the patient's life that events occurring in the analytic space have a mutative effect on the patient's internal object world. The internalized object world is created in the context of the relationship with parents, who are all-important to the child. The alteration of this inner world can only occur in later childhood, or adulthood, if the analytic relationship takes on something of this special quality.

CHILD TRANSFERENCE REVISITED

What are the implications of these object relations-based views for analytic work with children? Do the models of change presented here apply? At what age or stage does the internal object world become fixed or structured enough to speak of the analyst becoming an old object for the child? Is a child capable of the kind of balanced perception of the analyst as new and old object of which Greenberg speaks? Can an analyst or therapist assume a special, enhanced significance to a child?

As to structuralization of the child's object world, in normal development one expects some openness, some fluidity and flexibility in young childrens' perceptions of other people. It may be that the hallmark of psychopathology is when children are not open to the new experiences presented by each interpersonal encounter. It is when children are overly prone to constructing their interpersonal experiences in terms of danger, anxiety, frustration, and so on, that we are likely to see them in our offices and clinics. As with adults, we find with such children that they seem to seek out the very experiences that are problematic to them; they are also highly sensitive to the actions of others that can be interpreted as rejection, impingement, and so on. Children present to us what Fairbairn (1958) called "a closed system," just as adults do.

An analyst will likely become part of this closed system, and thus an "old object" to child patients. Can the analyst be a "new object" as well? My impression is that children make this aspect of our work relatively easy. Children seek out corrective experiences, second chances to work through problematic interactions with adults. For many children who are not in treatment, an uncle or aunt, a teacher, or some other adult is long remembered as a positive force, someone who was able to provide a counterbalance to the experience with the parents.

Furthermore, the tendency of children to use therapy as an opportunity to play creates an ideally conducive situation for the therapist to be both new and old object. In a play situation the therapist or analyst, as well as the self, can be assigned roles corresponding to internalized self and object roles. In play, as with transitional objects, there is a paradoxical intermingling of reality and fantasy that as Winnicott (1951) points out, cannot be resolved. The transitional object can be simultaneously felt to be the most important thing in the world and perceived as a dirty old blanket; in play, the doll or the analyst can be simultaneously known as persecutor, victim, frustrator, and so on, without losing sight of the fact that the analyst is also a middle-aged grown-up whom one goes to see on Monday afternoons after school. Play, then, by its very nature, creates the balance between analyst as "new" and "old" object of which Greenberg speaks.

Case reports in the literature make it clear that the analyst can assume the same enhanced significance in the lives of some children that occurs in the transference neuroses of some adults. Scharfman (1978) reports preschool age cases in which oedipal-stage feelings occurred in relation to the analyst before occurring in relation to the parents. He also mentions the crushes preadolescent children may have on adults, including analysts. From an object relations point of view, there is no reason to question the existence of transference manifestations in children, or the feasibility of working with transference therapeutically.

With the Freudian ego-psychological and object relations points of view in mind, let us now return to the case of Julia. From a drive theory standpoint, Julia's behavior reflects derivatives of libidinal and aggressive drives, the latter perhaps fueled by her many experiences of traumatic loss and deprivation. There is drive fixation or regression at the oral level, reflected in her concerns involving food and her generally demanding attitude toward the therapist. Ego deficits are evident, such as poor frustration tolerance and impulse control. The nature of the pathology makes an analytic approach quite problematic. The patient is unable to tolerate much abstinence on the therapist's part. She tends to act out by refusing to leave the session, requiring a response on the part of the therapist that compromises her neutrality. The therapeutic approach focuses on ego support, helping the patient to develop frustration tolerance that might some day make insight-oriented treatment possible. If one could get to that point with Julia, the goal would be for Julia to recognize her perceptions of the therapist as distortions, based on the carryover into the therapeutic relationship of conflicts with roots in the past.

Acting out or demanding food or more of the therapist's time, are not seen as reflecting ego deficits from an object-relational point of view. Nor are such behaviors seen as necessarily obstructive to successful treatment, but as the means by which the child inducts the therapist into his or her inner world. Let us consider the situation created when a child such as Julia refuses to leave at the end of a session. The therapist is likely to feel irritated and the child quickly comes to be perceived as a nuisance, especially if another patient is waiting. The therapist finds himself or herself rejecting the child. The rejecting object of the child's inner world has been projected into the therapist. If the rejected and angry child patient turns the tables on the therapist and refuses to talk, in the next session, the therapist will sample the child's experience of being rejected. In contrast to the classical view, no distorted perception of the therapist is seen to be involved here; a situation has evolved in which the child's anxieties, fears, and expectations of other people have become actualized.

In this manner, the therapist becomes an "old" object to the child. The child's problematic internalized object relations have become actualized in the therapeutic relationship. This is a necessary first step but not a sufficient condition for therapeutic change to occur. The therapist needs to be able to assume the role of new object as well. How does this occur? First, the therapist must, in Bion's (1983, p. 122) terms, "detoxicate" the child's projection. The therapist must be able to experience the role in which she is placed without acting the part. Here is where verbalization by the therapist may be useful. The therapist might say, "I think you want to see whether I will send you away as your mother and grandmother did." From an object-relational point of view, the purpose of such a verbalization is not only, or even primarily, to further the child's insight into the sources of her behavior, but to establish a position the therapist assumes in relation to the child. The therapist is commenting on the child's behavior but not retaliating. The exploratory or interpretive therapeutic stance is thus useful insofar as it does *not* entail a reinforcement of the closed internal object world the child brings to treatment.

There are also qualities in the child that facilitate or hinder the therapist's assumption of the role of "new" object. The ability to self reflect, a sense of humor, the capacity to play are all useful. Julia's letter, with which we started, seems to give evidence of these qualities. The therapist clearly has old object status, reinforced by the fact that the therapist is terminating the therapy, and not in response to the child's needs. At the same time, the child is responding with a sense of humor such as her reference to cleaning the therapist's ears. She seems to be using the therapy as a playground, or a stage, for the enactment of her inner drama. As in a theater, where there needs to be a "suspension of disbelief," the therapeutic relationship is serious enough to be meaningful, but has enough of an "as if" quality to allow for the taking of perspective, while the therapist's questions and comments serve a containing function. The old scenario of abandonment is being replayed, but with a different outcome. In the process, we hope, the child's sense of the possibilities in close human interaction, even when these interactions must end, have expanded.

TOM

Another clinical example: The patient, Tom, is a ten-year-old boy in twice-weekly psychotherapy. He is a big, freckle-faced, red-haired boy, who presents with an air of bravado. Sports are his life, or at least the most important part of his life. He has heroes in the sports world, especially Joe Montana, the "miracle man" quarterback of the San Francisco 49'ers. Play-acting sporting events often dominate sessions with him, facilitated by the fact that the therapy room has a basketball net in it, a small basketball and football, and a little space to move in. In a year and a half of therapy, many sessions with Tom consisted of Tom and his therapist being on the same team, playing against an imaginary opposing team. In other sessions, they played against each other. When the therapist made a mistake, e.g., dropped the ball, Tom taunted him. The sessions often had a driven quality, ostensibly in the service of a desperate need to beat the other team. After he had beaten his therapist in one session, Tom ran out of the room before the therapist could even attempt to engage him in conversation about what had happened. The therapist usually found it hard to get Tom to stop long enough to talk until he began to "interview" the players after each game, as if on television.

Tom had been in therapy from ages five to eight. When he was eight his father left his mother. Shortly thereafter, Tom's therapy terminated due to the departure of his therapist from the clinic he attended. A few months later, Tom's mother sought treatment for him again. The presenting problems now included generalized anxiety, especially fears at bedtime of kidnappers or of his mother dying. At school he was described as having difficulty with peer relationships because of bossiness, his insistence on having things go his own way. There were also reports of wetting or soiling himself at times. Tom had a 13-year-old brother who had also been in therapy on and off for several years, and was also described as "bossy"; the brothers, in evident rivalry with each other, competed for the same friends.

Following is clinical material from a particular session in the second treatment in which there was a dramatic shift in the "manifest content" of the session. The context in Tom's life at the time was that his remarried father, who had been taking Tom for two nights a week, was asking to reduce that amount of time, ostensibly because of crowded conditions now that there was a toddler, Tom's half-sibling, in the house.

Tom entered the playroom and complained that some playdough he had used in the previous session was "no good" any more, since it had been mixed with playdough of different colors. Then he assigned play roles to himself and to his therapist: he was Ms. Proper with a British accent (his father had a British accent). Ms. Proper has a restaurant. The therapist is to be a customer who enters the restaurant. The customer is to be rude, demanding and complaining. Ms. Proper responds to him with anger. She is replaced by "Rob," Ms. Proper's husband, who curses out the customer and calls in the butler to throw him out. The therapist is to enter the restaurant as "Mr. Nice Guy" who is briefly quite well behaved but starts to put his feet on the table becoming increasingly rude until he too is thrown out.

Before the next session, Tom's mother reported that Tom's father had told her of difficulty putting Tom to sleep on his previous visit, and that as a result he felt he could no longer have Tom stay at his place during the week. In the session that followed, Tom assigned to himself the role of Will Clark, a well-known baseball player. Will Clark is called out by an umpire and disputes the call vehemently, to the point of rushing the umpire and bumping him with his body. The umpire ejects him from the game. (Tom, discussing this interaction with his therapist, said that Will Clark felt he was going to lose the argument anyway, so he may as well get thrown out of the game.) Will Clark later gets angry at his manager because he's assigned to be the designated hitter (one who hits but doesn't have a position in the field). Tom says he's angry because it seems that his fielding ability is being disparaged.

In the next session, Tom's play involved being a rookie on the Boston Red Sox, the therapist to be his mentor, an older player. Before long, Will Clark appears on the Red Sox team, having been traded from the San Francisco Giants. Again he is angry because he did not want to be traded. Tom later took out his homework and asked the therapist to help him with it, as his father would have on their weekday visits.

From a Freudian or ego-psychological perspective, this clinical vignette reveals a boy with a generally intact ego, who can express his concerns and conflicts symbolically, without much acting out. If anything, he is quite compliant in the therapy. Many themes in his play revolve around oedipal issues: competition, cooperation, conflict with male authorities, and retaliatory rejection. There is some evidence of oral stage issues; for example, the scene with Ms. Proper is in a restaurant and has to do with a demanding attitude on the part of the customer. Anal issues are suggested by the wetting and soiling, and bossiness. Transference, in so far as it is present here, fits Anna Freud's category of "transference of current relationships:" Tom enacts, through his play with the therapist, the current rejection by his father. Oedipal rivalries with his father, as well as earlier concerns with deprivation, are awakened. The therapist's approach involves clarification of the feelings and impulses currently aroused in relation to his father, then interpretive linking of these impulses with the earlier oedipal, oral, and anal stage feelings and impulses.

From an object relations perspective, the focus is on the role into which Tom puts the therapist. On the level of symbolic play, the therapist is put in the position of the rejected customer, or the rejecting umpire. In symbolic fashion, the therapist is given the opportunity to experience and contain a bit of Tom's feelings of rejection, as well as the retaliatory anger that Tom presumably feels toward his father. On the other hand, the context of this play is a highly cooperative, mutual relationship. In this sense, Tom is using his therapist predominantly as a new object. Disappointed as he is with his father, he even engages the therapist as a sort of new father by doing his homework with him. The therapist takes on old object status mostly in the context of the roles he takes on in symbolic play. One might wonder whether the therapy would have maximum impact if Tom could also allow the therapist to assume old object status on the level of their actual interaction. The only hint of such a development in the session presented was Tom's comment that the therapist's play-dough was "no good" any more, implying that Tom was beginning to feel some disappointment with his therapist.

When we look at the cases of Julia and Tom together, they seem to be on opposite sides of the continuum described by Greenberg (1986). Julia reacts to the therapist more as an old object, while Tom reacts to the therapist more as a new object. While both seem to make good use of their therapists, in Julia's case the therapist struggles to be recognized as a new object, as someone with whom Julia can have a new experience. In Tom's case, the therapist might aim to bring into the therapeutic relationship some of the conflict and anger Tom experienced, presumably, in relation to his father.

To summarize, I try to articulate an object relations approach to analytic work with children, specifically with respect to the role of transference. I contrast this model with the classical drive-defense and ego-psychological model, in which the ultimate therapeutic impact is carried by insight, with ego support offered when necessary. The object relations model suggests a different way to conceive of the process of therapeutic change.

REFERENCES

Bion, W. R. (1959), Attacks on linking. In: *Melanie Klein Today*, Vol. 1, ed. E. Bott-Spillius. London: Routledge, pp. 87–101, 1988.
_____ (1983), *Transformations*. New York: Aronson.
Breuer, J. & Freud, S. (1895), *Studies on Hysteria. Standard Edition*, 2. London: Hogarth Press, 1955.
Burke, W. F. & Tansey, M. J. (1985), Projective identification and countertransference turmoil. *Contemp. Psychoanal.*, 21:372–402.
Eagle, M. (1984), *Recent Developments in Psychoanalysis*. Cambridge, MA: Harvard University Press.
de Folch, T. (1988), Communication and containing in child analysis: Towards terminability. In: *Melanie Klein Today*, Vol. 2, ed. E. Bott-Spillius. London: Routledge, pp. 206–217.
Fairbairn, W. R. D. (1959), On the nature and aims of psychoanalytic treatment. *Internat. J. Psycho-Anal.*, 39:374–385.
Freud, A. (1926), Introduction to the technique of child analysis. In: *The Psychoanalytic Treatment of Children*. New York: International Universities Press, 1946, pp. 3–53.
_____ (1936), The ego and the mechanisms of defense. *The Writings of Anna Freud*, vol. 2. New York: International Universities Press.
_____ (1946), *The Psychoanalytic Treatment of Children*. New York: International Universities Press.
Freud, S. (1909), Analysis of a phobia in a five-year-old boy. *Standard Edition*, 10:5–149. London: Hogarth Press, 1955.
_____ (1920), Beyond the pleasure principle. *Standard Edition*, 18:3–64. London: Hogarth Press, 1955.
Furman, E. (1957), Treatment of under fives via their parents. *The Psychoanalytic Study of the Child*, 12:250–262. New York: International Universities Press.
Gill, M. (1982), *Analysis of Transference*. New York: International Universities Press.
Greenberg, J. R. (1986), Theoretical models and the analyst's neutrality. *Contemp. Psychoanal.*, 22:87–106.
_____ & Mitchell, S. A. (1983), *Object Relations in Psychoanalytic Theory*. Cambridge, MA: Harvard University Press.
Grotstein, J. S. (1987), Making the best of a bad deal: A discussion of Boris's "Bion Revisited." *Contemp. Psychoanal.*, 23:60–76.
Klein, M. (1932), *The Psychoanalysis of Children*. London: Hogarth Press.

_____ (1946), Notes on some schizoid mechanisms. In: *Envy and Gratitude and Other Works 1946–1963*. New York: Delacorte, 1975, pp. 1–24.

_____ (1948), On the theory of anxiety and guilt. In: *Envy and Gratitude and Other Works*. New York: Delacorte, 1975, pp. 25–42.

_____ (1952), The origins of transference. In: *Envy and Gratitude and Other Works 1946–1963*. New York: Delacorte, 1975, pp. 48–56.

_____ (1955), The psychoanalytic play technique: Its history and significance. In: *Envy and Gratitude and Other Works 1946–1963*. New York: Delacorte, 1975, pp. 122–140.

Levenson, E. (1972), *The Fallacy of Understanding*. New York: Basic Books.

_____ (1983), *The Ambiguity of Change*. New York: Basic Books.

O'Shaughnessy, E. (1981), W. R. Bion's theory of thinking and new techniques in child analysis. In: *Melanie Klein Today*, Vol. 2, ed. E. Bott-Spilius. London: Routledge, 1988, pp. 177–190.

Ogden, T. (1986), *Matrix of the Mind*. Northvale, NJ: Aronson.

Phillips, A. (1988), *Winnicott*. London: Fontana Press.

Pick, I. & Segal, H. (1978), Melanie Klein's contribution to child analysis. In: *Child Analysis and Therapy*, ed. J. Glenn. New York: Aronson.

Sandler, J., Kennedy, H. & Tyson, R. L. (1980), *The Technique of Child Analysis*. Cambridge, MA.: Harvard University Press.

Scharfman, M. (1978), Transference and the transference neurosis in child analysis. In: *Child Analysis and Therapy*, ed. J. Glenn. New York: Aronson.

Sullivan, H. S. (1953), *The Interpersonal Theory of Psychiatry*. New York: Norton.

Winnicott, D. W. (1951), Transitional objects and transitional phenomena. In: *Through Pediatrics to Psychoanalysis*. New York: Basic Books, 1975, pp. 229–242.

_____ (1960), Ego distortion in terms of true and false self. In: *The Maturational Processes and the Facilitating Environment*. New York: International Universities Press, 1965, pp. 140–152.

_____ (1963a), The mentally ill in your caseload. In: *The Maturational Processes and the Facilitating Environment*. New York: International Universities Press, 1965, pp. 217–229.

_____ (1963b), Psychiatric disorders in terms of infantile mental processes. In: *The Maturational Processes and the Facilitating Environment*. New York: International Universities Press, 1965, pp. 230–241.

9

Attachment Research

An Approach to a Developmental Relational Perspective

DORIS K. SILVERMAN

The infant is a social being. Information from widely diverse sources, but especially from developmental researchers, is demonstrating this view. A similar emphasis on the underlying importance of social relatedness is evident in other fields. For example, social scientists have been revising their views of our ancestors. Since the 1960s an intriguing idea about the relationship between brain size and complexity and social organization has taken hold. It has increasingly replaced anthropologists' emphasis on the growth of a complex brain as a function of tool use, group hunting, and communication. Apes, monkeys, and lemurs live very involved social lives. From birth on they are part of an intricate familial and social hierarchy. They recognize parents, especially mothers, but also kin and close affiliative relationships. It is thought that the use of tools, group hunting, and the need for communication are all an outgrowth of the essential social lives of these primates. Superior brain development occurred alongside of complex social organization (Small, 1990). Brunner (1990) argues that there are inborn dispositions for socialization and the triggering responses for relatedness are "acts and expressions of others" (p. 73). He quotes the primatologist Roger Lewin who maintains that the criterion for evolutionary selection in higher primates is the requirement of living in groups. This view suggests that contemporary men and women, like their ancestors, are social beings; attachment behavior fosters survival.

Consistent with this point of view, Lewis (1987) maintains that social adaptation is the main focus of the infant and that skills and biological equipment make it feasible for social interactions to flourish. Thus, infants show greater discriminatory capacity for social over nonsocial stimuli (e.g. early recognition of speech sounds). They also have the ability to connect people's faces and voices, to distinguish between familiar and unfamiliar people, their distinctive odors and handling styles, to recognize gender and age differences, and to discriminate tonal and facial expressions. Brain differentiation occurs more readily in response to social stimuli. Diurnal wake–sleep patterns follow social interactions. Social stimuli evoke more interest and are more rapidly learned.

The focus of this chapter is to highlight the importance of representational experience derived from attachment patterns. I want to stress, however, the additional importance of representations derived from sensual-sexual and aggressive strivings, sometimes labeled as endogenous stimulation, reflecting its motive force originating in bodily experiences. These two patterns (attachment and sensual-sexual and aggressive strivings[1]) can be considered behavioral systems that can be activated and terminated. At times, one or the other may be the dominant behavior system activated; however, these two systems (as well as others,[2]) can be overlapping and intertwined in goal achievement.[3]

By sensual-sexual and aggressive[4] strivings, I am trying to capture the following aspects: 1) the desire to repeat bodily experiences organized around pleasures. 2) These bodily experiences (primarily of past sensual arousal but also aggressive activation) and their associated feelings of gratification or frustration eventually become organized into schemas (representations). 3) They are wishes and fantasy schemas since they are concerned with cognitive and affective experiences about thwarted or gratified pleasures. 4) The formation of these fantasies can be seen along the lines suggested by Freud's (1916–1917) concept of a "complementary series" (p. 347), that is, the

---

[1]Here I am linking sensual-sexual and aggressive strivings into one pattern. It might be more accurate to separate aggression from the sensual-sexual system as Lichtenberg (1989) does. He labels it the aversive system (p. 2).

[2]In this chapter I am focusing on two motivational systems, attachment and sensual-sexual and aggressiving strivings. A third is the need to maintain a stable self-organization. All three are significant organizers of mental experiences. This paper does not address the third. Silverman and Gruenthal's (in press) paper integrates the latter two motivational systems.

[3]I am extending Bowlby's ethologically constructed viewpoint of behavioral systems fueled by feedback information to include the more traditional notion of "drives."

[4]The motive power for aggression is problematic on two counts: both its sources in the body and its proactive or reactive nature bear further exploration (see also Lichtenberg, 1989).

inputs organizing these fantasies can be seen as on a continuum from those primarily self generated to those fantasies whose major influence derives from interactions with key people in the environment. Whereas attachment schemas can only evolve out of interactions, sensual-sexual and aggressive fantasy schemas while usually influenced by social interactions can also be shaped by endogenously generated sexual and aggressive motives. For instance, fantasies stemming from sibling rivalry may not be a veridical response to actual parental behaviors. The child's wishes to be the only child, or the best-loved one, may arise primarily from wishful ideas that reflect sensual-sexual and aggressive strivings. The fantasy of eliminating siblings can be a displaced oedipal wish to possess mother exclusively rather than one based primarily on attachment strivings. By contrast, sibling rivalry fantasies can be an outgrowth of actual dysfunctional mother–child interactions, producing a maladaptive attachment that is internalized and generates such fantasies (e.g., I can feel safe and secure next to mother because no one is impeding my way). I am describing systems representing different motives. One may be more prominent than the other, or they may be shifting motivational states, or both may exist simultaneously with relatively equal weight for any individual or at any point in time. Second, I am suggesting various shadings from primarily internal stimulation to mainly external-interactional contributions to fantasy. Sensual-sexual and aggressive strivings may show a greater reliance on internal-personalized ways of organizing experience than fantasies derived from attachment patterns. However, both types of fantasies become further elaborated by continuing social interactions. Eventually, both are intrapsychic experiences shaping and being shaped by each other and by external events.[5]

Winnicott in his typically evocative way has captured the uniqueness of these two dimensions of experiences. He writes:

> The phenomena I am describing (that is, basic secure personal relations) have no climax. This distinguishes them from phenomena that have instinctual backing, where the orgiastic element plays an essential part and where satisfactions are closely linked with climax. . . . Psychoanalysts who have rightly emphasized the significance of instinctual experience and reaction to frustration have failed to state with compa-

---

[5]Attachment patterns have elements in common with Freud's description of the self-preservative instincts. Freud initially saw these and libido as two major motivational considerations in mental life. (For a detailed presentation of the relationship between attachment patterns and self-preservation, see Silverman, 1991.)

rable clearness or conviction the tremendous intensity of those noncli-
matic experiences of relating to objects (quoted by Guntrip, 1971, p.
121).[6]

Some attempts at integrating dual and multi-motivational perspectives in psychoanalytic theory can be found in the work of Modell's
(1985) one- versus two-person psychology (see also Beebe and
Lachmann, 1988; and Ghent, 1989); Balint's (1979) ocnophilia and
philobatism; Blatt and Blass's (in press) anaclitic and introjective
orientation; Pine's (1990) drive, ego, object, and self; Gedo and
Goldberg's (1973) models of the mind; Mitchell's (1988) broad paradigmatic relational model; and Lichtenberg's (1989) multimotivational
theory. (See Blatt and Blass for a more comprehensive discussion of
these different trends and Silverman [1986] for a clinical example
utilizing different theoretical perspectives.)

Experience based on endogenous stimulation, while not an exclusive emphasis in Freudian theory, has been the major vantage point
of that theory in ordering and understanding the infant's representational world. There is considerable theorizing about infant development and the establishment of psychic structure from this perspective (e.g., Sandler, 1987). In this chapter I focus primarily on
interactional experiences initiated at birth that also contribute to the
structuring of experiences. I discuss research on patterns of attachment, the nature of their internalizations, and present some clinical
support for this point of view. In utilizing a clinical example, I hope
to demonstrate the relevance of both attachment and sensual-sexual
and aggressive strivings to the understanding of clinical data.

---

[6]Winnicott's quote reflects attempts to underscore an object relational orientation
whose motive power stems from representations of initial and ongoing interactive
experiences. In addition he addresses the more traditional emphasis on motives linked
to the concept of "drives." The object relational aspect of endogenously organized
strivings is more varied in Freudian theory. Whereas for Freud the linkage was at times
relatively loose – e.g., autoerotic behavior could gratify a sensual-sexual drive – even in
the Freud (1905) paper, clinical examples reflect the closer unity between drives and
objects. Loewald (1980) maintained there is never a drive without an object, and many
contemporary Freudians hold a similar view (e.g., Dowling, 1990; Sandler, 1987, 1990).
However, in this latter position, as I have suggested, the organization of the fantasy
may reflect minimal interactive input. This greater stress on the significance of
internally organized fantasy experiences, and less stress on the role of parent-child
interactions in organizing fantasy, may have contributed to the emphasis on increasing
autonomy and self differentiation in Freudian developmental theory. (I have suggested
elsewhere that it may also reflect a more male-centered theoretical perspective
[Silverman, 1987], as well as reveal values of Western societies [Cushman, 1991].)

ATTACHMENT: BOWLBY'S CONTRIBUTIONS

It was Bowlby's (1958, 1969, 1973, 1980) pioneering efforts to understand infants' struggles with separation, loss, grief, and mourning that led to his new motivational paradigm. He maintained that close observation of infants and young children demonstrates the power of an early attachment tie, and the effects on children when this tie is ruptured. This attachment is not libidinally organized. By that I mean it is not primarily pleasure and its satisfaction that promote powerful connections between infants and their mothers. Bowlby challenged Freud's view that it is nourishment and its need-satisfying aspect that leads infants to recognize caretakers as primary objects. Bowlby insisted that the need for proximity, closeness, and safety that mothers provide are exclusive factors motivating infants' connectedness.[7] Bowlby suggested that there are instinctual features demonstrated in infants' behaviors that foster attachment. For example, the infants' crying, clinging, and smiling are ways to facilitate mothers' physical presence, responsiveness, and care. Thus, there is in part a preprogrammed aspect to infants' behaviors, along with considerable learning that takes place as infants negotiate attachment experiences.

Bowlby (1988) defines attachment as "any form of behavior that results in a person attaining or maintaining proximity to some other clearly identified individual who is conceived of as better able to cope with the world. It is most obvious whenever the person is frightened, fatigued, or sick, and is assuaged by comforting and caregiving" (p. 26–27). Whereas in this chapter I focus on infants' attachments, it is clear that Bowlby does not limit this concept to young children. Rather he sees it as a life-long need and an essential aspect of human nature – to search out a significant other(s) – especially in critical times of stress and need.

Attachment behavior is a slowly evolving process occurring over the course of the first year of life. There are genetically programmed features of infants that permit them to engage, connect with, and discriminate their primary caregivers from others. Infants and their mothers are interacting before and at birth. Connections are established that continue to intensify and mature beginning with infants' prewired capacities for relatedness, the bond that is immediately established under optimal circumstances, the early configured inter-

---

[7]Bowlby's (1988) most recent statements suggest that attachment is not the sole motivational impetus for infant–parent connections, rather the one that he is interested in developing.

actions—face-to-face exchanges, synchrony of responses, mutuality of interchanges—all of which establish early social relations and subsequent attachments.

These early patterns of attachments eventually get internalized in what Bowlby calls "working models," or what in psychoanalytic theory has been designated as mental or psychic representations. This aspect of attachment behavior is a key to understanding the importance of Bowlby's challenge to traditional psychoanalytic theory. Working models suggest a pattern of behavior that eventually gets internalized. That is, from this theoretical perspective we are not dealing with only surface conscious behavior, the domain of much academic psychology research, but complex conscious and unconscious responses and interactions, which eventually get internalized and have their own motivational structure organized differently from those evolving from endogenously organized wish-defense compromises. Attachment patterns become habituated, and then can generalize to other interactions. When so established they can be considered schemas of interactional patterns. Whereas these representations occur over time, they are not rigid. New experiences can alter old patterns of interaction and their internalization.

Objections to the traditional Freudian developmental paradigm have arisen from the burgeoning infant research literature. (For reviews of the experimental literature challenging traditional Freudian perspectives see Lichtenberg, 1983, 1989; Stern, 1977, 1985; and Silverman, 1981, 1984, 1991). I will present data to highlight the infants' early awareness and connection to primary caregivers. I will then discuss Ainsworth and her co-workers' experimental work because it reflects the best research analogue to attachment behavior. Additionally, it has increasingly demonstrated strong predictions for subsequent development.

ATTACHMENT BEHAVIOR PRECURSORS: EARLY
MOTHER-INFANT INTERACTIONS

Pregnant women frequently discuss the baby growing with them, providing their fetuses with personality characteristics—describing their motility, their placidity or fussiness, their circadian patterns of activity—and initiating powerful psychic connections to them. In addition there are a host of physiological interchanges that prepare mothers for subsequent attachments. Fetal hormones increase mothers' responsiveness in utero and at birth (Bell and Harper, 1977). With birth the initial and continued physical closeness of infants and mothers is essential for healthy growth and adaptation of infants (Hofer, 1977, 1987). Recent findings (Barnes, 1988) suggest that "a mother's touch has real biological effects–it means growing and thriving" (p. 142). Depriving infants of maternal contact will lead to weight deficiency and damage normal development. Premature babies can overcome maturational lags and flourish through physical handling and solicitous care (Silverman, 1981; Barnes, 1988).

Babies, too, begin interactions with their primary caregivers at birth and even earlier. There are discriminating responses that fetuses make to their mothers in utero. When prenatally primed, they recognize their mothers' voice and can discriminate it from another (DeCasper and Fifer, 1980; DeCasper and Spence, 1986). They can identify tones previously presented to them in utero (Stern, 1985).

Initial neonatal behavior is dominated by social interactions. Sleep-wake regulation cycles in infants evolve through infant parent interactions (Lewis, 1987). Infants rapidly learn responses that provide auditory access to their mothers (Rovee-Collier, 1987). Infants show preference for high-pitched voices, and this is characteristic of mothers' speech to their infants (Osofsky and Connors, 1979). Olfaction develops in the first week of life as demonstrated by the neonates' discriminating their mothers' odor from others' odors (MacFarlane, 1975). Infants distinguish subtle kinesthetic, motoric, and interactive patterns between themselves and their primary caregivers and will demonstrate disruptive behavior when primary caregivers are replaced (Burns, Sander, Stechler, and Julia, 1972). This interaction can be demonstrated by the tenth day of the infants' lives.

The infants' perceptual apparatus develops rapidly and enhances social responsiveness (Aslin, 1987). Babies show early recognition and preferences for faces (Bushnell, 1982), and can discriminate their primary caregivers from others by five weeks of age (Lewis, 1988). By one to three months, infants have some understanding of the connection of voices and faces (Brazelton, Koslowski, and Main, 1974). Newborns focus best on an object when it is eight inches away; this is the typical and optimal distance between the infants' and mothers' faces during nursing or bottle feeding (Lichtenberg, 1983).

The presence of a social-interactional context facilitates learning. Emotional responsivity, interest, sustained attention, and visual exploration appear to be optimal in gaze behavior, that is, when infants are focused on human faces (Izard and Malatesta, 1987). Infants' smiling response to caregivers' faces (Spitz and Wolff, 1946) and voices (Wolff, 1966)–the latter noticed as well in blind children– and the caregivers' smiling response to their infants, suggest the genetically programmed adaptive importance of this bidirectional response. Children with minimal opportunities for social interaction show significant retardation in these discriminating capacities (Provence and Lipton, 1962).

An infant's appearance elicits responsiveness from parents. An infant's large forehead, small face, prominent eyes, chubby cheeks, small mouth and body attract adults (Bell and Harper, 1977; Kennell, Voos, and Klaus, 1979). Those prominent, large, round eyes engage mothers in gazing experiences. Extended eye contact is seldom terminated by mother and enhances connections between infant and mother (Stern, 1974, 1985). The prepatterned design of connectedness to infants is highlighted by the similarities in the initial approach and handling of newborns by parents from widely different cultures. These interactions are marked by a gingerly approach–touching infants' fingers, then hands, and finally their torso. Mothers typically cradle infants on the left side of their body (Salk, 1970; de Chateau, 1983). Correspondingly, infants prefer to turn to the right (de Chateau, 1987), giving them frequent opportunity to see mother's face.

Both infants and mothers bring qualities to the relationship that enhance adaptation for both. There may well be preprogrammed aspects in both participants as reflected for example in the left hand preference for holding babies for most mothers, regardless of their handedness. The infants thrive, smile, vocalize, and are reactive, and the average mothers' increasingly well-honed responsiveness demonstrates their mutual regulation. It is a jointly active interaction, each in turn eliciting responses from the other. When babies are in close physical proximity to their mothers, healthy growth and development have a better chance of being facilitated.

AINSWORTH'S THE STRANGE-SITUATION PARADIGM

Ainsworth designed a structured situation to demonstrate experimentally what Bowlby described as occurring naturally during the course of the first year. When distress or fear is stirred in the young child, it activates the attachment system in order to provide an experience of felt security. The Strange Situation consists of a number of episodes, with an emphasis on mothers' departures and reunions with their infants. This provides opportunities for studying how infants organize their attachment feelings and behavior under tolerable conditions of stress. The largest percentage of children are securely attached (65%–70%). Sroufe (1979) described this child in the following way:

When stress is minimal, the securely attached child can separate readily from the caregiver to explore. When distressed, however, by a brief separation, for example, the securely attached infant actively seeks and maintains contact until comforted, which promotes a return to play. Under other circumstances, or when the infant is older, a brief separation from the caregiver may not produce distress, especially if the baby is not left alone. If not upset, secure infants are nonetheless active in re-established contact [p. 838].

Mothers can be in physical or psychological contact. Thus, a smile, word, or supportive look can be effective.

Two other groups of nonsecure infants[8] have also been described, those labeled as avoidant (group A, 20%–25%) and those as ambivalent (resistant, group C, less than 10%). These two patterns of attachment behavior are not considered pathological. Rather they are thought of as styles of relating. They do not necessarily produce nonadaptive behavior nor are they necessary predictors of later maladaptive behavior in any linear fashion. Only in their extreme forms can these alternative styles of relating be seen as potentially flagging problematic subsequent adjustments. Nonetheless some consistent thematic patterns are becoming demonstrable. Avoidant children tend to be hostile and display unprovoked aggression (Kobak and Shaver, 1987). Ainsworth described these infants as not directly expressing their aggression toward mothers, but using "subtle ways," attacking objects or biting or hitting mother without any overt anger (Ainsworth et al., 1978, p. 129). Physically abused and neglected children demonstrate sometimes ambivalent (Egland and Sroufe, 1981) but, more typically, avoidant behavior (Lamb, Gaensbauer, Malkin, and Schultz, 1985). Children who victimize and exploit others are in the latter attachment category (Sroufe, 1988), as are those demonstrating depressive symptoms (Sroufe, 1988). Ambivalently attached children are thought to be preoccupied with their attachment figures. They tend to be the criers—crying a lot when separated from mother and crying for a long time upon reunion (Bell and Ainsworth, 1972).

There is variety and subtlety in attachment patterns. They seem to be culture specific (Lewis, 1987). Observations in other countries suggest different attachment configurations may be dominant. For example, a larger percentage of North German children were classified

---

[8]There are subtle divisions within the three categories: A (avoidant), B (secure), and C (ambivalent-resistant) as well as indications that a new category "D" (unstable-avoidance) may be necessary as a way of further refining classifications (Main, Kaplan, and Cassidy, 1985; Spieker and Booth, 1988).

as avoidant (A group) (Parke, Grossmann and Tinsley, 1981; Grossmann et al. 1985). Researchers implicate cultural differences. The avoidant classification reflects to some degree the German mother's emphasis on the child's early, independent, nonclinging, undemanding behavior. In Japan (Takahashi, 1986) more infants were classified as resistant (C group) than were their American counterparts. Different cultural and temperamental patterns were cited. Separations from mother are rare in Japan, and the novelty of separation in the Strange Situation heightens stress and irritability in Japanese infants.

INTERNALIZATION OF ATTACHMENT MODELS

These findings from attachment research have not yet been integrated within the traditional Freudian or relational paradigms of psychoanalytic theory (but see Aber and Slade, 1987, for a beginning effort in this direction). In order to enhance a developmental perspective for psychoanalysis, one needs to demonstrate that patterns of behavior become interiorized, automatic (i.e., relatively unconscious), and exert a motivational effect in mental life. In this section I will discuss the internalization of a working model of attachment from three points of view. The first draws upon recent research offering general information about the nature of perception, its transition to cognition, and the rudimentary existence of memory storage in infants. I describe how it is feasible to begin thinking about internalizations of attachment models during the course of the first year. The second line of inquiry addresses a generational pattern of attachment, that is, the relationship between mothers' attachment to their own mothers and the kinds of attachments infants demonstrate in the strange situation in their first year of life. Third, I will offer data demonstrating the predictive power of these attachment patterns. These converging themes, along with the data I have offered, demonstrate the adaptation-enhancing aspects of early social relatedness for infants and provide a picture of increasing internalizations and their structuring effects.

Infants have the capacities for representing their world at an earlier time in their development than was once considered (Mandler, 1990). By the second half of the first year, images and rudimentary conceptual thinking is established. This does not occur, as Piaget has suggested, through the long slow accumulation of sensorimotor schemas that eventuate in images and concepts. A primitive conceptual system probably exists at birth (Izard and Malatesta, 1987; Brunner, 1990; Mandler, 1990). In addition, infants rapidly learn to convert perceptual information into images and retain them briefly. Researchers have determined the existence of conceptual development by demonstrating infants' ability to find hidden objects after delays, or imitating a previously observed event, or more dramatically engaging in a novel action of an event they saw demonstrated. Thus, after a delay of 24 hours, infants could initiate an action of pressing a button that produced a buzzing sound after they had witnessed the experimenter manipulate the button. Two important points need to be noted here. One, infants can remember what they have seen earlier and reproduce it. Second and more important, the reproduction of a sensorimotor schema does not seem to be involved. The infant was not reperforming an earlier action schema. Rather the infant was engaging in an action he had seen before and understood conceptually in order to produce the sound. (This conceptual learning, of course, puts into question Piaget's ideas of how schemas develop into concepts).

Information garnered by infants from a variety of sensory sources is rapidly integrated and used to understand and remember their perceptual world. Thus, infants quite rapidly distinguish mothers from fathers and these people from others in their environment. As I have mentioned earlier, discrimination of gender and face differences occur in the first six months of life. Once again I am emphasizing the importance of personal, social stimuli for infants. We appear programmed and/or learn very rapidly to assimilate interpersonal events. This fosters an awareness of caregivers as vital sources of security and safety.

Early schemas of infants' perceptual world, alongside primitive conceptual schemas (the symbolic use of signs by infants whose parents use sign language, evidence of memory, Mandler, 1990), as well as the rapid transformation of perceptual schemas into conceptual ones (contemplation of objects, rapid comparison of objects with each other, contemplation and comparison of human faces), suggest the early and more rapid development of cognition in infants and therefore the capacity to internalize interactional experiences during the course of the first year of life.

Consistent with this early pattern of internalization are the precursors to later attachment—early interaction patterns between infants and mothers that predict subsequent attachment behavior at one year in the strange situation—face-to-face interactions (Blehar, Lieberman, and Ainsworth, 1977), feeding (Ainsworth and Bell, 1969), close bodily contact (Main and Weston, 1982), and crying (Bell and Ainsworth, 1979).

The second important source of data about internalized attachments are reflected in the work on mothers' working models of their relationship with their mothers (Main and Goldwyn, 1984, unpublished; Main, Kaplan, and Cassidy, 1985). Parents were assessed via a structured interview that can be reliably rated to evaluate attachment history. This history was based on the parents' current views of their attachment relationships. These ratings were compared to infants' Strange Situation behavior that had occurred five years previously. Parents demonstrated similar patterns of attachment to their infants; that is, most parents classified as secure had infants who had earlier tested as secure. Those parents who were dismissive of attachments had avoidant infants, and those preoccupied by past attachments had ambivalent infants. What is important about these data is that they reflect different patterns of attachment, and that these derive from different attachment histories, and that underlying these different patterns are internal representations of the relationship. Researchers, not wishing to impart more to the attachment data than is warranted, might agree with Main and Goldwyn (unpublished) that what is being described is both the internal state of mind of the infant in the Strange Situation and the current state of mind of the adults in the interview setting. This suggests that the infant has a primitive internal model of an attachment relationship; parents consistently and to a significant degree maintain a similar model and express it via their interactions with their infants.

It is reasonable to assume that adult behavior toward infants strongly affects the working models of infants' attachments (although I believe that certain characterological, temperamental, and/or inborn proclivities of the child can override attachment patterns). This effect appears to be lifelong. Attachment patterns affect the next generation. For example, parents who had reported experiencing rejecting parents also showed aversion to physical contact with their infants (Main and Goldwyn, 1990).

Attachment patterns, while stable, are also malleable. Secure relationships can become insecure as a result of parents' separations, divorce, or death. A stable marital relationship can enhance an attachment pattern (Sroufe, 1988). Main and Goldwyn (unpublished) offer these comments:

> It was the view of several of the parents of secure infants in our study that they had been (in essence) insecure as young children. Some indeed attributed change to a spouse. For others, changes in feeling and in understanding of the potentials of family relationships were attributed to the kindness of relatives whom they saw only occasionally, the parents of friends who provided alternative models of parenting

when they were very young, or teachers who took a personal interest. One father cited a cold night in early childhood when his visiting grandfather had gotten up to bring him an extra blanket: "Nobody had ever done anything like that for me before, and at that moment, I realized that not everybody was alike."

Some parents of secure children felt that they had changed in response to therapy. One attributed change to religious conversion, another to a moment of insight when a friend's child fell and broke an expensive vase and was not spanked. Upon recognizing that he was puzzled by the concerned reaction of the parents, and that he had expected the child to be punished, he realized that he had "several years of thinking to do" before he became a parent.

The third line of evidence contributing to the idea that attachment relationships are represented comes from predictive studies. These show differences for securely attached versus nonsecurely attached children through beginning latency. This is important because there is little from the first year of life that has predictive validity. Typical indices of functioning such as mental development, motor behavior, maturational achievements, and social responsiveness are not predictive for the first or even the first two years of life (see Silverman, 1981).

Attachment patterns demonstrate beginning coherence by the third month of life and can be demonstrated in "feeding, face-to-face interaction, responsiveness to infant crying, and close bodily contact" (Bretherton, 1987, p. 1080). Those infants judged secure during the Strange Situation can utilize their mothers as a comfortable base for exploration. Securely attached toddlers demonstrate more positive affect, enthusiasm, and persistence in problem-solving situations (Matas, Arend, and Sroufe, 1978). During nursery school and early childhood years they explore their environment more and score more competently on preschool tasks. They tend to be cooperative children and positively involved with their mothers and other adults (Ainsworth, 1979). These children also show greater flexibility in their thinking, engage in longer periods of planned symbolic play, and demonstrate greater differentiation of aspects of their environment (Aber and Slade, 1987). Sroufe (1979) described securely attached three-and-a-half-year-olds as "peer leaders, socially involved, attracting the attention of others, curious and actively engaged in their surroundings" (p. 839). By four to five years of age this group of children is described as demonstrating greater response flexibility (ego resiliency) and is resourceful and persistent in a preschool setting (Arend, Grove, and Sroufe, 1979). By six years of age emotional expressiveness and affect modulation exist (Bretherton, 1987). There is some beginning exploration of temperamental factors (Belsky and Isabella, 1988). However, these findings are inconclusive and on the whole neither temperament nor IQ predicts these differences.

Affect regulation among non-secure children is less optimal than in securely attached children. Avoidant children do not demonstrate affective distress when it is appropriate and are likely to express inappropriate hostile feelings in social relationships (Kobak and Sceery, 1988). The ambivalently attached child often vents heightened expressions of distress along with fear and anger (Kobak and Sceery, 1988).

In summary, I have presented what I hope can be thought of as intersecting data from a number of sources demonstrating the establishment and internalization of attachment patterns. Thus, the pre-wired perceptual and primitive conceptual system allows for the relatively rapid integration of repetitively experienced interactions. In this context, Stern's (1985) RIGs (Representations of Interactions that have been Generalized) is a useful conceptualization for understanding the establishment of mental representations during the first year of life (Bretherton, 1987). The representations I am referring to consist of an interactive pattern of behavior. The latter is demonstrated by consistent generational patterns manifested by parents toward their parents as well as toward their infants. Lastly, patterned attachment responses continue to demonstrate continuity in development as highlighted by research predicting increasingly longer effects—currently through early latency.

In addition to attachment behaviors and their development into working models, some theoreticians (e.g., Bowlby, 1988; Bretherton, 1987; Kobak and Shaver, 1987) have considered that once language and representational capacity exist, the beginnings of self- and object representations can be indirectly inferred from attachment behavior. Like representations of attachment relationships, this is an important theoretical construct for a developmental psychoanalytic perspective because it demonstrates the building of a model of personality organization. Kobak and Shaver (1987), for example, in stressing the importance of "felt security needs," offer a model based not only on the activation of attachment behavior but also on the initiation and development of self- and object representations. A child in a fearful or stressful situation, where activation of the attachment situation is likely, can be thwarted by an attachment figure who is ambivalent or rejecting of such needy behavior. This creates disjunctive emotional experiences within the child and leads to strategies of inconsistent or avoidant interpersonal relationships. In addition the child construes a negatively toned self-experience of a needy child. Interpretations of parental responses are subsequently internalized as well.

Whereas these are important concepts about how self- and object representations are initiated, there are some limitations that should be acknowledged. These ideas are more inferential than hypotheses concerned with patterns of attachment. Self- and object representations may be organized around the experience of responsive interactions to security needs. However, why should one assume that these interactions represent the *only* contribution to development and establishment of representations? In addition, this line of thinking presupposes a direct psychic representation of actual interactions without permitting the inclusion of the child's unique way of understanding parent-child interactions. The role of imagery, fantasy, defense, primitive guilt, and reparation are not considered. The establishment of representation, the development of language, experiences of play and fantasy development, all contribute to a personal-creative ordering of intrapsychic processes. Consistent with this latter point of view is Sandler and Sandler's (1987) position. They have described the often severe self-critical and self-punitive trends seen in children reared by benign parents. Given such parents, self-initiated aggressive fantasies produce guilty reactions and harsh, negatively toned self-representations. Here the Sandlers are referring to endogenously organized experiences that contribute to shaping self- and object representations and that these representations are not exclusively derived from actual parent child interactions.[9]

CLINICAL ILLUSTRATION

In the following I describe a maladaptive attachment pattern and its interaction with perverse sexuality. (The material comes from an analytic case I am supervising.) I hope to demonstrate the value of thinking about clinical material from the perspective of attachment motivation as well as from the more traditional vantage points of conflicted sexual and aggressive wishes.

---

[9]Bowlby (1973) assumed complex developmental sequences of a conscious and unconscious nature when he described how attachment relationships determine "what is perceived and what ignored, how a new situation is construed and what plan of action is likely to be constructed to deal with it" (p. 368). He also suggested there are multiple models of inconsistent and/or unconscious attachment relationships. Not only were these not explicated, but they are always derived from child-parent interactions. This is a limitation of attachment research as well.

Dr. A, a successful professional, is a shy, seemingly compliant, somewhat schizoid man who harbors painful memories of occasions of touching women's legs and engaging in voyeuristic activities. He describes experiences of being alone and lonely. He dates the theme of isolation, emptiness, and depression to spending time from infancy onward in child-care settings because his mother worked. He sucked his thumb until severely threatened at age ten and rubbed his ears so vigorously for so long that he eroded cartilage. Depriving mother-child interactive experiences appear to have led to compensatory, repetitive self-stimulation and care; in other terms, self-soothing and pleasure needs were often managed without the benefit of a caregiver and, at times, through distorted painful skin eroticism.

His description of his mother's inability to hold, cuddle, and be physically close with him suggests an initial maladaptive attachment relationship. His mother's incapacities were repeated in a similar manner with her grandchildren. This same pattern characterized his wife's relationship with their children. She held her babies at a physical distance, breast-fed them until they were six, and had them sleep between the parents. She was physically remote and non-sexual with the patient and was overly involved with the children.

His conflicted sensual-sexual and aggressive strivings have important roots in the lush soil of his maternal relationship. His mother was intrusive and seductive while simultaneously harshly condemning his sexual interests, setting the stage for his conflicted eroticism and aggression. He has memories from his later childhood of viewing her in her undergarments, her inappropriately showing him her surgical scars, making him her confidant in her sexual experiences, and uncovering and then inhibiting his masturbation in a traumatic fashion. His erotic wishes toward his mother were intensified by both her seductive enticements and her punitive responses to his sexual interests. It apparently produced experiences of sexual overstimulation for which he sought compulsive relief via his voyeuristic activities. Heightened sexual excitement and release were obtained through peeking at women through windows while they were disrobing.

One can speculate that the patient was an anxiously attached infant. His relationship with an intrusive, seductive mother produced an ambivalent, rather than avoidant, interactive pattern. His need for comfort-contact and his mother's inability to provide it led to the patient's conflicted struggles around touching, occasioning uncontrollable, impulsive touching. His wishes to be handled and touched as well as to touch others on parts of their bodies not only expressed proximity longings and needs for repetitive interactive care, but also served self-soothing functions, produced conflictual emotions around boundary differentiation (associated with intrusive, seductive parenting), and stirred sexual feelings regressively expressed in sadomasochistic merger fantasies.

He was occupied with fantasies of submission and dominance, weakness and power, femaleness and maleness, with a feared focus on each of the former in relation to women. His inhibited sexuality in intimate relationships developed as an accompaniment to his mother's coercive intimacy, her seductiveness, and her threats. His wife reinforced a similar pattern.

In addition, his father was viewed as a primitive, uncontrolled, philanderer—"He chased whores" and "couldn't keep his dick in his pants." His parents came from different religious backgrounds; the patient, looking more like his mother, represented the proper WASP. Both mother and son viewed the father as coarse, vulgar, loud, emotion-filled, sexually self-indulgent, and uncontrolled. The father at times acknowledged his guilty excesses and weaknesses, leading the son to feel contempt and intensify his unconscious conflictual identification with him as well as stir his oedipal guilt as the potential victor. To be a phallic, sexual male took on gross, repellent, crass coloration as well as threatened his attachment and conflicted sexual intimacy with his mother. To be his mother's obedient, clean, neat, well-behaved boy led him to feel castrated as well as merged with her—a "she-man," or, more accurately, a "she-boy."

The patient verbalized that his voyeuristic impulses also represented his wish to have his mother look at his buttocks and penis, examinations she performed into his adolescence around his various bodily "infirmities." His wish to unzip his fly and experience his mother's admiring glances were dealt with through displacement and reversal. Masturbating and peeking, he felt ashamed, dirty, and sick. His mother's admiration and appreciation of his phallic power could only be achieved through his weakened "she-boy" state. Voyeuristic distance from women also insured their safety against his violent aggressive, intrusive, insistent sexuality. During masturbation he was aware of his ownership of a penis, in contrast to the woman. He reexperienced his mother's seduction, but with the reduced threat of a merger: first with a displaced female, and second, one at some physical distance from him. His mother's inability to hold and cuddle him and satisfy sensual, erotic pleasures undoubtedly contributed to his negative fantasies about intimate sexuality. His conflicted sexuality was apparent in his voyeuristic needs and his wishes to touch; his wishes to receive the pleasures of sensual caregiving—the stroking, touching, holding, carassing, and fondling—are grounded in

conflict and can be gratified in the active, physically distant masturbatory experience of peeking at "maternal" figures.

He anxiously experiences repetitive transference configurations—
asking provocative questions, teasing and taunting his analyst to stir
her sexual responsiveness. At the same time, he is fearful of any
demonstration of her caring or sexual interest because it stimulates
oedipal guilt, castration anxiety, feared merger experiences, and
challenges to an old, familiar pathological attachment relationship.

A dual focus is useful in the treatment of this case. Each reflects
object relational configurations that the patient has internalized, but
each has different motivational considerations. The first addresses a
painful, compelling, need-seeking internalized object relation based
on a maladaptive attachment. The second recognizes repetitive
preoedipal and oedipal configurations. These two foci are interre-
lated. The patient's early minimal contact with his mother disturbed
his attachment relationships and distorted the manner in which he
pursued gratifying sensual-sexual experiences (not through intimacy
but through masturbatory gratification in which he satisfied his
insistent wishes to touch and peek at women). This activity diminished direct sexual engagements, thereby reducing possibilities for
contact-comfort, security and safety, and thus reinforcing his ambivalent attachments. I am suggesting that it is less beneficial clinically to
reduce one motive to the other. Clinical evidence is rarely compelling,
but this case material suggests that the patient's sexual difficulties
would not have been eliminated had the treatment focused exclusively on attachment issues; nor would an exclusive focus on sexual
problems have been sufficient. These are equally relevant and related
considerations and clinical exploration of both is essential.

SUMMARY

This chapter describes the social nature of infant experience, especially infant attachments. A study of prenatal, newborns', and
infants' responses during their first year suggest the various ways
they are adapted toward socialization and attachments. Whereas the
contribution of sensual-sexual and aggressive strivings are recognized
as important, I emphasize and focus on attachment research and
describe how such relationships are represented in the infant's
psychic life. Demonstrations of attachment relationships that are
internalized (represented) are essential to the building of a developmental model for psychoanalytic theory. The importance of immediate interactional experience between infant and caregiver, the

nature of their evolution—their stability, or change—as well as the eventual structuralization of these interactional patterns is relevant for a relational model.

A clinical example is offered demonstrating the importance of sensual-sexual and aggressive strivings and thwarted early attachment relationships. The interdependency of these two themes are considered.

REFERENCES

Aber, J. L. & Slade, A. (1987), Attachment theory and research: A framework for clinical interventions. Paper presented at a regional scientific meeting of the Childhood and Adolescence Division for Psychoanalysis of the American Psychological Association, New York, January.

Ainsworth, M. D. S. (1979), Attachment as related to mother–infant interaction. In: *Advances in the Study of Behavior*, eds. J. B. Rosenblatt, R. H. Hinde, C. Beer & M. Bush. New York: Academic Press, pp. 1–51.

_____ & Bell, S. M. (1969), Some contemporary patterns of mother–infant interaction in the feeding situation. In *Stimulation in Early Infancy*, ed. A. Ambrose. London: Academic Press, pp. 133–170.

_____ & Blehar, M., Waters, E. & Wall, S. (1978), *Patterns of Attachment*. Hillsdale, NJ: Lawrence Erlbaum Associates.

Arend, R., Gove, F. L. & Sroufe, L. A. (1979), Continuity of individual adaptation from infancy to kindergarten: A predictive study of ego resiliency and curiosity in preschoolers. *Child Development*, 50:950–959.

Aslin, R. N. (1987), Visual and Auditory Development in Infancy. In *Handbook of Infant Development*, 2nd ed. J. D. Osofsky. New York: Wiley, pp. 5–79.

Balint, M. (1979), *The Basic Fault*. New York: Brunner/Mazel.

Barnes, D. (1988), Meeting on the mind. *Science*, 239:142–144.

Beebe, B. & Lachmann, F. (1988), Mother–infant mutual influence and precursors of psychic structure. In: *Frontiers in Self Psychology: Progress in Self Psychology, Vol. 3*, ed. A. Goldberg. Hillsdale, NJ: The Analytic Press, pp. 3–26.

Bell, R. Q. & Harper, L. V. (1977), *Child Effects on Adults*. Hillsdale, NJ: Lawrence Erlbaum Associates.

Bell, S. M. & Ainsworth, M. D. S. (1972), Infant crying and maternal responsiveness. *Child Development*, 43:1171–1190.

Belsky, J. & Isabella, R. (1988), Maternal, infant, and social-contextual determinants of attachment security. In *Clinical Implications of Attachment*, ed. J. Belsky & T. Nezworski. Hillsdale, NJ: Lawrence Erlbaum Associates.

Blatt, S. J. & Blass, R. B. (in press), Relatedness and self-definition: Two primary dimensions in personality development, psychopathology and psychotherapy. In: *Psychoanalysis and Psychology*, ed. J. Barron, M. Eagle, & D. Wolitsky. Washington, DC: American Psychological Association.

Blehar, M., Lieberman, A. F. & Ainsworth, M. D. (1977), Early face-to-face interaction and its relation to later infant-mother attachment. *Child Devel.*, 48:182–194.

Bowlby, J. (1958), The nature of the child's tie to his parents. *Internat. J. Psycho-Anal.*, 39:350–373.

_____ (1969), *Attachment and Loss, Vol. 1*. New York: Basic Books.

_____ (1973), *Attachment and Loss, Vol. 2*. New York: Basic Books.

_____ (1980), *Attachment and Loss, Vol. 3*. New York: Basic Books.

_____ (1988), *A secure base*. New York: Basic Books.

Brazelton, T. B., Koslowski, B. & Main, M. (1974), The origins of reciprocity: The early mother–infant interaction. In: *The Effect of the Infant on its Caregiver*, ed. M. Lewis & L. Bosenblum. New York: Wiley, pp. 49–76.

Bretherton, I. (1987), New perspectives on attachment relations: Security, communication, and internal working models. In: *Handbook of Infant Development 2nd Ed.*, ed. J. D. Osofsky. New York: Wiley, pp. 1061–1100.

Brunner, J. (1990), *Acts of Meaning*. Cambridge, MA: Harvard University Press.

Burns, P., Sander, L. W., Stechler, G. & Julia, H. (1972), Distress in feeding: Short term effects of caretaker environment of the first ten days, *J. Amer. Acad. Child Psychiat.*, 11:427–439.

Bushnell, I. W. R. (1982), Discrimination of faces by young infants. *J. Exper. Child Psychol.*, 33:298–308.

Cushman, P. (1991), Ideology obscured: Political use of the self in Daniel Stern's infant. *Amer. Psycholog.*, 46:206–219.

DeCasper, A. J. & Fifer, W. (1980), Of human bonding: Newborns prefer their mother's voices. *Science*, 208:1174–1176.

DeCasper, A. J. & Spence, M. J. (1986), Prenatal maternal speech influences newborns perception of speech sounds. *Infant Behav. Devel.*, 9:133–150.

de Chateau, P. (1983), Left-side preference in holding and carrying newborn infants. IV. Parent holding and carrying during the first week of life. *J. Nerv. & Mental Dis.*, 171:241–245.

_____ (1987), Parent–infant socialization in several Western European countries. In: *Handbook of Infant Development*, ed. J. D. Osofsky. New York: Wiley, pp. 642–668.

Dowling, S. (1990), Fantasy formation: A child analyst's perspective. *J. Amer. Psychoanal. Assn.*, 38:93–112.

Egland, B. & Sroufe, L. A. (1981), Attachment and early maltreatment. *Child Devel.*, 52:44–52.

Freud, S. (1905), Three essays on the theory of sexuality. *Standard Edition*, 7:125–248. London: Hogarth Press, 1953.

_____ (1916-1917), Introductory lectures on Psycho-Analysis. *Standard Edition*, 16:243–463. London: Hogarth Press, 1963.

Gedo, J. E. & Goldberg, A. (1973), *Models of the Mind*. Chicago: Univ. of Chicago Press.

Ghent, E. (1989), Credo: The dialectics of one-person and two-person psychologies. *Contemp. Psychoanal.*, 25:200–237.

Grossmann, K., Grossmann, K. E., Spangler, G., Suess, G. & Unzner, L. (1985), Maternal sensitivity and newborns' orientation response as related to quality of attachment in northern Germany. *Monograph of the Society for Research in Child Development*, 50 (1–2, Serial No. 209):233–256.

Guntrip, H. (1971), *Psychoanalytic Theory, Therapy and the Self*. New York: Basic Books.

Hofer, M. A. (1977), *The Roots of Human Behavior*. San Francisco: Freeman.

_____ (1987), Early social relationships: A psychobiologist's view. *Child Devel.*, 58:633–647.

Izard, C. E. & Malatesta, C. Z. (1987), Perspectives on emotional development I: Differential emotions theory of early emotional development. In: *Handbook of Infant Development*, 2nd ed., ed. J. D. Osofsky. New York: Wiley, pp. 494–554.

Kennell, J. H., Voos, D. K. & Klaus, M. H. (1979), Parent-infant bonding. In: *Handbook of Infant Development*, ed. J. Osofsky. New York: Wiley, pp. 786–798.

Kobak, R. & Sceery, A. (1988), Attachment in late adolescence: Working models, affect regulation, and perception of self and others. *Child Devel.*, 59:135–146.

———— & Shaver, P. (1987), Strategies for maintaining felt security: A theoretical analysis of continuity and change in styles of social adaptation. Conference in Honor of John Bowlby's 80th Birthday. Bayswater, London, England, June.

Lamb, M. E., Gaensbauer, T. J., Malkin, C. M. & Schultz, L. A. (1985), The effects of child maltreatment on security of infant-adult attachment. *Infant Behav. Devel.*, 8:35–45.

Lewis, M. (1987), Social Development in Infancy and Early Childhood. In: *Handbook of Infant Development, Vol. 2.* ed. J. D. Osofsky. New York: Wiley, pp. 419–443.

Lichtenberg, J. D. (1983), *Psychoanalysis and Infant Research.* Hillsdale, NJ: The Analytic Press.

———— (1989), *Psychoanalysis and Motivation.* Hillsdale, NJ: The Analytic Press.

Loewald, H. W. (1980), *Papers on Psychoanalysis.* New Haven, CT: Yale University Press.

MacFarlane, A. (1975), Olfaction in the development of social preferences in the human neonate. *Parent-Infant Interaction* (Ciba Foundation Symposium), 33:103–117.

Main, M. & Goldwyn, R. (1984), Predicting rejection of her infant from mother's representation of her own experiences: A preliminary report. *Internat. J. Child Abuse & Neglect,* 8:203–217.

———— & ———— (unpublished), Interview-based adult attachment classifications: Related to infant-mother and infant-father attachment.

———— Kaplan, N. & Cassidy, J. (1985), Security in infancy, childhood and adulthood: A move to the level of representation. *Monograph of the Society for Research in Child Development.* 50 (1–2, Serial No. 209), pp. 66–104.

———— & Weston, D. (1982), Avoidance of the attachment figure in infancy: Descriptions and interpretations. In: *The Place of Attachment in Human Behavior,* ed. C. M. Parkes & J. Stevenson-Hinde. New York: Basic Books, pp. 31–59.

Mandler, J. M. (1990), A new perspective on cognitive development in infancy. *Amer. Scientist,* 78:236–244.

Matas, L., Arend, R. & Sroufe, L. (1978), Continuity in adaptation in the second year: The relationship between quality of attachment and later competence. *Child Devel.,* 49:547–556.

Mitchell, S. A. (1988), *Relational Concepts in Psychoanalysis.* Cambridge, MA: Harvard University Press.

Modell, A. H. (1985), The two contexts of the self. *Contemp. Psychoanal.,* 21:70–91.

Osofsky, J. & Connors, K. (1979), Mother–infant interaction: An interpretative view of a complex system. In: *Handbook of Infant Development,* ed. J. Osofsky. New York: Wiley, pp. 519–549.

Parke, R. D., Grossmann, K. & Tinsley, B. R. (1981), Father-mother-infant interaction in the newborn period: A German-American comparison. In: *Culture and Early Interactions,* ed. T. Field. Hillsdale, NJ: Lawrence Erlbaum Associates, pp. 95–113.

Pine, F. (1990), *Drive, Ego. Object, and Self.* New York: Basic Books.

Provence, S. & Lipton, R. C. (1962), *Infants in Institutions.* New York: International Universities Press.

Rovee-Collier, C. (1987), Learning and memory in infants. In: *Handbook of Infant Development, Vol. 2.* ed. V. D. Osofsky. New York: Wiley, pp. 98–148.

Salk, L. (1970), The critical nature of the post partum period in the human for the establishment of the mother–infant bond: A controlled study. *Dis. Nerv. System,* 1(suppl.):110–116.

Sandler, J. (1987), *From Safety to Superego.* New York: Guilford Press.

———— (1990), On internal object relations. *J. Amer. Psychoanal. Assn.,* 38:859–880.

———— & Sandler, A-M. (1987), The past unconscious, the present unconscious and the vicissitudes of guilt. *Internat. J. Psycho-Anal.,* 68:331–342

Silverman, D. K. (1981), Some proposed modifications of psychoanalytic theories of early childhood development. In: *Empirical Studies of Psychoanalytic Theories, Vol. 2.* ed. J. Masling. Hillsdale, NJ: The Analytic Press, 1986, pp. 49–71.

_____ (1984), New perspectives on development and their implications for psychoanalytic treatment. *Psychoanal. Psychol.*, 1:257–266.

_____ (1986), A multi-model approach: Looking at clinical data from three theoretical perspectives. *Psychoanal. Psychol.*, 3:121–132.

_____ (1987), What are little girls made of? *Psychoanal. Psychol.*, 4:315–334.

_____ (1991), Attachment patterns and Freudian theory: An integrative proposal. *Psychoanal. Psychol.*, 8:169–193.

_____ & Gruenthal, R. (in press), Fantasy: A consolidation. *Psychoanal. Psychol.*

Small, M. F. (1990), Political animal, social intelligence and the growth of the primate brain. *The Sciences*, 30:36–42.

Spieker, S. J. & Booth, C. L. (1988), Maternal antecedents of attachment quality. In: *Clinical Implications of Attachment*, ed. J. Belsky & T. Nezworski. Hillsdale, NJ: Lawrence Erlbaum Associates, pp. 95–135.

Spitz, R. & Wolf, K. (1946), The smiling response: A contribution to the ontogenesis of social relations. *Genetic Psychol. Monographs*, 34:57–125.

Sroufe, L. A. (1979), The coherence of individual development: Early care, attachment and subsequent developmental issues. *Amer. Psycholog.*, 34:834–842.

_____ (1988), The role of infant-caregiver attachment in development. In: *Clinical Implications of Attachment*, ed. J. Belsky & T. Nezworski. Hillsdale, NJ: Lawrence Erlbaum Associates, pp. 18–38.

Stern, D. (1974), Mother and infant at play: The dyadic interaction involving facial, vocal and gaze behaviors. In: *The Effect of the Infant on Its Caregiver*, ed. M. Lewis & L. Rosenblum. New York: Wiley, pp. 187–213.

_____ (1977), *The First Relationship.* Cambridge, MA: Harvard University Press.

_____ (1985), *The Interpersonal World of the Infant.* New York: Basic Books.

Takahashi, K. (1986), Examining the strange-situation procedure with Japanese mothers and 12-month-old infants. *Devel. Psychol.*, 22:265–270.

Wolff, P. H. (1966), The causes, controls, and organization of behavior in the neonate. *Psychological Issues*, Mongr. 5. New York: International Universities Press.

10

Secrets in Clinical Work
A Relational Point of View

NEIL J. SKOLNICK
JODY MESSLER DAVIES

Psychoanalysis has always been concerned with secrets. Indeed, by their very nature, secrets implore psychoanalytic speculation. They are an infinitely rich, complexly textured, and inherently intriguing phenomenon. They involve the seen and the unseen, the verbalized and the unspoken, the involvement of others as well as their exclusion. It is surprising, given the nature of psychoanalytic investigation, with its emphasis on uncovering and revelation, that more has not been said about secrets. Yet from the inception of psychoanalysis as a theory and a practice, secrets have been a tacit concern of psychoanalysis, whether or not they have been addressed directly.

Implicit in Freud's earliest attempts at a "cathartic" cure was the premise that the extraction of an unconscious and noxious secret wish, idea, or experience could be mutative, if not curative. Subsequent speculation about secrets has by and large paralleled the evolution of and divergences within psychoanalytic theory. The proposed meanings and functions accorded secrets have been considered from a purely drive perspective (Gross, 1951), an ego-psychological approach (Margolis, 1966, 1974), and an object-relations point of view (Khan, 1978; Winnicott, 1971; Meares, 1976). Each respective theoretical treatment has tended to draw new bottom lines, placing the psychic meaning of secrets into a paradigm that gives special weight to a limited focus, be it the drives, ego functions, or object-relational concerns. In this paper, we first present a brief historical overview. We then argue for an updated consideration of secrets that includes a description of different types of secrets and, more importantly, an attempt to understand secrets from a primarily relational perspective. To accomplish this, we rely on clinical material to illustrate our points.

Gross (1951), a drive theorist, places the motivation underlying secrets squarely in the realm of an unfolding sequence of psychosexual concerns. Impressed by the temptation of the owner of a secret both to surrender its content and to retain it, he suggests that there might be in our unconscious a complete identity between the secret, on one hand, and bodily excretions on the other. He finds partial support for his hypothesis in the etymology of the Romance languages; the literal meaning of the Latin word *secretum* is "that which has been secreted, or secretion" (p. 38). He then makes an important distinction between the content of a secret and its function. The importance of this distinction is underlined by his contention that the secret undergoes certain changes over the course of development. At certain points in time, its content holds its meaning; at other times, its function. It is at the anal stage, Gross claims, that the content of the secret, its quality as a possession, holds most explanatory sway, whereas at later psychosexual stages it is the quality of its function that is more important. Specifically, as the genital stage approaches, with its increase in a tendency toward external effectiveness, the secret is placed in the service of exhibition (e.g., making oneself seem important by hints about a secret), and later it can be employed as a potential gift to initiate friendships, and ultimately as an aid to wooing a love object.

As psychoanalysis shifted its focus from the contents of the repressed psyche to the agent of repression, the ego, so too did discussion of secrets shift from what was kept secret, and why, to the mechanisms of the ego involved. As Sulzberger (1953) put it, "the keeping of a secret is not just simply an easy act of omission, but rather constitutes a task, involving the whole ego" (p. 43). Margolis (1966, 1974) presents the most comprehensive attempt to describe secrets from the perspective of the functioning of the ego. Indeed, he likens the keeping of a secret to the very process of repression itself. Building on what Sulzberger (1933) called the "confession compulsion," he claims that the more important a secret is, the greater the energy charge it acquires and the stronger its push to reemerge. Margolis (1974) concludes:

> [C]onscious secrets thus obey many of the laws of unconscious secrets (secrets which a person keeps from himself). There is continued pressure for them to express themselves just as there is continual pressure from unconscious id impulses and the repressed for expres-

sion (the return of the repressed), requiring in both cases constant counter-pressure to keep them contained [p. 291].

For ego psychology, not only does secret-keeping resemble the process of repression, but it is actually a precursor to repression itself. Ego psychologists hold that all the contents of the repressed unconscious involve issues, events, wishes, etc. of childhood that the child first decides to keep secret from his or her own superego and its predecessor, the child's parents. Furthermore, "the formation of neuroses proceeds from conscious secret-keeping by the child to keeping things secret from his or her own superego and ego" (p. 292). Psychoanalysis is, then, held to be a process by which patients reverse this course of events by revealing conscious secrets to the analyst and no longer having to hide unconscious secrets from their own ego and superego.

Khan (1978) promoted a radically different perspective on secrets in his conception of them as potential space. According to Khan, no longer are secrets considered to be in the province of repressive forces, ego defenses, or similar processes designed to negotiate the balance between expression of the drives with the demands of the external world. Secrets, as potential space, are now accorded a life-affirming role in the development of the self. Borrowing the concept of potential space[1] from Winnicott (1967), Khan spoke of secrets as a place where one could go to absent oneself, both from one's own internal world and from the traumatizing aspects of one's external environment. As opposed to *hiding* oneself in symptoms, a secret provides a potential space where a part of the self is absented, placed in suspended animation. The secret, Khan (1978) maintains, carries a hope that one day the person will be able to emerge from it, "be found and met" (p. 266) and thus become a whole person, sharing life with others. Like others before him, Khan emphasizes that the content of the secret is not what is important, but that the *act* of creating and maintaining a secret is what is meaningful. For him, however, it is meaningful because it tucks part of the self away for safekeeping. Of significance is that this piece of the self is no longer available for elaboration or alteration. It is not that the person has a secret hidden within; on the contrary, the person infuses a secret with

---

[1]In his paper "The Location of Cultural Experience," Winnicott (1967) states: "From the beginning the baby has maximally intense experience in the potential space between the subjective object and the object objectively perceived, between me-extensions and the not-me. This potential space is at the interplay between there being nothing but me and there being objects and phenomena outside omnipotent control" (p. 100).

part of the self, which then becomes frozen in time and exists apart from ongoing development. Khan describes the case of a child who, by hiding a pair of candlesticks, absented herself into a secret when her ongoing life with her mother broke down, when "her growth in mutuality with her mother had been disrupted" (p. 268). He states further that a secret will be shared only when there is an opportunity for mutuality with an object—when one perceives that someone out there is available to respond and adapt to one's needs.

The secret, then, as Khan conceived it, becomes a maneuvering by the self for protection and control when the outer world ceases to be responsive to the needs of the child. This conceptualization places secrets in a relational frame. They are born of failures in the interpersonal matrix, sustained by hope of a more hospitable environment in the future, and relinquished when a person perceives the opportunity for mutuality with an object.

Implicit in the discussion of secrets as potential space is that secrets can be appreciated for their developmental function. They can be created adaptively to protect the developing self from trauma. Perhaps their adaptive function can provide, in a more ongoing fashion and in a less pervasive manner, a means to negotiate the everyday failures of the significant object to rise to and respond to a child's needs. Meares (1976) takes steps in this direction when he proposes that some secrets can be distinguished as being "creative secrets." He suggests that the attainment of the idea of secrecy is an important feature in a child's development, specifically in its contribution to forming personal relationships. His idea is that secrets become the "coins of intimacy," shared with others as a means of establishing a close bond. Furthermore, he claims that they are related to the child's growing ability to distinguish between inner and outer worlds and establish a boundary between them.

To summarize thus far, we have attempted to outline a historical perspective of the treatment of secrecy in psychoanalytic theory. Originally conceptualized as rooted in the conflict between the drives and reality, the secret has been considered from an ego psychological approach and an object relations point of view. We find value in both approaches, particularly as they can be helpful in informing the theoretician as well as the clinician; we do not feel that any one approach has been sufficiently comprehensive to understand the multifaceted concept of a secret, with its many forms and functions, as well as the complexities of its role in the clinical process. To begin to explicate a more comprehensive viewpoint, we have chosen to approach the issue of secrecy from a clinical/developmental point of view.

We approach the secret from a relational perspective, which regards it not as a valuable gem to be excavated and carefully unearthed, but as a developmental/relational phenomenon involved in the growth and maintenance of the self and its inner world and in the relationship of that inner world to external reality. We expect that the secret will emerge clinically as an essential aspect of the characteristic interplay between analyst and patient. The secret is a defining element of the process by which patients induct us into their private world, make us acquainted with the internal cast of characters, and reveal through transference–countertransference paradigms their particular ways of relating to each of these internal figures, as well as to the specific developmental arrests that impinge on all these relationships in characteristic ways.

We suggest a particular typology of secrets based on the different ways in which secrets can emerge in clinical work. Each, we believe, places emphasis on very different yet equally significant developmental issues and on the relational matrices specific to their emergence in the transference–countertransference processes. We include (1) secrets meant to be shared with others; (2) secrets that are announced to the therapist but whose specific content is withheld; (3) shameful secrets; and (4) secrecy as a pervasive character style.

SECRETS MEANT TO BE SHARED WITH OTHERS

We consider this particular use of secrecy to represent the developmentally optimal use of the process in that it represents the most adaptive and successful negotiation of object-relational tasks.

All analysts have found themselves in the situation of being presented with a special parcel of information. This bundle, which we now refer to as a "secret meant to be shared," is typically a highly valued and affectively charged piece of information about the patient or the patient's internal world that not only is shared with the analyst, but is identified as a secret being shared exclusively (or almost exclusively!) with the analyst. "You are the only one I've ever told this to" and "I'm relieved just to tell someone" are phrases commonly heard preceding these types of revelations. The statement is usually made in the spirit of conspiratorial playfulness, with the obvious motive of engaging the analyst.

Our contention is that it is primarily within the relational matrix that evolves from the sharing of the secret that its importance and ultimate meaning is to be found. We consider the offering of the secret to be an invitation to another to share, notice, acknowledge a piece of one's inner subjective world. Furthermore, it is an offer of a potential type of bond, which, if successful, will result in a sought-after intimacy or mutuality. It can be likened in a sense to a scout who is sent into unknown, potentially dangerous waters in advance of an exploratory expedition. Is the expedition safe to proceed? Will the group be welcomed, acknowledged, and appreciated? Or will it meet with hostile forces looking to absorb the group or, worse, destroy it? This type of secret appears to be a way of initiating a bond with someone in the external world, or more precisely, with an external object's internal world (subjectivity), by roping off a piece of one's own internal subjective world and sending it out, not unlike a trial balloon.

We place this type of secret in the realm of transitional phenomena as described by Winnicott (1951). Winnicott referred to transitional phenomena as illusions set up to mediate and negotiate the distinction between internal and external realities. They are used to relinquish gradually the omnipotence a child experiences over his or her external reality and to be able gradually to distinguish between an internal reality and the limits of an external reality that is much less under psychic control. A secret, if negotiated successfully, represents a step in the relinquishing of omnipotence. By revealing an inner subjective reality (a secret) to someone out there, one is clearly making a distinction between separate inner and outer realms. But by labeling it as a secret, the person is still maintaining or attempting to maintain control over the content of the internal package as it ventures outside.

The most successful outcome of such a venture is that the other person will accept the secret and acknowledge both its importance and *its secrecy*. Thus the two people enter into a bond that gains its strength from the mutual recognition of the secret as a transitional phenomena. Both now hold the secret precious in their internal worlds, yet both recognize that some control has been relinquished in the sharing of the secret. This relinquishing of control implies a mutual trust, at least for the moment, that one's internal world is separate and safe from both the external world and the internal world of another. Omnipotent control over the external world has been momentarily suspended and placed into the hands of another.

The two also enter into a shared world of intersubjectivity that can exclude others, thus defining their own safe interpersonal reality separate from the rest of the external world and remaining under their shared control. This process can be observed in pairs of school children of five and six who delight in forming secrets that are kept from others. The content of their secrets, often in fact freely revealed, seems much less important than the experience of having shared a secret with another. Later, these twosomes are expanded into secret groups and clubs that appear to have the same function.

Of course, the best outcome, a mutual bond, is not always the case. The list of potential snags is endless; they range from betrayal, to nonacceptance, to a lack of recognition, to many other pitfalls in the process. Children who have had some relative degree of success relinquishing omnipotence and distinguishing internal and external worlds, will merely pull back their trial balloons, pack up their toys, and go elsewhere, looking for other uncharted territories to explore. Our point is that they *will* go elsewhere and continue to engage others in this process. We wish to stress this point because it implies that these types of secrets, secrets-meant-to-be-shared, are a manifestation of a normal and regular course of events. They can be utilized in the lifelong struggle to negotiate boundaries; and furthermore, given an environment that is reasonably safe, these types of secrets can be imbued with delight and pleasure as they are used repeatedly in establishing intimacy in relationships.

This view of secrecy has implications for the treatment setting as well. It can become all too easy to regard a patient's announcement of a secret as a defensive process, aligned with the forces of repression to maintain information out of conscious awareness. There are many ways in which an analyst might regard the offering of such a secret as a form of resistance or defense. Those more classically inclined might regard it as the acting out of a wish rooted in a libidinal or aggressive drive. Is the patient being seductive? Or overly familiar and possibly demeaning? Others might hear an intent to idealize the analyst. Still others might attend to self-deprecating undertones. While, of course, these inferences might be accurately perceived nuances of the analytic interaction we hold that there is a risk that the analyst may be missing the patient's attempt to establish a bond or mutuality with another, that the offering of a secret represents an initial step in establishing a safe, intersubjective tie.

We offer as a clinical example a character in a recent movie, *Europa Europa*, based on a true story. The movie revolves around a major secret, that of a 16-year-old Jewish boy's attempt to survive the atrocities of World War II Germany by pretending to be non-Jewish. In situation after situation, for example, his being sent to an elite school for Aryan Hitler youth, he lived in perpetual fear that his secret would be unearthed and result in almost certain death. His world revolved around his efforts to keep his true identity a secret. At one point in the story, the boy reveals his secret to a member of the enemy. He exclaims through tears, "I just had to let someone know." The audience's suspense at this moment hinges on the fate of his revelation. Will he immediately be revealed, resulting in almost certain destruction? Or will his secret be safe within the confines of a newly established mutuality? Indeed, not only is his secret accepted, but the sharing of the secret fuels the development of a powerfully intimate bond between the two. This example, while extreme, beautifully illustrates the relational needs embodied in a secret meant to be shared. It is an invitation to share one's subjective world with another, motivated by the hope for a bond with the other in which one's subjective safety and integrity is upheld.

ANNOUNCED SECRETS WHOSE CONTENT IS WITHHELD

In contrast to secrets that are meant to be shared is the type of secret whose existence is announced by the patient, although the content continues to be withheld. Here the patient describes being "not quite ready," "too embarrassed," "not sure what you'll think of me," to reveal the content of the secret, though he or she clearly wants the therapist to know that the issue exists. Although this type of secret emerges periodically in almost every treatment, it can, for some patients, emerge as a predominant transferential paradigm, giving a particular coloration to the therapeutic relationship. In contrast to the mood of paralyzing humiliation evoked by shameful secrets (to be discussed later), the atmosphere here has an almost playful, tantalizing, "catch-me-if-you-can" quality. The therapist, caught up in this play, clearly wants to know, discover, and understand what the patient is so engagingly offering up, for there is little as truly engaging as a secret announced but withheld.

Classical analysis has, traditionally, regarded such an announced but withheld secret as a resistance to the reemergence of forbidden libidinal wishes; a defense against the patient's demand for drive gratification, usually within the transference; essentially, a disruption in the free associative flow of the hour. Emphasis has been on interpreting and working through these transference resistances in order to uncover the true meaning of the secret that lies embedded and encoded within the content of what is withheld. Beginning with Freud's (1913) basic description of the "fundamental rule" of psychoanalysis, the very idea that a patient could consciously withhold information from the analyst has been viewed as antithetical to the entire analytic agenda.

Freud stated:

> [I]t is naturally impossible to carry out our analysis if the patient's relations with other people and his thoughts about them are excluded. . . . It is very remarkable how the whole task (psychoanalysis) becomes impossible if a reservation is allowed at any single place [pp. 135–136].

Greenson (1967) includes a special section on consciously held secrets in his chapter on analyzing resistance. His position, fundamentally consistent with the classical one, stresses the need ultimately to uncover the content of the secret by patiently analyzing why the patient feels the need to withhold it. Greenson says,

> our basic attitude is that there shall be no concession about secrets. They have to be analyzed. . . . The analytic attitude is that we shall attempt to analyze secrets as we would any other form of resistance. We are just as determined and just as patient. We may be aware that a patient has a conscious secret, but we know that it is the unconscious factors that have to be analyzed, before the patient can reveal the secret. The patient knows the content of the secret, but he is unconscious of the important reasons which make it necessary to maintain the secrecy [p. 130].

We propose here that patients who characteristically engage their analysts with a series of withheld secrets are attempting to accomplish a particularly important development shift, one that has either failed to occur or has only partially occurred. We find it most useful to define this shift in the Winnicottian mode of facilitating new capacities. The psychic shift we refer to here is thus indicative of the capacity to regard oneself self-reflectively, that is, to adequately cordon off and respect the existence of a separate, private, and entirely subjective inner reality. Implied here is the capacity to move between this entirely subjective inner reality and a field of intersubjectivity without fearing undue penetration and influence by another or the omnipotent, rageful, potentially destructive impact of oneself.

What, then, of patients who routinely organize their interpersonal relationships around a series of tantalizingly withheld secrets? It is our contention that these patients have arrived at a level of ego organization and object relations that has established the potential for preliminary trials with intersubjective experience, but that certain developmental issues preclude further maturation in this realm. By announcing the existence of encapsulated pieces of inner reality that may or may not be available for sharing, the patient defines the field on which these issues will be played out. On this field, through the transference-countertransference constellations, the specific lacunae in ego development and self/object representations will be highlighted, and the patient's avoidance of open disclosure in an intimate setting will be analyzed.

The following case vignette highlights some of these issues.

Jesse was a 29-year-old, white, southern woman, the youngest of three children. She had two brothers, five and eight years older than she, respectively. Jesse's parents owned and operated the local bar in her hometown, and this fact, coupled with the age difference between the patient and her brothers, meant that much of her early childhood had been spent alone or in the homes of neighbors and friends. In fact, loneliness was far and away the most potent affective residue of this woman's childhood as she began treatment. Also significant in her early memories was the experience of needing to fit into the homes in which she was cared for in as unobtrusive and invisible a way as possible. There were few childhood friends, and the patient reported spending most of her time in a rich, highly developed, and well-articulated internal fantasy world. Though she seemed in most instances to distinguish this world from her actual life and claimed that she never experienced any confusion as a child between what was real and what was "make-believe," it was clear that the patient retreated to this fantasied place as a source of comfort, soothing, and emotional sustenance. No real relationship evoked within her the same experiences of warmth, wholeness, and safety that her imagined world had.

Jesse remembered her parents' relationship as alternately calm, deadening, and passionless, or actively engaged, volatile, and emotionally abusive. She recalled her father as a rather depressed, withdrawn, almost schizoid man, and her mother's way of making contact was to become provocative and inflammatory until both appeared out of control. Jesse recalls that her parents related to her as they did to each other. Father was withdrawn most of the time, although a certain level of coquettish flirtation could be counted on to "elicit a wan smile." Mother was most often not at home, but when she returned Jesse recalled a subtle yet insidious demand for compensatory experiences of intense emotional and physical contact. "She would literally swoop down upon me; wrapping me up in herself; wanting to know about every minute of my day; expecting me to return her need. I felt numbed; I couldn't be with her the way she wanted."

At the time she entered treatment, Jesse was a bright, vivacious, and engaging woman; she was professionally and academically successful. She had a somewhat promiscuous history with men, moving from one relationship to another as soon as the man became serious about her. She was at the time involved in a serious relationship with a young man she described as gentle, passionate, and emotionally available. The patient was eager to preserve this relationship but was only too aware of what she called her "pattern of restless wandering."

Jesse entered treatment in a most striking and dramatic way. She announced at the beginning of her first session that although she felt committed to an analysis, there was one event in her life about which she would never speak and about which the analyst must promise never to ask. She would say nothing other than to reassure the analyst that her "secret" involved no illegalities about which the analyst need feel concerned. It was "simply a private matter." The analyst responded that for such a private matter, the patient certainly felt compelled to announce its existence rather precipitously. The analyst went on to wonder aloud whether the patient had certain concerns about her capacity to keep a secret and might not be setting that as one of the goals of the analysis; after all, being able to "keep someone out" is a prerequisite for the decision to "let them in." Toward the end of this initial consultation, patient and analyst agreed that revealing her secret would never be made a precondition for Jesse's continuing the analysis; however, the analyst insisted on maintaining the right to refer to Jesse's secret and its possible relevance during the course of the work. This condition was acceptable, and the analysis began.

Clearly, this unusual situation raises certain clinical issues relevant to our topic. For although the contents of this secret were sure to be pointedly meaningful on a symbolic level and were, eventually, to assume some importance within the analysis, the specific content of the secret was essentially peripheral to the exploration of its place and function within the analytic relationship. By using the metaphor of "her secret," the patient was able to represent externally and highlight certain areas of intrapsychic vulnerability: the richness of her inner world as compared with the emptiness and isolation of her actual life; her difficulties with a guilty and intrusive mother who was unavailable for extended periods and alternately was invasive, controlling, and disrespectful of her daughter's needs for consistent boundaries and privileges of privacy; a depressed and withdrawn father in relationship to whom the patient's "secrets" represented attempts to actively master his essential indifference to her (she had no secrets from him, for he showed no interest in her inner life). In the analysis, exploration of the patient's efforts to maintain the boundaries around her secret, her ambivalence about doing this, her fantasies about the analyst's curiosity or lack thereof, and her less conscious attempts to engage the analyst in pressing for disclosure of the secret, all emerged in different aspects of transference–countertransference engagements.

This clinical example highlights one of the therapeutic "choice points" that often make interventions based within a relational framework incompatible with those stemming from more traditional, instinctually driven models. To the extent that the analyst focuses on "resistances" to revealing this secret, implying that the patient must comply with the analytic standard of uninhibited free association, exploration of the vital issues surrounding separateness, boundaries, privacy, impingement, autonomy, submission, and the like will be unavoidably discouraged or even foreclosed.

Of particular interest here is that two years into the analytic work, the patient's "secret" emerged in undisguised form in a dream she reported to the analyst. Having told of a dream where she was dancing "topless" in a small disco, Jesse turned to the analyst, shrugged with a smile, and said simply, "I suppose I was ready to have you know." The patient then began her own analysis of the special meaning that this event had played in her life. Placing the secret within a relational frame did not, therefore, prevent analyzing the content of this secret but did attempt to understand its broader meaning as a transitional bridge between Jesse's internal and external object worlds and her complex relationship to both.

SHAMEFUL SECRETS

These are conscious experiences, usually occurring in childhood, that patients have chosen to keep to themselves for many years. Although these may at times overlap in their phenomenology with secrets in other subtypes, they do have enough special features to warrant separate consideration. We are not referring here to those fleeting experiences of shame that often accompany the revelation of new material in psychoanalysis, but more specifically to those secrets which have been kept for so long and with such a commitment of energy that they become core aspects of the identity and self-representation of the patient, although they are known to no one. The secret itself comes to serve a characterological function for the patient, and when its defensive function is challenged by revelation within the treatment setting, varying degrees of regressive disorganization may ensue.

Shameful secrets have to do mostly with childhood experiences of a traumatic nature – incest, child abuse, or illegal, antisocial acts occurring outside of a predominantly psychopathic character structure. In most of these cases, the secret is an attempt to maintain a homeostatic balance in the inner object world, that balance which allowed the child to survive in a world where parents abandoned, betrayed, or failed in other ways to protect from paralyzing overstimulation. Although this type of secret involves behavior that is almost never the young child's fault, the manifest content that emerges during analytic hours involves experiences of intense shame and mortification, as well as the conviction that the analyst will certainly reject that patient if his or her behavior is revealed. Symptomatically, one often sees compulsive self-abusive behavior and intense self-hatred. In following the patient's associations, we are often led to interpret, along more traditional lines, the content of the secret as a manifestation of guilt over unconscious gratification of unacceptable wishes. From a self-psychological point of view, the likelihood is that this gratification has been incorporated by the patient into a system of compensatory grandiose fantasies. For example, it is not uncommon for the adult survivor of child abuse to express, in the analytic context, the belief that as a child he or she revealed some special quality that made him a particular target of abuse, and that, furthermore, by exhibiting this quality, the patient could provoke and control outbursts of parental abuse. The passive experience of parental abuse and betrayal thus comes under active control and is used as a way to refortify the child's sense of omnipotent control of his or her very dangerous world. The secret could, then, be viewed as a defense against both the exhibitionistic urges that might reemerge in the treatment situation and the overwhelming terror and fear of annihilation that would be reexperienced were the true passivity of the original trauma to be recalled by the patient.

It has been our experience, however, that an approach that focuses exclusively on the unconscious guilt of the patient or on the split-off, grandiose fantasy is often insufficient to render the secret open for association and analysis and end the patient's intense self-hatred and abuse. Although a patient may accept these types of interpretations and may begin to deal with the content of the secret during analytic hours, the shame itself remains virtually untouched. The patient's experience is one of being "worn down," and though he or she may come to understand the symbolic meaning of the secret, the shame, fear, and self-hatred continue. The interpretive process, thus conducted, may become a retraumatization itself.

That the shame, humiliation, and self-hatred often prove to be the most immutable aspect of this clinical picture is in itself an interesting paradox. For it is clear that this kind of secret, once revealed, is almost never anything for which the young child was himself responsible. Most often the secret concerns something that was "done to" the child by a person of some significance in his or her life. The importance of keeping the secret, then, stems not only from the guilt and shame processes already described, but, on a fundamental level, from a primitive, primary identification with the painful object in its aggressive or abandoning aspects. It is, in fact, the very blamelessness of the patient in the context of a struggle with powerful ties to bad objects that provides the most powerful motivation for maintaining the secret. It is the child's need to protect himself or herself from the crushing experience of betrayal and aloneness that is operative. The assumption of guilt and shame reflects the idea that it is safer to think oneself a bad person, deserving of punishment, in an otherwise good world, than a blameless victim, abandoned and surrounded by evil (Fairbairn, 1952). One is reminded here of Fairbairn's classic description of a patient whose dream reflected a choice between eating poisoned pudding or dying of starvation. The child, helpless and dependent, cannot choose aloneness; therefore, the tie to the object is established, the evil internalized and converted to shame, and the patient's continued security maintained. As Fairbairn himself put it,

> The essential feature, and indeed the essential aim of this defense is the conversion of an original situation in which the child is surrounded by bad objects into a new situation in which his objects are good and he himself bad . . . [p. 68].

There is, then, a danger in approaching such a patient either from a classical Freudian perspective, which would stress the patient's unconscious guilt over the gratification of unacceptable wishes, or from a self-psychological model, which would emphasize the therapist's empathic bond to the helpless and victimized child. In our opinion, the crucial clinical question asks: which approach to this patient will allow for all the more classical and self-psychological issues to be analyzed, and at the same time set the stage for the emergence onto the clinical scene of the sadistic/abandoning introject? It is only, we believe, when this introject is given full reign to act upon the therapist and to understand through the therapist how he

or she acts upon others in the world that the vicious projective/
introjective cycle of abuse–counterabuse, and self-abuse can be broken.

The secret, ultimately, is a secret co-existing on many levels:
libidinal, narcissistic, and object related. The working-through process is long and complex; it entails gratification of unconscious
wishes, compensatory omnipotent and grandiose fantasies with
external idealizations of sadistic figures, and finally the attempt to
make real and therefore analyzable the early sadistic introject. The
last of these tasks is the most formidable because the process involves
something of a therapeutic paradox. On one level, the patient works
through several different defensive positions: I was abused and am
bad; I was abused, but I am not bad; I was a victim and should not
continue to punish myself. However, a parallel process also begins to
emerge: I am a part of someone who would abuse/abandon a
blameless child, and that someone is a part of me. If I deny that
contact, I am a part of no one, and anyone who is a part of no one
must truly be bad after all.

SECRECY AS A CHARACTER STYLE

We now turn to a discussion of a type of secret we believe accompa-
nies the experience and functioning of a more pathological level of
adjustment. This type of secrecy occurs frequently in those patients
presenting with severe character disorders, whom we refer to today
as borderline or narcissistic and whom the British object relations
theorists commonly referred to as schizoid. Rather than a delineated,
discrete secret, or series of secrets, we are referring to a pervasive *style*
of secrecy that casts its shadow over large areas of a person's
experience, behavior, and functioning. The person acts as though
guided by an imperative to relegate a wide spectrum of his or her
experience, actions, or thoughts to the realm of secrecy. Nothing is
spared. Mundane, routine events can be included, as can symptom-
atic behaviors such as bulimic episodes or compulsive rituals. Even,
and sometimes especially, major triumphs and successes are shielded
by secrecy. Clinically, this type of secrecy can manifest in many ways.
Lengthy, withholding silence can signal such a style, or perhaps
glaring omissions, as when a patient announces some future event
that, the therapist realizes at some later point in time, has never been
mentioned again. At times a belated announcement of a major
incident or event, leaving the therapist wondering, "Why am I just
hearing about this now?" can signal such a process. Sometimes it is

announced directly, as in the case of a severely reclusive and narcissistically impaired man who stated several years into treatment, "I have a fantasy of getting better, living a rich, full life, and keeping it all a secret from you."

This man did, in fact, keep much of his life shrouded in a veil of secrecy. From a very early age, he would keep not only his needs, wants, and actions, but also his successes and failures from his family and others. It became apparent that he relished his world of secrecy. It was not a world to which he retreated, but rather it was a world that contained and protected his self *and* his self in relation to the world of others. It was a world in which he could interact with others safely and not include them at all. Paradoxically, the only available, safe, and acceptable means of interacting with others did not include them. In the continual struggle to define the boundaries between inner and outer realities, objects in the outside world were brought into the inner experience and related to, acted upon or reacted to through the vehicle of secrecy.

The realm of secrecy does not represent a divorce or retreat from reality, but rather a harnessing of what is perceived to be an unbearable and uncontrollable reality. Thus, we are not describing a retreat to a fantasy world. Secrecy, as we understand it, involves real people and actions. Contact with reality is maintained. It is, therefore, unlike the world of psychotic experience, in which reality is generated from and dictated to by an internal fantasy world and its contents. Indeed, the reality that is brought into this secret world probably is composed, to a large extent, of an array of part-object representations, rather than fully integrated wholes, and to that extent reality testing may be somewhat impaired. Furthermore, since much relating to others (these part-object representations) occurs in a safe and secret world, the constraints and limitations of *real* others are rarely confronted, thus perpetuating unrealistic knowledge of others and a further need for secrecy. So a sense of reality is maintained, but reality testing may never be given adequate opportunity.

The motive to hide oneself also does not appear to emanate from shame or embarrassment, nor does it appear to represent a libidinally rooted tendency to withhold. While shame, embarrassment or withholding can be operative, they are not the primary motivating force and are better understood as derivatives of a type of failed object relationship that seems to underlie this tendency toward massive secrecy.

It is our contention that where secrecy becomes a pervasive style, there has been a severe disruption in an early relationship with a primary other. Either severely depressed or markedly focused on their own narcissistic needs (or both), the parents are physically present but severely detached and unavailable. Often, issues of control may dominate. Furthermore, we have noted powerful, usually unconscious, murderous desires occurring in the parents toward the child. The external world provided by such parents is extraordinarily frightening and unsafe. This creates a situation in which the normal use of secrets as transitional phenomena is radically aborted. As noted, we maintain that secrets can be utilized for the developmentally necessary task of relinquishing omnipotent control, initiating intersubjectivity, and gradually achieving a more realistic sense of one's own limitations and the limitations of the external world. In the situation we are describing here, the child experiences his or her world as massively unsafe, and attempts at transitional phenomena are met with either no response or a murderous (disavowing, unconfirming) response. Omnipotence, then, is not gradually relinquished but, rather, tenaciously retained. Illusions of omnipotence, both about one's self and one's objects, are not given the opportunity for disillusionment. One's objects are maintained as dangerous and potentially destructive, to be reckoned with only within the confines of a safe, removed, and secret world where one can omnipotently control all the contingencies.

Crucial to understanding this form of secrecy, and indeed secrecy in general, is that a secret, or secret world, does not exist without an object. A secret is a piece of experience *kept from somebody*, and the object is inherently and inextricably involved in the phenomenology of keeping the secret. For a person who creates a world of secrecy, objects are abundant. Actual interactions with others need no longer occur; the person need no longer be frustrated, or worse, destroyed, by a world of others who are either absent or harbor murderous impulses. These others are brought into the internal subjective world by virtue of their exclusion from it, without an opportunity to act, react, destroy, or control. The resulting pervasive style of secrecy represents a contact with the outside world that, for purposes of safety, control, and even survival, remains tucked inside of an illusion.

Consider the case of a 28-year-old woman who entered treatment (with a supervisee of one of the authors) after having been evicted from a prior therapy. Her previous analyst, reciting a litany of complaints, had become uncontrollably enraged at this patient and found that she could no longer tolerate the patient's antics, particularly her unremitting, relentless efforts to stalk the therapist. The patient, a high-achieving medical resident, would repeatedly walk or drive by her analyst's house and office, calculating when she might catch a glimpse of her, however briefly. She always remained inconspicuous, hiding unobtrusively in the shadows, never allowing her presence to be known. Faithfully, however, at the next session she would reveal, in exquisite detail, the nature of these stalking expeditions. The patient's repertoire of enraging behavior was not limited to her stalking. During most sessions, she was childlike and provocative, taunting her analyst with personal questions and persisting even as limits were set or an analytic frame was reinforced. The analyst became increasingly unable to tolerate what she referred to as the patient's "acting out." She decided her countertransference reaction (primarily rage) precluded the opportunity for further treatment, and she transferred the patient.

Two aspects of this woman's initial presentation were immediately apparent. One was the enormous disparity between her regressive, childlike demeanor in the therapy situation and her high level of functioning elsewhere. She had successfully completed an Ivy League education and medical training; she had friends and was engaged to be married. While it is not uncommon for patients to present with similar inconsistencies (though not always as extreme or immediately apparent), an additional feature was puzzling. There was a playful quality to her antics, an almost tongue-in-cheek shading to her "bad" behaviors. Indeed, her stalking, manipulating, provoking, or generally enraging behavior had a compulsive quality and was distressing to her; but she exercised a noticeable degree of control in that she never got caught, never actually crossed boundaries (i.e., she would call the therapist at home only when fairly certain no one would be there), and she faithfully confessed to all her transgressions. She engaged in many of the same behaviors that characterized her previous therapy.

The analyst's initial stance was to enlist her cooperation in exploring the meaning of what she did and to set limits on what was intolerable (i.e., stalking the analyst's house). The patient proceeded to figure out the analyst's work schedule and purposely lingered at certain places hoping to see the analyst without being seen. This was accomplished at the expense of tremendous time and energy, as when she would traverse town, in the middle of a work day, and circle the office block for up to an hour. She became obsessively ruminative about all aspects and every corner of the analyst's life, attempting to smoke out every activity, every acquaintance. One particular ritual she performed provided valuable insight into the nature of what was going on. After figuring out which car belonged to her analyst, she would routinely pass the car en route to sessions, hoping to catch a glimpse of something, anything, in the car, that might provide a clue about the analyst's life or recent activities. The analyst, in turn, repeatedly found himself surveying the car for artifacts of his recent out-of-office-life (a map, a car seat, a candy wrapper). He was struck by the enormity of the power, the outright omnipotence, she was attempting (at times successfully!) to wield. While typically experiencing anger or rage in response to such a patient's omnipotent machinations, the analyst remained amused, feeling he was being drawn into something that could be stopped at any time, perhaps some form of play.

What did gradually emerge was that this woman had an enormous secret world in which she revelled and from which little in her life was spared. She delighted in erecting and maintaining secrets from the major cast of characters in her life. For example, when she and her husband bought a car, she named the car after her analyst and delighted in this secret name and secret knowledge. Indeed, by far, the most encompassing secret in her life was her therapy. Since adolescence she had been involved in a series of therapies in which she lived an entire existence parallel to, apart from and outside her life. These worlds were her special secret, and she carried them around with her perpetually. She was master of these worlds; she created them, ruled over them, determined their edges, and filled in their substance. They gained much of their significance not just from the power she wielded, but from being kept secret from others. The others—her parents, husband, colleagues—populated her secret world by virtue of her keeping the secrets form them and lording the secrets over them in her thoughts.

Her secretive existence began early in childhood. Her mother was an extremely controlling, narcissistic, and erratic woman, prone to wild, unpredictable, and explosive tantrums. Her younger brother was labeled the "bad" one of the family, and she repeatedly observed her mother physically strike him. She developed a compliant "good" self, which she defensively erected and presented to her mother and the world. Her father appeared to be well meaning but was largely absent and unable to control her explosive mother. Neither parent seemed able to set effective, consistent limits and enable her to feel protected from her own impulses and omnipotent desires. While presenting her "good" self to the world, early on she secretly harbored her "bad" self, a world composed of her own impulses and identifications with her impulsive mother, as well as her more spontaneous wishes and desires, which could not be expressed in her mother's controlling world. This self was cordoned off and expressed increasingly in the safety of her secret world. First it was expressed privately (i.e., secret eating binges), then in her play, and eventually in her therapies. For her, therapy represented an invitation to another to participate in her secret world. She, of course, was the master of ceremonies, and the therapist was to be at the mercy of her omnipotent control. It became clear that whether the analyst allowed her antics (e.g., her stalking) or protested, becoming enraged like her previous therapist, or benignly set limits did not actually matter. In all eventualities, the analyst was responding to her omnipotent demands.

The way out of this morass was for the analyst to respond to her secretiveness as an illusion of control existing in a transitional space. More and more the analyst approached her secret world as a parent might a transitional object. She had set up this world to maintain the omnipotence that had never been disillusioned in either her own internal world or that of her mother. In the therapy her secretive control became more of a transitional game. The analyst could recognize it, even allow it, but also remind her of its limits. Thus therapy became an arena wherein she could use transitional phenomena (her secret world) not just to maintain her omnipotence, but gradually to relinquish it. Therapy provided an opportunity for a safer exploration and discovery of an intersubjective world and allowed for a diminution of a need for a secretive style of existence. She began to chance real encounters with both her analyst and the major people in her life and recognized the limits, boundaries, and subjectivity of each. She could increasingly tolerate the controls on her wishes mandated by the realities of another's internal world. She felt freer to risk revealing her inner world to others without fearing destruction. With an increasing tolerance for the limits of her control, and of others', she could venture out from her secretive world.

We have presented this case in order to illustrate a pervasive style of secrecy, as well as to emphasize the importance of taking a relational perspective to inform the treatment. The patient had been evicted from a previous therapy. Did her enraging stalking behaviors represent an expression of sadistic, destructive impulses? Were they aimed at a therapist who could no longer tolerate her own rage and the threat to her own omnipotence evoked by the seemingly uncontrollable acting out? While we do not discount these formulations, we believe that a relational perspective can expand our understanding. It appears that the patient succeeded in transforming her first therapist into her explosive, murderous mother with the ultimate expression of this transference–countertransference enactment being her eviction from therapy.

It is our contention that the first therapist was unable to recognize and respond to the patient's attempt to negotiate an intolerable situation with her own mother by creating a world of secrecy in which all who entered were held under her omnipotent sway. The patient, by inviting the therapist to participate in this secret realm, was attempting to maintain omnipotent control and at the same time chance relinquishing the same control. Her secret world, then, operated on the level of transitional phenomena (Winnicott, 1951) in which she could maintain illusory control over external others, in this case the analyst, while struggling to acknowledge the limits of that control. Once the second analyst was able to recognize the transitional nature of her secret behavior, he was able to respond to her antics with the tolerant distance of a parent observing and occasionally participating in a child's play enactments. While the *content* of her secret world may indeed have included sadistic, exhibitionistic, and self-destructive wishes, the treatment was endangered as long as the analyst failed to recognize the relational configurations to which those impulses were brought.

CONCLUDING REMARKS

We have argued for a conceptualization of the secret that places relational configurations at the heart of our understanding of this ubiquitous phenomenon. We have described several core relational commonalities of secrecy that, at times, emerge from the background into the foreground of analytic work. So encapsulated, such phenomena can imply the normal unfolding of developmental processes, aberrations of psychopathology, or significant transference–countertransference patterns. We have demonstrated how they can be constructed and maintained as part of a lifelong effort to support the requisites of self-development and continuity. They can be employed as an aid to the discovery and experience of intersubjective bonds, as transitional phenomena providing an opportunity to relinquish primitive omnipotence, and as a vehicle for the establishment of safe, secure boundaries between inner and outer, between self and others. In pathology, they can be adaptively erected to negotiate severe environmental trauma. We do not discount that drive impulses or strictly defensive concerns may be implicated in the complex meanings and textures of a secret.

We do not, however, agree with the heretofore held conceptualization of secrets as serving the sole purpose of keeping forbidden instinctual wishes out of consciousness. Rather, we view impulses embedded in secrecy to be of secondary importance to and a product of the developmental/relational concerns we have attempted to explicate.

REFERENCES

Fairbairn, W. R. D. (1952), *Psychoanalytic Studies of the Personality*. London: Routledge & Kegan Paul.

Freud, S. (1913), On beginning the treatment, *Standard Edition*, 12:121–144. London: Hogarth Press, 1958.

Greenson, R. (1967), *The Techniques and Practice of Psychoanalysis, Vol. 1*. New York: International Universities Press.

Gross, A. (1951), The secret. *Bull. Menn. Clin.*, 15:37–44.

Khan, M. M. R. (1978), Secret as potential space. In: *Between Reality and Fantasy*, ed. S. A. Grolnick, L. Barkin & W. Muensterberger. New York: Aronson.

Margolis, G. J. (1966), Secrecy and identity. *Internat. J. Psycho-Anal.*, 47:517–522.

_____ (1974), The psychology of keeping secrets. *Internat. Rev. Psycho-Anal.*, 1:291–296.

Meares, R. (1976), The secret. *Psychiat.*, 39:258–265.

Sulzberger, C. F. (1953), Why it is hard to keep secrets. *Psychoanal.*, 2:37–43.

Winnicott, D. W. (1951), Transitional objects and transitional phenomena. *Through Paediatrics to Psychoanalysis*. London: Hogarth Press, 1958.

_____ (1967), The location of cultural experience. *Playing and Reality*. New York: Basic Books, 1971.

_____ (1971), *Playing and Reality*. Middlesex, Eng.: Penguin Books.

11

Money Matters in Psychoanalysis

LEWIS ARON
IRWIN HIRSCH

The subject of money has generally been overlooked in the psycho-analytic literature, and it has taken almost a century of psychoanalytic practice for the topic to begin to be openly discussed. It is for this reason that Kruger (1986) aptly entitled his book about money, *The Last Taboo*. In many ways, money has replaced sex as the great secret in the family, in the analytic situation, and even within the society of psychoanalysts.

Freud (1908) was well aware of the significance of money matters in psychoanalysis, and he emphasized the sexual meanings of the patient's "money complex" (p. 173). He wrote:

> An analyst does not dispute that money is to be regarded in the first instance as a medium for self-preservation and for obtaining power; but he maintains that, besides this, powerful sexual factors are involved in the value set upon it. He can point out that money matters are treated by civilized people in the same way as sexual matters—with the same inconsistency, prudishness and hypocrisy. The analyst is therefore determined from the first not to fall in with this attitude, but, in his dealings with his patients, to treat of money matters with the same matter-of-course frankness to which he wishes to educate them in things relating to sexual life [Freud, 1913a, p. 131].

The classical psychoanalytic literature examines money as a symbol focusing on the sexual and especially the anal erotic significance of money and on the unconscious equation of money, gifts, feces, baby, and penis (Freud, 1917a, p. 128). However, the classical literature has neglected the interpersonal meanings of money within the analytic bipersonal field.

We are emphasizing a shift from a study of money within the context of a "one-person psychology" to an investigation of money within a "two-person," relational matrix (Aron, 1990). We believe that analysts need to carefully examine their own conscious and unconscious attitudes, beliefs, feelings, concerns, and conflicts about money, and in addition they need to analyze their patients' perceptions of the analyst's attitudes regarding money and the ways in which their behavior with the patient around money issues affects the development of the transference.

In Freud's most famous case histories, money matters are given a great deal of attention. However, Freud focuses exclusively on the intrapsychic meanings of money and rarely discusses the impact of his own money issues on the patient. This is true in spite of the fact that Freud was regularly concerned with referrals and income and often got personally involved in the financial circumstances of his patients' lives. He was often generous with money and was known to treat needy patients for free or to reduce his fees. He was also known to prefer American patients, specifically because they could pay in hard currency (Gay, 1988).

In the analysis of the Rat Man, Freud describes how the Rat Man translated all of his concerns about money matters into the language of rats, "rat money." For example, Freud (1909) wrote that when he told the Rat Man his hourly fee, the patient had the silent thought "so many florins, so many rats" (p. 213). Much of the analysis concerns the patient's conflicts about money and its anal erotic significance.

In the analysis of the Wolf Man, Freud (1918) said that the patient had become very wealthy through inheritances passed on from his father and uncle, and that he attached great importance to being seen as rich. Money matters for the Wolf Man had meanings that were beyond conscious control, and much of the analysis aimed to elucidate these meanings. During his second period of analysis, when he encountered severe financial problems, the Wolf Man was treated free of charge.

Freud (1913b) presented the case of a woman whose analysis revolved around the significance of money. As a child, this analysand had been witness to a secret sexual liaison between her nursemaid and a doctor, and she was given a few coins so that she would not reveal this affair to her parents. In spite of accepting this bribe, the little girl had betrayed her nursemaid by playing ostentatiously with the coins in front of her mother. Just a few years later, a central event in the patient's life occurred to cause her humiliation and mortification when it was discovered that she had lied to her parents about stealing a few coins from her father. Freud interpreted the meaning of this episode as an expression of her wish to receive money from her father because receiving money had symbolically become equated with sexual seduction. Freud observed that for this woman, taking money from anyone took on the meaning of a physical surrender to an erotic relationship.

Nevertheless, when the analysand's husband, who was not living in Vienna, failed to provide financial support for her in the course of the analysis, Freud offered to lend the woman money and made her promise to accept his help. The woman refused his offer, saying that she could not accept money from him. Freud did not indicate that this interaction between him and the patient would have implications for the treatment; the case was presented to illustrate the dynamics of lying in children, and was not intended as a treatise on technique or on the handling of transference. Therefore, it is possible that Freud pursued the analysis of the meaning of this event for the patient as well as its influence on the transference. However, it remains striking to the contemporary reader of Freud that he makes no mention of the significance of this event. As Gill (1982) has argued with regard to the Rat Man case, it is hard to believe that Freud would not have reported the results of the analysis of this transference–countertransference interaction if he regarded it as significant. Freud was interested in the intrapsychic dynamics of the patient and in the symbolic meanings of money in the patient's unconscious life; he was less focused on the systematic exploration of the meanings of the actual analytic situation.

Ferenczi (1928) was one of the very few analysts to call attention to money matters in psychoanalysis. He wrote, "Psycho-analysis is often reproached with being remarkably concerned with money matters. My own opinion is that it is far too little concerned with them" (p. 93). To illustrate a patient's conflicts regarding paying the analytic fee he told the following joke. A patient began a consultation by telling the analyst, "Doctor, if you help me, I'll give you every penny I possess!" The doctor replied, "I shall be satisfied with 30 kronen an hour." "But isn't that rather excessive?" the patient unexpectedly remarked.

A SUMMARY OF CONTEMPORARY RELATIONAL PERSPECTIVES

From a two-person relational perspective, the analyst is viewed as neither neutral or as a blank screen but as an unwitting participant-observer or observing-participant. Hirsch (1985, 1987) and Aron (1991) speak in terms of a technical focus on analyzing the patient's experience of the analyst's subjectivity. Hoffman (1983) views the patient as an active interpreter of the analyst's experience and argues against a view of the patient as a naive observer of the analytic interchange. These authors view the fiction of analytic anonymity (Singer, 1977) as a self-protective stance on the analyst's part.

Freud, despite his early inclination toward an interpersonal psychoanalysis (the seduction theory), developed a one-person psychology. The aim was to isolate the intrapsychic world of the patient and keep it free from contamination by the analyst's psyche. Psychoanalysts were thereby schooled to believe that they indeed could be neutral to the patient and therefore were able to observe an almost pure culture of intrapsychic experience. Psychoanalysis was defined as the study of the intrapsychic reality of the patient, whereas, in contrast, the nonparticipating analyst was seen as representing objective reality.

Within a two-person psychology, the analyst, as well as the patient, must be the focus of examination, for it is only natural that the analyst's own personal psychology enters the analytic field. The analyst must strive to be aware of both personal character traits and personal reactions to the patient and how they are enacted in the dyad (see, e.g., Hirsch, 1988). It is important to note that the term "enacted" is used instead of "experienced." From this viewpoint, the analyst as person and/or respondent directly influences the patient and the analyst can never totally control affect to the point that it is kept invisible and restricted to the analyst's internal feeling states.

Some classical analysts have also come to this conclusion (Jacobs, 1986). Despite efforts at neutral exploration of the patient's life, the analyst's own personal psychology actually enters the analytic field. In the two-person model the analyst must always strive to be aware of his or her personal self and how it comes into play in all analytic contexts. The patient is enlisted to help the analyst become more aware of his or her own participation, which can thus make the analyst a better analyzing instrument (Searles, 1979). The analyst must also be alert to the inclination to become enmeshed in the interactional world of patients and to repeat with them facsimiles of early and current internalized relational patterns (Levenson, 1972; Sandler, 1976; Mitchell, 1988). If the analyst does not invite the patient to openly and freely illuminate the analyst's coparticipation by encouraging the patient's constant observations, the analyst runs the risk of overly influencing the patient with the analyst's own psychol ogy, or repeating without resolving the patient's old and internalized interactional patterns (Gill, 1982; Mitchell, 1988).

MONEY MATTERS

Since money must be dealt with in some manifest way, the analyst is always exposing elements of his or her own greed or dependency as well as a wide array of other feelings. Indeed, in our culture money is associated with power and strength. This theme has been deftly satirized in the popular novel *Bonfire of the Vanities* (Wolfe, 1987). Analysts usually do not wish to expose neediness and dependency to the patient, for traditionally it is the patient who is thought to be dependent on the powerful analyst. It is very clear, however, that this does not escape the patient's scrutiny. The analyst is inevitably exposed with respect to money. There is no way to entirely avoid the subject, because money always plays a part in any analytic transaction. Analysts can act as if their own personal relationship to money is well hidden but this can only be an illusion. Patients can and do frequently help analysts perpetuate such self-deception by protecting the analyst from the patient's perceptive scrutiny.

Analysts, therefore, frequently avoid picking up allusions to the transference around such matters, as a way of trying to hide. In other professions these qualities (greed, dependency, weakness) can be exhibited but the lawyer or internist does not encourage the patient/client to "say everything which comes to mind." In the psychoanalytic profession we must face the embarrassment of exposure of these qualities, unless the analyst colludes with the patient to suppress clarity. Under ideal analytic conditions, because of the genuine encouragement to tell all, anonymity is lost and the analyst stands exposed in many sensitive areas. This is especially so in the relational model being described here, where we can never assume that the patient is projecting and instead must assume that he or she is responding to some actual participation on our part (Hoffman, 1983; Hirsch, 1985). As Levenson (1975) has noted, "We are paid to be vulnerable".

To highlight the significance of money matters, an anecdote that made a lasting impression on one of us is recalled. It refers to a wise, older, civil liberties lawyer, married to a psychologist. After not seeing him for a number of years I (Hirsch) ran into him and told him I was now in full time practice. He quickly asked how analysts help people get better, since ending treatment means losing income. Is that not a stark conflict of interest? I mumbled something about satisfied clients who refer new ones but acknowledged that it was a real problem. Relentless, as lawyers can be, he replied that he just said it was a real problem: "What is your answer?"

Twelve years later we still do not have a satisfactory answer. In fact, we consider this the single biggest practical problem today in the field of psychotherapy and psychoanalysis. To be specific, we are referring to the competition for income from private practice among what appears to us to be a very large pool of therapists and analysts in full but mostly part-time practice.

We here summarize four ways in which greed and economic dependencies on patients can readily lead to trouble. Though we are focusing on these two countertransference feelings, there are many others that may readily interfere with optimal analytic functioning.

1. The reluctance to terminate successfully.
2. The willingness to continue unproductive treatment instead of referring elsewhere.
3. The failure to confront, challenge, or raise certain issues for fear that the patient may leave.
4. The wish to be liked by the patient, for the same reason.

We are here raising the issue of prolonged, unproductive treatment. We are suggesting that among numerous possible reasons leading to this not uncommon phenomena are the analyst's desire to keep the patient, partly out of attachment to the patient and partly out of economic need. As in all such matters, the interesting analytic question is the nature of the participation of both parties. That is, why do patients help their needy analysts by remaining "sick" or by getting better and remaining longer than they need to? This is prime analytic material but the analyst must be prepared to acknowledge it to himself or herself and to raise it as an issue. If done, this could be most helpful to the patient but if suppressed, the analyst is repeating rather than trying to work through. We think of Searles's (1979) article, "The patient as therapist to his analyst" and his and Singer's (1965) thesis that most psychopathology is caused by children's efforts to aid their troubled parents. Ties of love and loyalty lead to reluctance to emerge from embeddedness in the family (Fromm, 1964), causing personal stagnation and a narrowing of one's life. If this issue can be exposed in the transference instead of being interminably played out, the patient stands to experience love or loyalty and perhaps does not need to display it via the route of sacrifice. However, like parents, analysts must be prepared to sacrifice loss of dependence upon the patient, and this is where the analyst is faced with repeated personal and professional dilemmas. There exists an ethical responsibility to promote growth but analysts may hold back the very growth they are hired to facilitate. There are three choices, if you will: strive to remain unconscious of this dilemma; become conscious and do nothing about the conflict in order to satisfy personal desire; become conscious and use this consciousness to either control greed or address the dilemma directly with the patient. At some point or another, we think all analysts are guilty of the first and second alternative.

The rationale for not referring out when a therapy or analysis seems stagnant is that the stagnancy itself is meaningful and must be analyzed. It could reflect the patient's ambivalence about change, the patient's stubbornness or negativism, the patient's desire to destroy the analyst's esteem, the patient's desire to preserve an angry and dependent relationship. Because all of these and many other possibilities are quite plausible, it is genuinely difficult to determine among them, sometimes resulting in the prolongation of an unproductive or no longer productive dyad. We are usually inclined to try to weather difficult periods because we believe in the psychoanalytic lore: never trust an analysis that is going well. Analysis should be difficult because change is so very difficult. However, in examining counter-transference experience, the analyst must always be willing to entertain the possibility that this is not an impasse but a mismatch, at least at that particular point. This is especially so when there are long periods of plateaus in analyses lasting five, six, seven years and upward. Once again, the patient may be staying to protect the analyst and the analyst may collude because of economic or other dependencies on the patient. Additionally, if the analyst acts out prolonging treatment in either instance, the result is inevitable self-hatred for the analyst.

A corollary to the dependency-based prolongation of treatment is the analyst's reluctance to face certain transference issues for fear that the patient will become angry or feel too exposed and leave. We can always justify caution since the cliche "the patient is not ready" has permeated our profession from the beginning. We are more prone to agree with Singer (1968), who attributed the reluctance to interpret as a countertransference problem often based on the therapist's fear and not the patient's fragility. Analysts are frightened by many different sorts of exposure and consciously or unconsciously conspire to suppress the patient's observations. For instance, it is not unusual to avoid responding to the patient's subtle or indirect hostile or critical feelings for fear that if they are recognized the patient will leave treatment. Similarly, analysts also may hold back on challenging some form of transference acting out and allow the patient to continue this as a bribe for remaining in treatment. Delicate or sensitive areas for the patient may be neglected for fear that his or her anxiety may lead to flight. It is quite common to overlook the patient's references to the analyst's dependent needs or weaknesses, again for fear that the patient will recognize that the analyst needs the patient, perhaps as much as or more than otherwise. We believe unequivocally that any matter that remains unaddressed compromises an analysis, yet we recognize how frequently this occurs.

Regarding the wish to be loved by patients, analysts may act out in ways to provoke positive responses from the patient. That is, the analyst can actively strive to influence the patient to like him or her even though such influence runs against the grain of the analytic attitude. The "therapeutic alliance" may be rationalized, but the motive may be the therapist's desire to be liked and/or the therapist's economic need to hold on to the patient. Despite much literature to the contrary, an analyst may feel that the patient's negative transference can be suppressed without leading in some way to acting out of such feelings. Sometimes the patient must leave treatment because the analyst cannot hear, in any other way, the patient's negative feelings toward him or her. More problematic, however, are the situations when the patient remains in treatment and suppresses negative feelings in order to protect the analyst. This repetition of sacrifice for the parents can lead anywhere from stagnation to self-destruction. The analyst must be willing to feel the full fury of the patient's hatred and risk premature termination. Bird (1972), in his classic paper on transference, wrote that such hate and destructiveness are inevitable in any successful analysis and says that at some point both parties come very close to "throwing in the towel." An analyst's economic anxieties can readily interfere with full exposure of the patient's hateful affect.

A case example by one of us (Aron) is presented to illustrate some issues related to the contribution of the analyst in the acting out of money matters in the analytic interaction. We believe that further case reports are needed in this area.

CASE EXAMPLE

Ms. M very "graciously" let me know that I had mistakenly undercharged her on the previous month's bill. She had carefully gone over her records and noted that she had attended three additional sessions that did not appear on the bill, and consequently I had undercharged her. I asked her what sessions she had in mind, and she cited three

Friday sessions. I pointed out to her that we had not met on those three Fridays, because I had previously cancelled those sessions. She then said that in that case she must have overpaid me. I assured her that I would double check my records. At the beginning of the next session, I told her that she had paid me the correct amount. She realized that, although she initially thought I was mistaken in the dates, she now thought that I had included three other dates, which were incorrect, and so both mistakes had cancelled each other. In any case, she now realized that none of this was my fault and that in fact it had all balanced out; we were even. I commented on her belief regarding the series of mistakes about the bill and asked her what she thought that had been about. She was sure it was just a simple mistake. "Nothing to analyze!" It angered her that we spent our time talking about these petty details, instead of moving on to the "real" issues. "Analysis is expensive," she reminded me.

She had spoken with people and had concluded that $60 or $70 was a typical Manhattan fee. Since she was paying $90 she began to wonder whether she was subsidizing other patients. Although she understood sliding scales, she could not help but wonder what I would do if she "went broke" tomorrow. She doubted that I would insist on continuing to charge the same fee. She was sure that I would be more sensitive than that! Parenthetically, she told me that Mr. R, another patient of mine, who had referred her to me and who paid only $60, had asked to know her fee. She had not told Mr. R because she resented his intrusiveness. Because their relationship was distant and they saw each other infrequently, she had always felt that Mr. R envied her and her income. She remarked, "He has a thing with me, you know, you make all this, and I make shit!" I found myself wondering whether in some more or less subtle way I had conveyed my own envy to the patient.

Based on her series of miscalculations, one might not guess that Ms. M is a high-powered and successful litigation attorney and that her professional life involves constant dealings with money and complicated business negotiations. Moreover, she deals with considerably larger sums of money than any psychoanalyst would in a professional practice, and her financial negotiations indeed make our discussions of money seem "petty." It is certainly not in keeping with her character or professional life to make such slips regarding a bill.

Ms. M continued that she remembered that Mr. R once told her that he was paying $60, "But you said $90 and I said O.K." Why hadn't she questioned the fee, protested, or negotiated? "I guess I was too anxious. I don't mean that I was desperate. After all, I figured that I bill out for consultations at $200 an hour." Ms. M went on to wonder whether I would have lowered my fee if she had said something. She questioned whether she should have negotiated with me.

Some might argue that I should not have accepted a referral from a patient who was still in treatment, particularly of someone he knew and with whom he had contact. Although it was my understanding that they were only acquaintances and had little contact with each other, clearly even this relationship did lead to complications. (Perhaps it is relevant to note the compromises we make because of the economic realities of practicing psychoanalysis in New York in the 1980s.)

I asked Ms. M why she did not remember clearly what Mr. R was paying. Would this not have been interesting to her? What was her doubt and hesitation about? How did she feel confronting me with this apparent inequity and injustice? Why did she think I charged Mr. R less than her? Ms. M was not ignorant of the realities of running a business; she imagined that at an earlier point in my practice I might have been more eager for patients. Did the higher fee indicate something about my success and therefore lend me prestige? Was she perceiving me as greedy and seeking to take advantage of whatever I could get? She noted that she lived in a rent-controlled building where rents vary and thus she supplemented other people's lower rents. Did I use a sliding scale by which I charged wealthier patients higher fees? Whose treatment was she subsidizing? Who would subsidize her if she needed it? What did she imagine was my motive in subsidizing the poor? Her father was an active communist who argued for socialized medicine but who could not manage his own financial or business affairs. What did she imagine about my relation to money: Was I stingy, cheap, extravagant, greedy, hoarding? How did I manage my accounts? Was I competent or incompetent? Did I have a "depression" mentality?

The next session was cancelled because Ms. M was flying around the country "negotiating business deals." I later heard that she had "made a killing!" The question emerged between us as to who would have killed whom if she and I had negotiated the fee?

In the following session, Ms. M complained that she was dissatisfied with her recent raise. She was feeling "nickel and dimed" at work. Changing the topic, she told me that she had not yet paid her landlord for the month's rent. He had not kept up the building in the condition that he should, and she was leading the tenants in a rent strike.

What would it be like for Ms. M to negotiate with me over money? She said it would change everything! She explained that we both had self-interests here. "I want the money in my pocket and you want it in yours, we both can't have it. Once you negotiate, it changes everything; the ultimate threat is that you have to terminate the relationship and I don't want to do that." For Ms. M, once you negotiate and you put all your cards on the table, there is no pulling back; after a confrontation the relationship changes. She said that either she feels that she is "steamrolling" someone else into doing whatever she wants or that she is a "chump" being taken and abused. She often feel that "it's like playing poker with a shitty hand, and you keep throwing money in the pot." Ms. M had lost one of her closest friends after a fight they had years ago. She now recalled that she had lent her friend money, and when her friend returned the money Ms. M thought that she had not returned the full amount. Ms. M was angry that her friend was cheating her, but was even more disturbed because she had not kept any written record. She had been "pissed" that she had to do any accounting at all. Ms. M did not spontaneously connect any of this with the recent dispute with me about the bill.

At about this time, Ms. M won the battle with her landlord, and repairs in the building were being made. Her mother had called and asked for some help in managing her investments. This would involve her in a complicated position in relation to her father who disagreed with her mother's handling of finances, and so Ms. M tried to stay out of it.

Ms. M understood that she had to pay for all missed sessions. It annoyed her, and she did not think it quite fair, but for the time being she considered the work we were doing "profitable." Talking about the money is annoying, she said, "It's not worth spending 15 minutes on 15 cents," an expression her father often used. "But if I don't pay attention to every nickel and dime, and you do pay attention to every nickel and dime, then pretty soon you'll have more nickels and dimes than I do."

Ms. M missed a session because she had to be out of state with a client. She resented that she had to miss a session because of this business and felt inconvenienced. She admitted guiltily that she charged an additional dinner to the client's account. She was also sorry that she had "inconvenienced" me because she had been unable to call and let me know she would not make the session but added, "That's what I pay you for." Still, she continued, she hates waste.

In the next session, Ms. M remembered a "traumatic" car accident she had caused. When she was in her late teens she had borrowed a friend's car and had smashed it into a tree. She later told her friend not to worry, that she would pay her what she owed for the damage to the car. They agreed that the car had been worth about $400. Ms. M had not negotiated with her friend; she had felt, "You have me over a barrel." Ms. M gave her friend $200 but then began to resent the agreement. She avoided the friend until much time had gone by, and she never paid the remaining money. She had always felt guilty and uneasy about this incident. I found myself wondering in what ways she would express her resentment toward me, and in particular alerted myself to how promptly she would pay the monthly bill.

This material, gathered from only a few sessions in the course of an analysis, is a relatively benign example of how money issues may come up in treatment. In this case, we should not be surprised to learn that money matters played an important role in her family of origin. Ms. M's parents fought over money with each other and with everyone else. Even now, her parents live with incompletely repaired plumbing because her father had a fight with the plumber over the bill, and the disagreement was never resolved. She described her only sister as unable to handle finances and as belonging to "credit card anonymous." From the beginning of her analysis Ms. M complained about the inefficiency of the analytic procedure. She would say, "I don't like waste. Time is money. I hate waste." She described her family as frugal and said she had grown up in a home with a "depression mentality." In fact, her father had been seriously depressed for a number of years in her early adolescence and was unemployed much of this time.

Ms. M said that when not depressed her father was a colorful and charismatic "character." He had returned from fighting in World War II dedicated to liberal values, to an egalitarian society, and to communism. His devotion to communism led him into serious difficulty at work, since he had a semipolitical career.

While many issues might be raised by this material,[1] we would like to focus specifically on the ways in which money matters both to the patient and to the analyst and how it is an issue between them. The reality of the analyst's beliefs, values, attitudes, and desires has an ongoing effect, not only on the "therapeutic alliance" or on the "real relationship" between patient and analyst, but on the transference itself (see Gill, 1984). In this case, Ms. M established a transference based not only on her own needs, fantasies, desires, and past

---

[1]In the clinical material presented there are numerous associations to waste, shit, and dirt, and the analysis of the "money complex" in terms of its anal erotic significance would be revealing and enlightening. We do not mean that the patient's concern with money would be reductively interpreted as a derivative of a biological drive associated with the anal erotic zone. Rather, following Fromm (1941), we believe that the underlying anal fantasies and concerns are important because they inform us about the development of the patient's character and of "the specific kind of relatedness toward the world which is underlying them and which they express" (p. 293).

experiences concerning money and interactions around money, but also on her perceptions of my attitudes about money and her observations of my handling of money matters between us.

It seems to us that it is not a matter of indifference to the patient that the analyst does have real economic concerns and pressures, which in subtle and not so subtle ways are communicated to the patient. Say the patient, for example, fails to pay on the first session of the month, when this has been the ongoing arrangement. Does the analyst bring this up immediately, at the beginning of the session or at the end, or only after two or three sessions have gone by? Does the analyst raise the issue immediately and directly, such as by saying, "I notice that it's the first session of the month and you haven't mentioned anything about payment"? Does the analyst wait for the patient's associations to lead to some relevant topic and then say, "Perhaps this is in some way connected to your not paying me this week?" Does the analyst wait patiently until the issue surfaces in the patient's associations? True, all these approaches could be taken by different analysts in a more or less heavy-handed way, our point is that subtle differences in tone, wording, gesture, and style might very well convey to the patient aspects of the analyst's feelings, attitudes, anxieties, and conflicts.

To return to Ms. M, for the first time since we began the treatment, she gave me a check that was returned by the bank for insufficient funds. At the beginning of the next session I raised the matter with her. Note how much ambiguity there is in my saying that "I raised it with her." Analysts might vary considerably in how and with what tone they would raise this issue, and these differences matter a great deal. I handed her the check and said that it had been returned by the bank. I caught myself before I referred to it as having "bounced." In my mind, the colloquial word "bounced" would have been more offensive and embarrassing to the patient. Thus I was made aware of my need to defend against my desire to retaliate for the "bounced check" by humiliating the patient with it. Ms. M was very apologetic and obviously embarrassed. She experienced any questioning of the meaning of the bounced check as an attempt to humiliate her.

We discussed her profound embarrassment, including her fantasy that I would think she was trying to "rip me off" and that she might not want to pay me. The possibility arose that she might get into a squabble with me over the payment, which would lead to a fight and an attack by me. Most important, from my point of view, we discussed her experience of my questioning the meaning of the bounced check as my "rubbing her nose in it." I asked Ms. M if she could imagine what I must have thought and felt toward her at the moment when I opened the bank statement and found her name on the returned item. This question led her to discuss her intense fears that I would throw her out or attack her violently. We were back to her parents' fights over money and to her father's real physical abusiveness. But just as significantly, the patient and I both knew that we were involved in a real transaction in which she did something to me that had an adverse financial effect, and now I was making her "pay for it."

She asked me whether I would redeposit the check or if she should write a new one. I told her that I would prefer she write a new check and include the $5.00 bank fee. We were back to nickels and dimes.

The analyst is always maintaining some balance between participating in and observing the interaction, including observing his or her own participation in the interaction. When it comes to the monetary transactions between analyst and patient, the analyst is a very real participant, and this puts additional strain on his or her capacity as an observer.

How does the analyst feel analyzing the patient's money issues when the patient earns more money than the analyst? This is after all not uncommon. How comfortable is the analyst with feelings of greed, envy, and competitiveness? How much attention has the analyst paid to his or her own money complex? Might these issues be less emphasized in a training analysis where the patient will be entering the same field as the analyst, so that in some way they will be in the same financial boat?

It matters that, in our society, money paid in salaries and fees provides an important measure of the society's order of value. In our society people often value themselves to the degree that other people are willing to pay for their labor and services. Are psychoanalysts so well analyzed that they stand above all of this? Are they exempt from the American fascination with and worship of money? Are analysts so uncompetitive and so secure in their self-esteem that they can not be moved by these pressures? Can they remain so neutral, so anonymous and unrevealing that their patients do not pick up real cues as to their attitudes concerning money?

One day Ms. M said that she had been planning to pay me in cash, but her cash machine was out of order. She began to write a check but hesitated because she thought it better to wait and give me cash the next time. "It would be better for you in April!", she said.

Is it unrevealing, anonymous, or neutral for the analyst to remain silent? Do you tell patients that you accept only checks or that you prefer cash? Do you say that patients should pay as they prefer? Do you make explicit that patients have the fantasy that you intend to withhold income on your tax returns and that they want to ingratiate themselves to you by an illegal collusion that must remain secret between patient and analyst? Or are patients accusing you of immoral and illegal clandestine acts, putting you on the spot by condescendingly implying that they know what lowly finagling you are up to? Does the analyst's tone convey a sense of moral superiority and indignance in response to this offer by patients? How many psychoanalysts follow Langs's (1982) directive that patients should pay exclusively by check and that analysts should stamp the check "for deposit only" so that there can be no question of its being deposited into a professional account? The reality of the analyst's attitudes and behavior concerning money inevitably comes across to patients. It is not just a matter of their affecting the "working alliance." We are arguing that whether or not the analyst reports all of his or her income may very well affect the development of the transference.

The analyst's response is always a participation with the patient, and there is no way to hide behind anonymity. As discussed earlier, it is a basic premise of the relational model that the analyst is always a "participant-observer," in Sullivan's (1954) terms, or an "interventionist" to use Fairbairn's (1958) phrase. Greenberg (1986) has clarified that these do not refer to prescriptions for technique but are, rather, statements of fact from a particular philosophical point of view. From a relational or interpersonal perspective, the analyst cannot help but be both a participant and an observer.

Ferenczi (1914) described the development of the interest in money in terms of libido theory. Children show a natural interest and pleasure in defecating and in holding back their stool. The retained feces are the first savings and the first toys. In moving toward an interest in mud, the child gives up the anal-erotic pleasure in the smell of the feces. "Street-mud is, so to speak, deodourised dejecta" (p. 322). Next the child gives up the pleasure in the moisture and interest shifts to sand. Later interest shifts to pebbles and stones and later to marbles and buttons. "The attributes of evil odour, moisture, and softness are represented by those of absence of odour, dryness, and now also hardness" (p. 325). Finally, interest is shown in coins, and, as cognitive development proceeds, coins are replaced by stocks, bonds, and abstract figures. "Pleasure in the intestinal contents becomes enjoyment of money, which, however, after what has been said is seen to be nothing other than odourless, dehydrated filth that has been made to shine" (p. 327).

In our experience as analysts, we have become aware of a developmental line in the meaning of fees, although this phenomena may be idiosyncratic to us. When we began practice we had to struggle with setting a fee that had some relation to that of our own analysts. Fee setting was complicated by the fact that we both had paid a reduced fee for some time. Raising fees above what was our analysts' fees for us led to issues of competitiveness, outdoing, greed, and oedipal rivalry. During the next career phase, fee issues revolved around comparison with peers. How much were friends charging? Who would be the first in the group to raise the fee? What would supervisors think if they knew what we were charging? In peer supervision groups we often found ourselves focusing on fees. Cases were presented, and time after time questions emerged about money. What does the patient pay? When was the last time the fee was raised? How much does the patient owe? Why did you agree to a reduced fee? How do you negotiate to raise it? The local gossip had it that one peer study group had stopped talking about patients altogether and now concentrated on real estate and investment strategies, something that none of us social science types had been taught in school. The first shift from oedipal issues to peer issues was followed by yet another development. As life progressed and supporting a family became a priority, realistic economic issues became prominent. Fees were no longer only issues of rivalry, status, and adequacy, but were related powerfully to the responsibilities of professional and personal adulthood and maturity. Development is not linear or final, however, and many motivations continue to operate in our handling of all money matters.

Why all this preoccupation with money? Should we not be more concerned with providing a needed service to as many people as possible at a low or moderate cost? Should we not at least try to rise above the worship of Mammon to analyze our greed, envy, and rivalry? Many of the early generation of pioneer psychoanalysts were rebellious intellectuals with broad liberal, cultural, political, and social commitments. Many were radicals and rebels (Jacoby, 1983). Many psychoanalysts have been and continue to be humanitarians. Psychoanalysis should not become a clinical specialty so professionalized and insular that it serves only an affluent clientele. Freud (1917b) recognized and bemoaned the fact that "the necessities of our existence limit our work to the well-to-do classes" (p. 166), and he dreamed that, one day, either the state or private charity would enable psychoanalysis to become available "for the wider social strata, who suffer extremely seriously from neuroses" (p. 167). Inspired by Freud's reminder of the social obligations of psychoanalysis, Simmel and Eitingon set up the Berlin Institute to provide psychoanalysis to the poor (Jacoby, 1983). Many years later, Eissler (1974) advised that psychoanalytic societies should suggest to their members to analyze, gratis, at least one patient at a time. He believed that this would not only serve a social purpose, but would also broaden the analyst's knowledge of social structure and the effects of socioeconomic conditions on the individual. Fromm and many others also worked toward the establishment of free psychoanalytic clinics.

We are not calling for an unqualified acceptance of greed, nor are we advocating any particular fee structure. We are arguing that money matters to all of us—to analysts just as much as to patients. None of us can escape our social and cultural milieu, and money stirs up powerful emotional forces in all of us. However analysts choose to deal with their own money matters, ethics, values, and conflicts, it is bound to effect their treatments. In a series of studies Lasky (1984), has demonstrated the pervasiveness of psychoanalysts' ambivalence about fees and has highlighted the lack of training in our field about money matters (see also Kruger, 1986). We are recommending increased professional discussion of these complex and sensitive issues and increased recognition by analysts of the ways in which their realities contribute to the coconstruction with the patient of the transference–countertransference integration.

REFERENCES

Aron, L. (1990), One person and two person psychologies and the method of psychoanalysis. *Psychoanal. Psychol.*, 7:475–485.
_____ (1991), The patient's experience of the analyst's subjectivity. *Psychoanal. Dial.*, 1:29–51.
Bird, B. (1972), Notes on transference: Universal phenomenon and hardest part of analysis. *J. Amer. Psychoanal. Assn.*, 20:267–301.
Eissler, K. R. (1974), On some theoretical and technical problems regarding the payment of fees for psychoanalytic treatment. *Internat. Rev. Psycho-Anal.*, 1:73–101.
Fairbairn, W. R. D. (1958), On the nature and aims of psycho-analytical treatment. *Internat. Rev. Psycho-Anal.*, 39:374–385.
Ferenczi, S. (1914), The ontogenesis of the interest in money. In: *First Contributions to Psycho-Analysis.* New York: Brunner/Mazel, 1952.
_____ (1928), The elasticity of psycho-analytic technique. In: *Final Contributions to the Problems and Methods of Psychoanalysis.* New York: Brunner/Mazel, 1955, 1980.
Freud, S. (1908), Character and anal eroticism. *Standard Edition,* 9:168–175. London: Hogarth Press, 1959.
_____ (1909), *Notes Upon a Case of Obsessional neurosis. Standard Edition,* 10:153–318. London: Hogarth Press, 1955.
_____ (1913a), On beginning the treatment. *Standard Edition,* 12:121–144. London: Hogarth Press, 1958.
_____ (1913b), Two lies told by children. *Standard Edition,* 12:303–310. London: Hogarth Press, 1958.

_____ (1917a), On transformations of instinct as exemplified in anal eroticism. *Standard Edition*, 17:126–133. London: Hogarth Press, 1955.

_____ (1917b), Lines of advance in psycho-analytic therapy. *Standard Edition*, 17:158–168. London: Hogarth Press, 1955.

_____ (1918), From the History of an Infantile Neurosis. Standard Edition, 17:3–122. London: Hogarth Press, 1955.

Fromm, E. (1941), *Escape from Freedom*. New York: Holt, Rinehart & Winston.

_____ (1964), *The Heart of Man*. New York: Harper & Row.

Gay, P. (1988), *Freud: A Life for Our Time*. New York: Norton.

Gill, M. M. (1982), *Analysis of Transference*, Vol. I., New York: International Universities Press.

_____ (1984), Transference: A change in conception or only in emphasis? A response. *Psychoanal. Inq.*, 4:489–524.

Greenberg, J. R. (1986), Theoretical models and the analyst's neutrality. *Contemp. Psychoanal.*, 22:87–106.

Hirsch, I. (1985), The rediscovery of the advantages of the participant-observation model. *Psychoanal. Contemp. Thought*, 8:441–459.

_____ (1987), Varying modes of analytic participation. *J. Amer. Acad. Psychoanal.*, 15:205–222.

_____ (1988), Mature love in the countertransference. In: *Love, Psychoanalytic Perspectives*, ed. J. Lasky & H. Silverman. New York: New York University Press, pp. 200–212.

Hoffman, I. Z. (1983), The patient as an interpreter of the analyst's experience. *Contemp. Psychoanal.*, 19:389–422.

Jacobs, T. (1986), On countertransference enactments. *J. Amer. Psychoanal. Assn.*, 34:289–307.

Jacoby, R. (1983), *The Repression of Psychoanalysis*. New York: Basic Books.

Kruger, D. W. (1986), *The Last Taboo*. New York: Bruner/Mazel.

Langs, R. (1982), *Psycho-therapy*. New York: Aronson.

Lasky, E. (1984), Psychoanalysts' and psychotherapists' conflicts about setting fees. *Psychoanal. Psychol.*, 1:289–300.

Levenson, E. (1972), *The Fallacy of Understanding*. New York: Basic Books.

_____ (1983), *The Ambiguity of Change*. New York: Basic Books.

McLaughlin, J. (1981), Transference, psychic reality, and countertransference. *Psychoanal. Quart.*, 50:639–664.

Mitchell, S. (1988), *Relational Concepts in Psychoanalysis*. Cambridge, MA: Harvard University Press.

Sandler, J. (1976), Countertransference and role responsiveness. *Internat. J. Psycho-Anal.*, 3:43–47.

Searles, H. (1979), *Countertransference and Related Subjects*. New York: International Universities Press.

Singer, E. (1965), *Key Concepts in Psychotherapy*. New York: Basic Books.

_____ (1968), The reluctance to interpret. In: *The Use of Interpretation in Treatment*, ed. E. Hammer. New York: Grune & Stratton, pp. 181–192.

_____ (1977), The fiction of analytic anonymity. In: *The Human Dimension in Psychoanalytic Practice*, ed. K. Frank. New York: Grune & Stratton, pp. 364–371.

Sullivan, H. S. (1954), *The Psychiatric Interview*. New York: Norton.

Wolfe, T. (1987), *The Bonfire of the Vanities*. New York: Farrar, Straus & Giroux.

12

On the Occurrence of the Isakower Phenomenon in a Schizoid Patient

PHILIP M. BROMBERG

In a now classic paper, Isakower (1938) described a relatively rare but intriguing complex of sensory phenomena recalled and reported by certain of his patients as occurring in the twilight state of consciousness just prior to their entering sleep. These phenomena, taken together, appeared so closely to recapitulate precognitive elements of nursing at the breast that they were considered by Isakower, and thereafter, as parts of a single experience. The predominant theme in the subsequent psychoanalytic literature on the subject has been an effort to establish more precisely the psychodynamic nature and etiology of this hypnogogic event by examining the personality structure of those patients who, during the course of an analysis, either report it as a childhood memory or reexperience the event itself.

The Isakower phenomenon, as it is referred to, is characteristically remembered or reexperienced by the individual as the visual sensation of a large, doughy, shadowy mass, usually round. As it comes nearer and nearer to his face, it grows larger, swelling to a gigantic size and threatening to crush him; it then gradually becomes smaller and moves farther away. Often there is an indistinct perception of a purplish shape like the nipple area of the breast. The approaching mass slowly seems to become a part of the person, obscuring the boundaries between his body and the outside world

An earlier version of this chapter appeared in *Contemporary Psychoanalysis* (1984), 20:600–624.

and blurring his sense of self more and more. All this is typically accompanied by sensations of tactile roughness on the skin and inside the mouth, and a milky or salty taste in the back of the throat. Often there are feelings of floating or loss of equilibrium. In some people there is, interestingly, a memory of voluntarily producing the experience or prolonging it.

Lewin (1946, 1948, 1953) and Rycroft (1951) believe there are several modified manifestations of this event and that the Isakower phenomenon, the "dream screen," and "blank dreams" are essentially equivalent experiences; whereas Stern (1961) holds the view that all these should be considered variations of a more inclusive category of perceptual disturbances, which he calls "blank hallucinations."

Case histories and reviews of the literature have described the phenomenon from a variety of clinical and theoretical perspectives— oral hunger, oral frustration, a defense against unmet oral needs, a defense against primal scene memories, a character manifestation of passive aims, an early representation of the mother's face rather than the breast (Garma, 1955; Sperling, 1957, 1961; Stern, 1961; Dickes, 1965; Fink, 1967; Easson, 1973; Blaustein, 1975). It has also been reported as occurring in people whose development seemed to be normal (Heilbrunn, 1953); it does not, then, appear to be in itself a pathological phenomenon.

Each of the interpretations of the phenomenon, informative within its own metaphor, reduces its context to a circumscribed developmental crisis or trauma, a defense against such trauma, or an expression of a particular level of psychosexual conflict or interaction between levels. From a review of reports of the phenomenon, however, what appears quite conspicuous is that although it has a clear core of consistency across individuals (which is the aspect that different authors have been attempting to explain), it also has a large idiosyncratic component that tends to be discarded as random "noise" in the system. Some people, for example, report it as a benign, even pleasant experience. Some describe it as terrifying. Some report instances of both. Certain experience it passively, while others make a determined effort to control it.

I am going to discuss these issues in the context of my work with an anxiety-ridden, schizoid man, whose seven-year analysis began with a recollection of the Isakower phenomenon as a memory from early childhood and was marked at about its midpoint by the direct occurrence of this event during the course of a session. It is my view that, at least in his case, the appearance of the Isakower phenomenon did indeed relate to oral conflict, to passive aims, to a defense against primal scene experience, and to a characterological vulnerability to traumatic anxiety—but not to any one of these as the defining concept for best understanding it. All those perspectives are framed by something more comprehensive. I believe the appearance of this event signaled the reemergence of an early, unsuccessful struggle to deal creatively and adaptively with potentially catastrophic interpersonal experience prior to the development of an impenetrable character structure that had shielded him from the realities of human relatedness. I hope to demonstrate that, for this man, the significance of the Isakower phenomenon can best be understood by looking at it not simply as a libidinally derived symptom, but as a map of his capacity for human relatedness, reflecting, as did his dreams, daydreams, and schizoid life style, his unique patterning of interpersonal mental representation at a given point in time.

The schizoid character structure is a tightly regulated balance between relatedness and detachment. As a personality disorder it embodies a mode of living that I have described in a previous paper (Bromberg, 1979) as a "psychopathology of stability," allowing the person to manipulate fantasy in the service of securing a sense of control over his inner world, his place of primary residence. Guntrip (1969) views this cramping of the self into itself as enabling the person to live his life by establishing what he calls "the schizoid compromise" in the struggle to maintain an ego.

> The schizoid person, because of his fears, cannot *give himself* fully or permanently to anyone or anything with feeling. . . . This makes life extremely difficult, so we find that *a marked schizoid tendency is to effect a compromise in a half-way-house position, neither in nor out.* . . . Yet in this compromise position people live far below their real potentialities and life seems dull and unsatisfying [pp. 59–62].

The issue of a "schizoid compromise" is particularly relevant to how one manages the treatment process with such a patient because it really goes beyond what would typically be called a character resistance. It becomes the fundamental quality of the working alliance itself. At one level it can be seen as a chronically blocked analysis or therapeutic stalemate. At another level it expresses the schizoid patient's sense of stability and security and is thus the only pathway to growth. The analysis itself, in other words, often serves the purpose of an ideal schizoid compromise—a way of retaining the security of a relationship that does not involve a full emotional response even while this very issue may be the subject of verbal exploration in the content of the sessions (see Bromberg, 1984). For both the analysis and the patient to emerge ultimately as alive and real, the analyst must work toward engaging the patient directly, in the immediate moment, as content and process simultaneously, while taking into account that this can happen only if the overall ambiance of the treatment generates sufficient anxiety to allow the patient an increasing sense of mastery in regulating it, but not so much anxiety that it evokes a sustained reliance on character detachment as the primary mode of defense. In this regard, how one conceptualizes the interrelationship between earlier and later phases of ego development is particularly significant for schizoid patients in whose history traumatic anxiety appears to have been a central issue.

Let us say that somewhere in the domain of prelogical experience in infancy—before the development of language and higher order symbolic processes—serious psychic trauma occurred consistently. The memory traces laid down by the prevailing sensorimotor organization of experience will tend to remain symbolized in precognitive form as body sensations and as global apprehensions that become phobically linked to aspects of the real world. Regardless of one's theory of personality development, I think it can be postulated that this state of affairs will influence and reverberate with subsequent developmental phases and will contribute to the shaping of adult character. I believe it is also reasonable to hypothesize that it will become a particularly difficult problem when interpersonal experience with significant figures during later stages of development do not lead to identifications that facilitate the structuring of a sense of self cohesive and active enough to "heal" the earlier precognitive wound. In such cases, derivatives of the early trauma would tend to be avoided at all costs, and the individual will learn to structure his life so as to minimize the possibility of such encounters. The shame and anxiety surrounding this course of behavior will gradually lead to the motivation behind his life style becoming unconscious and will further reduce the likelihood of his engaging in interpersonal experience that might successfully promote maturation and an ability to feel fully in the world with a sense of mastery. Often the best that is achieved is an increasing withdrawal into his inner world and a futile, counterphobic struggle to behave "as-if" he felt autonomous but that masks a perpetual longing for the moment when he is released from the demands of living and is permitted to be at peace.

For the most part, the person has no way of dealing with the entirety of this situation in a human relationship that could potentially lead to a synthesis of his ego functioning with interpersonal security. Despite his forays into the real world, he always feels alone inside himself. The external world—ordinary day-to-day life and its routine pressures—remains represented as a potential preverbal horror that continues to haunt him in dreams, physical derivatives, and sometimes hypnogogic states, appearing in its most threatening form in those contexts where there is the least verbal and cognitive structuring.

The phenomenological experience for the person is, in daily life, that of being endangered by something that cannot be handled and may cover a broad range of derivatives. "A party I give may be dull, and I will feel humiliated; I may not know the answers on a test; I may step on someone's feet if I have to go the bathroom while in a theater, so I better make sure to sit on the aisle; I may have nightmares if I go to sleep; I may not be able to perform sexually if someone is willing to go to bed with me; I may go into a panic on the subway and might not be able to get out."

It seems to me that to comprehend most fully a person in such a state and to work most usefully with him in a psychoanalytic setting, no single theoretical perspective should be applied as an attempt to encompass all levels of meaning. There are issues of self-esteem to be considered, precisely in the way that Sullivan (1953) viewed the interpersonal nature of anxiety; but with patients such as the man I discuss here (who will be referred to as Mr. C), raw feelings are frequently felt as sources of anxiety in the way Freud conceived of it, because their potential expression is not under the command of the cognitive patterning of the self-representation. In such people, the feelings are global, undifferentiated, and "not-me." They thus remain as alien forces and potential sources of anxiety in their own right.

THE CASE OF MR. C

For Mr. C, any internal or external experience with the potential to lead to a situation that could not be regulated in a predictably secure manner was felt as a threat not only to his self-esteem but to the stability of his core identity. Something as innocuous as the ticking of a clock, the sound of his own heartbeat, or the falling of raindrops upon him when he did not have an umbrella would produce enough anxiety to resomatize the precognitive channels and snowball into either a panic or a state of mild depersonalization.

The force acting against the threat that these states might unexpectedly occur was the security of feeling able to prevent them or escape from them. Thus, passivity was his hallmark. In reality, it was a caricature of passivity that served as an active and ever-present screening device against the imperatives of both the external world and his inner life — work demands, sexual demands, sleep demands, intense affect, etc. His life-style was "passive" interpersonally because initiative and assertiveness failed to develop as a dimension of his self-representation linked to his functioning in the real world. Initiative and assertiveness are also *unlikely* to have developed because he then would have had to commit himself wholeheartedly to a person, duty, responsibility, or goal from which he was then not free to escape without reproach. Inasmuch as full emotional involvement meant turning some control over to the outside, it evoked, in a variety of forms, feelings of potential helplessness, enslavement, and burial by the crushing force of a sadistically perceived other.

Thus, character detachment became a primary means of avoiding panic states and acute anxiety symptoms associated with his felt inability to regulate self-esteem in everyday life. He clung to a self-generated reality of weakness and ineptness that no encounter with the external world could disprove. Passive behavior became a security operation designed to maintain the "schizoid compromise." That is, it became a means of avoiding the state of normal ego passivity that involves a certain degree of regression through which partial ego control can be trustingly surrendered to both the outside world and to one's own feelings and in which mutuality, love, a sense of being fully alive, and the ability to enjoy peaceful sleep can all find their place.

If a feeling of one's own humanness in a human world has not fully developed, then any situation in which regression occurs or is anticipated is potentially fraught with anxiety. In the regressed state of Stage IV sleep, for example, Mr. C was particularly vulnerable. He had a childhood history of enuresis, sleepwalking, and pavor nocturnus—those cataclysmic eruptions of somatized anxiety into terrifying dreams which continue to be felt as real even after one is fully awake and which the mind and body cannot shake off for a long while.[1] In the process of falling asleep, when control is normally surrendered gradually, there was an elaborate presleep ritual as well as the partially structured event of the Isakower phenomenon that allowed some degree of ego participation. In waking situations, where surrender of control was voluntary but was felt as unavoidable—such as being a passenger in a car—the anticipation of the event would elicit heart palpitations that could themselves threaten to generate into a full-blown panic state.

Mr. C, a verbally gifted, unmarried man of middle-class, Protestant background, entered treatment in his late 30s. He was unusually tall and, despite an insatiable appetite, was slender to the point of

---

[1]The studies of Fisher et al. (1970, 1974) and Broughton (1968) present an informative and conceptually thoughtful treatment of the psychoanalytic and psychophysiological aspects of Stage IV sleep phenomena and their associated pathologies.

looking undernourished. Thick hornrimmed eyeglasses he had worn since childhood partly masked the tenseness in his face while giving the impression of his peering down at you through binoculars. He worked as a free-lance speechwriter at the local political level. As is often true of extremely bright people with severe character pathology, he was in many ways quite astute at looking at himself while feeling hopeless that his insights would ever lead to change. He was well aware, for example, that his choice of career was somehow tied to his difficulty in finding a voice of his own and that speaking through another person was a comfortable compromise.

He had been claustrophobic and an insomniac and for most of his life had suffered from various manifestations of anxiety ranging from somatic symptoms to panic attacks. His relationships felt unreal and always stressful; he had a constant expectation that they would end at any moment. He felt very little hope of any of this changing. The one positive relationship that felt genuine and stable was with his only sibling, a married sister six years younger than he. He entered analysis to try to cure the problem that was for him the most immediately real and inescapable: sexual impotency with a woman he had begun to care for. Treatment was established on the basis of three sessions a week with Mr. C on the couch, a combination of conditions that was for him as initially frightening and then rendered as unreal as the rest of his life.

As an infant, hungry or not, he had been breast fed on a rigid schedule for the first six months of his life. Between ages one and two he was unable to sleep through the night and cried inconsolably. His parents disagreed on how to respond to this behavior, and a pattern emerged in which he was allowed to cry to the point of hysteria, at which juncture, depending on which parent prevailed, either his mother would take him from the crib and carry him around, or his father would come to the side of the crib and shout. If neither procedure stopped his crying, they would take him into their own bed where he would eventually fall asleep between them. He slept in his parents' bedroom until age six, a situation structured around the same power struggle between the parents as to whether he should be forced to grow up and sleep alone in another room or should be allowed to feel "comfortable" and be permitted to sleep in their room until he grew up.

This pattern of relating to him was consistent throughout his history with his parents and was replayed in different forms in different situations at different times in his life. His parents fought constantly over how to rear him and showed little more respect for one another's identity than they showed for his. Unable to relate to peers in any way other than either a pampered child or a bullied victim, he became a loner, hiding his envy and isolation behind a mask of congeniality, false humility, and verbal manipulation of reality. The one aspect of his life that was mutually respectful and mutually supportive was his closeness to his sister, the person whose birth demanded that he finally leave the parental bedroom.

The broad objective during the early part of Mr. C's analysis was the development of more fully individuated self- and object representations and their integration into those areas of his ego functioning that were either mechanical and dehumanized or were filled with dread. The goal was to enable him gradually to surrender his attachment to his inner world as the embodiment of reality and to engage the external human environment in new ways experienced as genuine, if not always pleasant. His ability to relate to me was limited mainly to my role as a potential bridge between one of his various disconnected experiences of himself and another and depended on my own ability to have a direct impact that would increase over time. In the back of my mind was always the question of whether I was making my presence felt in a way that increased his ability to sustain the representation of a reliable external figure who was not simply supportive, or whether the analytic situation remained at its core just another schizoid compromise—an ongoing test of his facility in writing verbal cadenzas to his analyst's compositions. For the most part, although my feelings about my impact were mixed, I did not have a sustained conviction that anything palpably changed between us during the first three years. My deepest experience was that the impact of my presence was an illusion I had created to keep from feeling hopelessly helpless, but it was only by my ability to accept this experience and communicate it that any genuine impact was possible at all.[2] It was primarily through my own helplessness that I was able to convey my experience in the context of his own feelings of helplessness and convey my own sense of "falseness" as part of the overall "falseness" that framed the ongoing interaction. For brief periods of time he was able to respond in a way that seemed to be more immediate, credible, and involved, but I was seldom sure how my words were being processed in the deeper domain of trauma and trust.

We were just starting our fourth year of work when something quite unexpected occurred. While on the analytic couch, Mr. C directly experienced the Isakower phenomenon, which he had reported early in treatment as a childhood memory from ages three to

---

[2]Feiner (1979) has creatively developed this same point from a theoretical base that places the *countertransferential* issue into clinical and historical perspective.

six and which had not been mentioned since. It occurred at about the halfway point of the second of his three weekly sessions, following a rambling, uninvolved discourse on the previous day's events; he then fell silent. He had of late been indulging in long periods of silence with even greater determination than usual, as a transferential affirmation of his right to retain his use of detachment as an ego-syntonic character trait and in secret defiance of my efforts to make him aware of it on his own. I had not perceived that anything out of the ordinary was going on during the silence because it appeared to be simply another of his routine phases of somnolent reverie. In reality, his mental state had changed while he was lying silently, and he had let himself drift into the twilight state of consciousness that precedes sleep. It was at this point that he experienced the Isakower phenomenon and continued to remain silently in this hypnogogic state, eyes almost completely closed as he actively engaged it. After what he later estimated to be two or three minutes of this experience, he brought himself out of it and reported it. His description of the sensory aspects was, except for one addition, identical to his early memory, but his affective experience was totally different.[3] It was not frightening nor did it feel like something completely outside of his self-experience. He was not helplessly at its mercy, as he had remembered it from his past. He described the reexperience as pleasurable: pushing the mass away, letting it ap- proach, pushing it away again, and continuing this push and pull as though playfully wrestling a ghost from his past—a ghost he no longer experienced as an enemy, but not yet as a friend.

His early memory of the event had been of visual and kinesthetic phenomena only, with no mention of any sensation referring to the skin, mouth, or sense of taste. In the reexperience, the one addition he reported was of a rough and tingling feeling on the left side of his face, a sensation he had no recollection of from childhood. (No tactile sensations in the mouth or unusual tastes were mentioned.) That the description of this addition was volunteered (not elicited by question- ing) made highly unlikely any possibility that Mr. C was either con- sciously or unconsciously "putting on a performance" for me by cre- ating an event, the details of which he already knew would interest me. His earlier description of the event, which he reported as a child-

---

[3]His childhood memory reported during the initial interview had been of lying in bed and seeing a large, "soft" grey shape (sometimes round and sometimes amorphous) with a blurry protuberence in the center, slowly descending upon him while he tried to hold it away; he recalled also growing more and more panic stricken until he opened his eyes and sat up, usually in a state of dizziness.

hood memory during the initial interview, had evoked no special interest on my part and very little on his, other than his listing it along with his many other symptoms and jokingly referring to it as "a big tit that came to me in the night." I had never questioned him regarding the unreported aspects associated with the phenomenon, so until the session in which it was reexperienced he had no reason to view it as anything other than idiosyncratic and possessing no greater significance than any of his other dramatic symptoms. In other words, the addition of the skin sensation during the reexperience was a manifestation that was, to the best of his recollection, completely new and a total surprise. It was, however, immediately associated by him with the fact that he could fall asleep only if he was lying on his left side, with his own arm cradling the left side of his face.

The event can be conceptualized theoretically from a number of vantage points, but the overriding quality, as Mr. C described it, was that of a very young child using a newly discovered physical capability and seeing how far he could safely and creatively go with it. In one sense, it was reminiscent of Silberer's (1909) experiments in producing and observing hypnogogic hallucinations in himself as an act of scientific discovery. Winnicott's (1971) notion of "playing" as a bridge between fantasy and reality and Mahler's (1968) description of the "practicing" subphase of the separation-individuation process capture further aspects of it in overlapping but different ways. In the context of Mr. C's specific life experience, it could be conjectured that he was at that moment, with a feeling of relative security, allowing himself to regress to an interpersonal position he had attempted to master as a young child but lacked sufficient ego strength to utilize in the service of his own growth. In the act of "playing" with the Isakower phenomenon during his session, he let himself reencounter a direct facsimile of an early interpersonally traumatic situation and play with it hypnogogically while "playing" with the previously frightening analytic situation itself in a simultaneously identical manner. In other words, what frames this event conceptually is not simply its intrapsychic locale, but that it took place in the context of a relationship that felt secure enough at that point to enable him both to let the event occur and to use himself that way in my presence—to "play" with it and with me at the same time.

He later stated as part of his background experience that he had been aware that he had to make a choice between reporting it and letting it happen and that he chose to keep it going until he had had enough. He further stated that unlike previous sessions, in which he was afraid I might become angry if he fell asleep, he was not focused on what my response might be and just "let himself go."[4] Interestingly, the event was in this regard more important to me than it was to him. He was actually a bit amused by my excitement, in part because I had never witnessed it before whereas he had, but mainly, I think, because he was starting to become interested in something other than his own ability to be an object of adulation. I am referring to something more fundamental emerging in him, of which this experience was a symbolic, albeit dramatic, expression: his growing sense of feeling real in the real world and the existence of a state of mind in which he could acknowledge my presence without loss of his own. It was as if at this moment his precognitive and cognitive domains of experience were being given one more chance to synthesize under the umbrella of a newly emerging sense of self that he knew about but that I felt as only illusory.

In the next session, this "half-dead" man with his history of lively symptoms revealed that when watching television he always turned away when people kissed and would simultaneously remove his eyeglasses. He had, however, become aware the night following the "Isakower session" that he was not performing those two acts at a moment when they would usually have been automatic, and he reported that this awareness felt somehow important to him. Not a very dramatic piece of material for someone whose calling card was inscribed with chronic insomnia, depression, night terrors, and claustrophobia and who just the previous session had captured my intense interest with a dramatic hypnogogic phenomenon. Unlike in the preceding phase of his analysis, his self-experience in response to the "Isakower session" was organized not simply in terms of what he had exhibited or "shown"—his ability to exist through making an impression—but also in terms of what he "gave"—his having determined on his own when and how he relinquished total control over the experience and "gave" it to me through the reporting of it.[5] In

---

[4]Tauber and Green (1959), expanding on Silberer's (1909) position that hypnogogic phenomena occur at the point of tension between drowsiness (a passive condition) and the effort to think (an active condition manipulated by the will), state: "It is thus a struggle between these two antagonistic conditions that elicits what Silberer calls the autosymbolic phenomenon. . . . It is essential, he asserts, that neither of these two conditions outweigh the other. . . . The prevailing of the first condition would lead to sleep, the prevailing of the second to ordered normal thinking" (p. 42).

[5]I refer here to Fairbairn's (1940, pp. 19–20) view that the inner uncertainty of self-experience in schizoid persons leads to an interpersonal stance in which "showing" rather than "giving" is the dominant mode of relatedness, because giving feels too much like self-emptying. In Mr. C's dream that concludes this paper, this issue will surface once more as a self-image in the process of accommodating a wish to prepare a satisfying meal for his friends while poignantly mourning his diminishing exhibitionistic power.

other words, it was an event (his television-watching behavior) that had significance in its own right and engendered curiosity in himself from a vantage point other than having given an interesting performance.

His associations to this change in his television-watching behavior, and the analytic work that followed, centered on his recalling and working through vivid primal scene material that had appeared in derivative form throughout his treatment in dreams and symptoms, but that had been hollow and intellectualized or overly dramatized by him whenever it was addressed by me. This aspect of his early life and the issue of its impact on his personality development was now alive and real to him and interlocked with the parallel appearance in his character of a greater degree of forthrightness in his manner of relating both to me and to people in his outside life. This new "directness" included the disappearance of the sexual impotency problem that had originally brought him to treatment. His ability to recall the act of turning his eyes away from the television while removing his eyeglasses, and to engage this issue actively on his own while in my presence, had a greater impact on him than his ability to impress me with the Isakower phenomenon.

It is important to note, however, that the sexual issue itself had significance only in the context of his level of psychological individuation and interpersonal relatedness. Although Mr. C's sexual conflict was profound, for the largest part of his treatment it was only tangential as a point of leverage in my making contact with him. Until this pivotal point in his development, it was in my ability to understand the act of turning away – not what he turned away from – that the therapeutic action of psychoanalysis existed. Only now did his impulse life, erotic and otherwise – as well as his fear of it – become real enough as part of his self to be genuine analytic material. He had indeed been "tuning out" to kissing on television for many years. But he also tuned out to nonsexual aspects of real life; for example, when in conversations with friends the topic turned from politics to something "real" like how to invest one's money, or interesting restaurants to try, he would stare vacantly into space. The common denominator was not the content of what he was trying to hide from, but the act of hiding itself. It was this investment in ego detachment that shaped his personality structure and the variety of archaic mental states that were a lifelong part of it. The process of chronically and automatically "turning away" from full emotional involvement with the external world led to a pathology of both his internal world and his perception of real life. The act of averting his eyes and removing his glasses had been until now simply one of many expressions of his failure to integrate the two worlds. In this sense it paralleled his wish to stay asleep in the relative security of his fantasy life and to avoid being pulled too sharply awake by some aspect of reality perceived as a harsh voice demanding that he face an interpersonal setting that he felt as totally alien and once again play act participation while concealing his overwhelming hopelessness.

The session of the Isakower phenomenon was special to me because it was such an unusual mental state to witness for the first time. From a broader vantage point, the session was special because his behavior during the twilight state was structured by the manner in which he was interacting with me as it was going on. By his own self-authorization, he had actively pushed me away until he had "had enough" on his own terms and reported this act of self-assertion without deference or anxiety. This was the significance to *him* and from that perspective might be viewed as both a verbal and a preverbal beginning of a working-through process. In this context his behavior during the "Isakower session" could be seen as a creative act, much as proposed by Tauber and Green's (1959, p. 42) suggestion that hypnogogic phenomena demonstrate the creative function of imagery.

But how did it happen? What combination of factors permitted him to have this experience during a session at this particular instant in time, to grasp the moment and take it as his own, and to then use the experience as a transition point in his growth? Although I can say little that might qualify as an answer to these questions, two issues are relevant as speculations. For one thing, it had already become increasingly difficult for him to use his inner world as a secure hiding place. Our ongoing struggle over his detachment during sessions was becoming an internalized experience from which he could not escape but had not yet fully addressed with me. My approach of underlining his moments of greatest detachment had already begun to accomplish its aim, leaving him no longer able to retreat into a reverie state and remain peacefully unconflicted with regard to his silence.[6] At this point he had already begun to process his own silences as violations of his stated agreement to try to disclose all his experience as it occurred, regardless of its nature, and he could not free himself from the *internal* imperative of this task by using my silence as tacit

---

[6]The approach to which I refer here is the subject of an earlier paper (Bromberg, 1984) on schizoid processes and the value of Freud's basic rule of free association as the patient's "absorbing errand," which gradually requires him increasingly to engage the immediate transferential context as a voluntary act, rather than being "pulled" into it as a continued schizoid compromise maintained by a pseudoexploration of content.

permission to avoid experiencing his own. In other words, because he was now unable to detach from my presence emotionally when he needed to avoid anxiety, he was forced to confront my existence as a real person within his inner world and thereby felt his own existence as violated and diminished—an inner drama in which one of us had to submit to the will of the other.

This scenario of forced submission followed by self-righteous indignation had recently been a powerful theme through which our relationship was represented in his unconscious fantasy life but until now had been played out only in disguised form (through his dreams). More recently, however, it had emerged directly in the transferential relationship itself as a consequence of the diminishing effectiveness of his detached state as a means of avoiding the here-and-now. He had stated his own view of the matter a short time earlier as follows: "I resent the fact that you can just sit there knowing that I can't stay silent, and that I now have to think about the fact that I'm not saying anything. Anything I can think of to say is so trivial it's embarrassing, but it's now also embarrassing not to say anything. I even resent saying *this*." In this light, the Isakower session might justifiably be seen as a continued working-through of the same issue, but at a level that reactivated and integrated some of the earliest and most deeply buried aspects of its mental representation.

Why, then, did it play itself out in a manner that freed him to exist as a person in his own right, instead of taking the form of an act of rebelliousness or subtle exhibitionism? Looking back on that session, I suspect that a gradual shift in the transference had already occurred of which I was unaware at the time and that this shift enabled him to trust both me and my genuine regard for his autonomy despite my "tough" analytic stance. The relationship providing the wellspring for this transition that comes most readily to mind is the one with his younger sister and even raises the possibility that something as seemingly minor as my own "innocence" during the Isakower session might have played a major role in shaping its meaning for him as a turning point. On that occasion I was the wide-eyed, naive child, and he the sophisticated expert, helpful and playfully amused by my genuine amazement. It was one night later that he noticed he was no longer behaving like the innocent child, averting his eyes from the television screen. If this element of my "innocence" was indeed significant, perhaps it reaffirms not only the importance of maintaining a consistent attitude of curiosity, but also that the most genuine definition of analytic technique may be what I have called "hindsight in the service of the ego."

DREAMS, DAYDREAMS, AND REALITY

During the remainder of Mr. C's analysis, much of what had been worked on in the earlier phase of treatment surfaced again in a richer, more integrated context and as an active, analyzable aspect of the transference. He was a prolific dreamer and had flooded the analysis with dreams for a long time. The self-protective function of the delugelike quality in his dreaming had been much explored, as had the expressive function, but the work in this area typically felt as unalive and as unconvincing as the man himself. The dreams, in contrast, were alive to the point of bursting, filled with shimmering meaning and begging to be analyzed. Early in treatment they seemed to be the only channel Mr. C could use to structure his unformulated experience of our relationship in an ongoing way. What we did with each other as we dealt with his dreams in one session became the latent content of his dream life in the next session, with never a direct or overt sign that he consciously registered an interaction going on between us other than in his dutiful responses when I would probe for one. During this period of work, the dreams seemed more a source of raw material through which reality was to be constructed than a channel through which it was revealed.

His earliest dreams in treatment were traumatic, chaotic, archaic, and often bizarre, filled with images of his severely damaged sense of self and his terrifying vulnerability to the world as embodied in the strange situation called psychoanalysis. There were dreams of gouged-out eyeballs speeding past his field of vision, calves whose throats had been cut out by the milkmaid but who were unaware of what had happened to them, and radio programs that suddenly became real, leaving him nowhere to hide. Night terrors were not infrequent—all too real dreams of being devoured by cats, which had been peaceful house pets on a beautiful tropical island but without warning became creatures out of hell. In one ghastly metaphor after another, the voice of the dreamer screamed in terror as it received sadistic, talionic self-punishment for attempting to reveal the existence of dissociated reality in Mr. C's past and personality. It was as if the dreamer were signaling: "To preserve my sanity and emotional survival, the dangerous organs of seeing, knowing, and speaking shall be once again torn away." In fact, that is precisely what began to take place.

As this phase of treatment progressed, Mr. C's schizoid defenses against his dissociated sadistic rage became more pronounced. It was then that the analysis began to take the form of what Guntrip (1969) has described as a "schizoid compromise." The nature of his character structure, not the uncontrollable and traumatically sadistic quality of his reality, became the core of his dream imagery. Dreams of watching movies abounded. Dreams of prisons and concentration camps were frequent, but always created with guards who looked the other way while he briefly escaped. As he put it: "It didn't matter that I would eventually have to go back; the fact that I got out *at all* was rubbing their noses in it, and that was the real freedom." During this period of the analysis, it was difficult for me to manage my continued feeling of helplessness in response to his somnolent state of consciousness without becoming overly active in order to feel alert and productive. My words were taken in by him readily and hungrily, but they entered only his "false mouth"—an invisible anatomical lining within his real mouth, created in one of his dreams. His mouth was actually "false" in both meanings of the word; it was false both in what it emitted and in what it appeared to receive.

It was the reexperience of the Isakower phenomenon that seemed to usher in a new stage of the analysis. Even his dreams took on a different character. They were clearly recognizable as belonging to no one but Mr. C, but now *he* was alive as well as the dream content. He spoke openly and spontaneously of his wish to remain "asleep" on the analytic couch so as to avoid direct contact with me, and of his fear of revealing his anger (not yet brought into sessions) at having to follow *my* rules in such matters as the use of the couch and payment for missed hours.

His wish to be able to return to his formerly schizoid state of half-deadness and his inability to do so were represented by a dream in which he decided it was time to die, but when he lay down in his grave he did not feel as if he were dying. In the dream he became afraid that the cemetery caretaker (a figure resembling me) might cover him with dirt while he was still alive, so he got up out of the grave and began to walk toward a distant town. I had no difficulty in empathizing with either my own role as the caretaker who heaps words on his passive body or with his role of wishing he could deaden himself when he wanted to—particularly when he mentioned that the date of his death inscribed on the tombstone was April 15, the date income taxes are due.

As in his real life, Mr. C's progress in the analytic process was characterized at this point not by a sudden or dramatic shift from a state of half-sleep to a state of full engagement, but by a lengthy transitional period during which he did with me what he did with the Isakower phenomenon: lying on the couch in a half-awake state; playing with my potentially smothering ideas as they approached him, pushing them away, looking at them from different perspectives, challenging them with ideas of his own; and gradually using the total interpersonal context in a creative act that more and more felt as if it belonged to both of us. In this manner the analysis approached what could be considered the final phase, in which the "false mouth" and his use of detachment to avoid life were felt by him as ego alien. In his outside life, his relationships both personally and professionally had become richer and more fulfilling, and he anticipated marriage to a woman with whom he had been living for more than a year. With regard to the analytic process, he had reached the point where he could not only take in my words without anxiety, but also no longer attributed any magical power to them. His own use of language was therefore employed less as a shield to neutralize the other person's potentially traumatic impact (cf. Sullivan, 1973, pp. 229–283) and became more available as a genuine expression of his own personality in the context of full emotional involvement in the external world.

His daydreams, for example, became alive to him and a subject of his own curiosity. "I became aware over the weekend, while taking a walk," he said, "that my daydreams really prevent me from seeing what's around me, and I realized that I don't daydream when I'm at home. It struck me that my daydreams perform the function of screening out the outside world in the same way that reading or watching T.V. does it when I'm home. The reason I don't need the daydreams when I'm there is that I'm already in my apartment with the blinds down. In my daydreams I'm usually exploding at some situation in the real world that I might get into, and I'm full of righteous anger at being taken advantage of, and I'm telling them off. Its like walking down the street writing somebody's political speech except that the speech is in me. I also thought that my daydreams might have the same purpose as my dreams at night. I can deal with the real world in my head but still stay asleep to it out there and not have to really get involved with anybody."

This insight was achieved and articulated by Mr. C while he was in the midst of recovering some very early primal scene memories and disclosing some vivid fantasies associated with them. It struck me shortly thereafter that what Mr. C was attempting to deal with there in bits and pieces resonated closely with Lewin's (1950, 1952, 1953) conceptualization and description of the function of dreaming and the relationship between the primal scene and what he refers to as the "oral triad"—the wish to eat, to be eaten, and to sleep. In claustrophobia, Lewin (1950) suggests, "the fantasy of being within the mother's body, there to eat and sleep, is a displacement downward and inward of the wish to eat and sleep at the breast." He states:

I propose an additional, and perhaps essential factor: namely the wish to sleep is a repetition of nursing and a defense against the disturbance of the primal scene. . . . Because the primal scene interferes with the course of sleep, it reactivates the whole oral triad. This may be studied in certain insomnias. The sleeplessness can be traced back to the primal scene experiences, but the problem of going to sleep is expressed in oral terms. The patient manifests a continual hunger of one sort or another. . . . and the insomnia of the primal scene is equated unconsciously to the sleeplessness of an unfed baby. The patient wishes to eat so that he may sleep, and the insomnia of the primal scene gets put into the terminology of the nursing process. . . . The first line of defense against the primal scene stimuli at their origin is sound sleep, a complete repetitive success of the oral procedure of nursing. The secondary defense, after some penetration of the stimuli, would be a dream, a guarding of sleep by the oneiric neutralization of the intruders [pp. 120–121].

Mr. C's bedtime pattern had been to eat until he felt bloated—he was unable to sleep if he felt the least bit empty—and then enter his bed and fixate on the television screen until he was totally exhausted. At other times he would fight sleep with obsessive rumination until he finally succumbed to overwhelming fatigue. The transitional period between the waking state and sleep had always been harnessed with the tightest rein possible and until this point in his life was designed as an experience in which looking without seeing would lead to sleeping without falling asleep.

THE PRIMAL SCENE AND THE TERMINAL SCENE

For Mr. C, the "seeing" issue was the last to be resolved during the course of a stormy and confrontational termination phase. The question of termination had emerged in a way he perceived as overly authoritarian on my part because the subject had been overtly initiated by me rather than by him. He felt that for me to raise the issue first was equivalent to a "command" that impinged on his right to leave when "he felt ready." At about this same time he had paid several visits to an optometrist to replace his thick eyeglasses with new, more flattering contact lenses. He had come to view the old glasses as a kind of prosthesis—an artificial addition to his body, similar to his metaphorical "false mouth"—which made him look harmless and thus served the function of protecting him from potentially harmful people whom he could not clearly see. The contact lenses, however, were quite another matter. They were openly associated with the wish to see as a statement of potency, sexual attractiveness, and manifest sexual initiative.[7] It was in the context of having the lenses made that the wish to see, to be seen, and to act became, in his sense of self, compatible with the developmentally earlier triad—the wish to eat, to be eaten, and to sleep. He experienced, for the first time while in treatment, intense anger toward a male figure of authority while in that person's presence. Mr. C felt that there was something wrong with the lenses and with my raising the issue of termination, and that in both cases he was being prevented from "seeing" as well as he potentially could. His anger was directed simultaneously toward the optometrist and toward me, and, in this final phase of the work, its previously uncontrollable and sadistic quality was gradually worked through and integrated as normally assertive, authoritative self-expression. He was able, in each relationship, to feel his own impact on resolving the issue with the other person to a conclusion that he was able to accept even though he felt it as less than "perfect."

Transferentially, the same elements were operating here that had been at issue all along—oral conflict, erotic wishes, and fear of parental authority—but now there was a sense of self that was sufficiently individuated to enlist his anger in the service of his own growth. It was even possible now to see the interplay between the various levels of conflict as expressed through his relationships with each parent and with his sister. At the level of oral deprivation, he was the infant who felt that his being was in control of a maternal figure who was unresponsive to it, not an ungiving maternal figure, but one who disregarded his unique identity and gave when she decided something was needed. It is in this sense that the Isakower phenomenon is, of course, the breast, but it is also an interpersonal phenomenon, as in Mr. C's symbolic and creative effort to master his early precognitive experience with his mother around the *act* of feeding. His lifelong hopelessness paralleled his chronic feeling of impotency in his interchanges with the external world. At the oral level, the world embodied a mother who, if he was not self-protected and self-fed, would suffocate him when he was already full because she felt he should be hungry or would starve him when he was empty

---

[7]Fink (1967), reporting on one of her own patients who experienced the Isakower phenomenon five times during analytic sessions, mentions the striking fact that "the first two reports of the phenomenon came in two consecutive sessions in which the patient wore his contact lenses in the session, something he rarely did, and which he associated with potency and sexual looking" (p. 238). Like Mr. C, the patient described by Fink subsequently elaborated a rich associative context of primal scene fantasies and memories.

because she felt he should not *still* be hungry. This level of experience was vivid in his perception of me around the issue of termination and in his perception of the optometrist around the issue of whether the lenses still needed further correction.

At the level of oedipal experience and primal scene fantasy, the two male figures were seen by him as replicating the way in which he had felt treated by his autocratic, insecure, competitive father. "I know what's best for you" was the communication he heard again, but at this level he heard it as a retaliation for the way he was using his new visual clarity. He was using it both sexually and aggressively and had started to look at me and say what he saw, in the same way he perceived me using my own vision. What had made the primal scene so singularly terrifying for Mr. C was not simply that he had slept in his parents' bedroom for the first six years of his life; it was that he could organize what he saw and what he fantasied only into a rigid interpersonal frame of reference that had nothing to do with two people doing something together that was fun, exciting, and mutually satisfying. Nothing in Mr. C's relationship to either parent would have led him to believe that something mutually respectful of one another's identity was going on. Since in his experience one person had to be submitting to the will of another, his oedipal fantasies would be inevitably terrifying because he already felt "preoedipally castrated" as a person. Trauma was built upon trauma, with no developmentally secure interpersonal context except the relationship with his younger sister, whose birth had probably provided the nexus for therapeutic hope.

Regardless of the inviting developmental smorgasbord that was always available in the content of the sessions, the crucial dimensions of meaning were, during the early phase of the analysis, structural rather than dynamic. What mattered in his personality growth had been determined not simply by phase-specific psychosexual conflict defined by unmet oral needs or oedipal castration anxiety. What most influenced his early development as well as the course of his analytic treatment was the question of what structural level of mental representation existed in which new phase-appropriate interpersonal experience could be accommodated. For a long time this instability in his representational world framed the degree to which he could process and own a full range of human emotions without burying himself in the only source of security he trusted—his inner stage and the dyadically structured scenario it provided (cf. Balint, 1968).

The end of Mr. C's treatment can be summarized by a dream he reported three months prior to the agreed-upon date of termination. Like the analysis itself, the dream did not tie up all the loose ends but conveyed his new sense of hope, potency, and security in the outside world, as well as his resentment that he had to surrender his old sources of self-aggrandizement in order to achieve it. It also conveyed a genuine feeling of sadness at the loss of our relationship.

> He was being visited in his apartment by some important childhood friends whom he wanted to both impress and cook dinner for, but his apartment was too dimly lit. Accompanied by his friends, he went out in search of a brighter light bulb and encountered a variety of obstacles, which they, as a group, were able to deal with successfully and aggressively. At last, dirty but exhilarated, they returned with the bulb. He replaced it, and the apartment was filled with light and looked lovely. But by this time the friends had run out of time and could not stay for dinner. They were happy to have seen him and to have gone on this adventure with him but were now ready to go about their own business. ("There was this terrible frustration," he commented in session, "that they were going to leave and couldn't stay for dinner. I wanted so much for them to be there longer. I went through all this stuff to let more light in, but when I finally did it, it was too late. By that time the people from my past were beyond being impressed.")

During the final three months before the agreed-upon termination date, each of the "old" themes resurfaced with an uncanny realness, as though he were living out a shadowy replica of the same uncertainty that had characterized his parents' conflict about how to do the "right thing." Was the termination perhaps premature? Was I, like his friends in the dream, "leaving too soon," perhaps to preserve my role as the analyst who, except for rare and dramatic occasions, is "beyond being impressed"? If so, was I unwittingly enacting the father's unconscious wish to "throw him out" of the bedroom just as he was becoming old enough to see me clearly and challenge me? Or was I perhaps playing out the role of the mother who wished to keep him around only as long as he validated her significance as his ego support; and once I had helped him achieve a full sense of separate identity was I then ready to receive a "new baby" to take his place? Should this uncertainty have been resolved before termination? Could it have been? By my own standards as well as his, the analysis had been a success. Why, then, did his termination process recapitulate the past with such vividness?

Levenson (1976), from the vantage point of what he calls "the aesthetics of termination," proposes that

> one might expect that a patient would terminate more or less in the configurational style within which he operates. One would hope that

the improvement would be evident in that the configuration would be markedly extended and modulated. . . . I would say that it makes no more sense to ask when to terminate than to ask when to die. It is a natural event in the course of therapy [p. 341].

In Mr. C's case, this metaphor is, I think, both apt and ironic. For most of Mr. C's life, asking when to die had indeed made perfect sense to him. Death had always been unconsciously experienced as under his control through his ability to remain detached from life and thus to feel that "living" had not in itself yet begun. As in the dream in which he entered his grave to await his death, it was only in the act of climbing out and seeking the real world, that death, like the eventual culmination of his analysis, could become for better or for worse, part of the natural configuration of life.

REFERENCES

Balint, M. (1968), *The Basic Fault*. New York: International Universities Press.

Blaustein, A. B. (1975), A dream resembling the Isakower phenomenon: A brief clinical contribution. *Internat. J. Psycho-Anal.*, 56:207–208.

Bromberg, P. M. (1979), The schizoid personality: The psychopathology of stability. In: *Integrating Ego Psychology and Object Relations Theory*, ed. L. Saretsky, G. D. Goldman & D. S. Milman. Dubuque, IA: Kendall/Hunt, pp. 226–242.

_____ (1984), Getting into oneself and out of one's self: On schizoid processes. *Contemp. Psychoanal.*, 20:439–448.

Broughton, R. J. (1968), Sleep disorders: Disorders of arousal? *Science*, 159:1070–1078.

Dickes, R. (1965), The defensive function of an altered state of consciousness: A hypnoid state. *J. Amer. Psychoanal. Assn.*, 13:356–403.

Easson, W. M. (1973), The earliest ego development, primitive memory traces, and the Isakower phenomenon. *Psychoanal. Quart.*, 42:60–72.

Fairbairn, W. R. D. (1940), Schizoid factors in the personality. In: *Psychoanalytic Studies of the Personality*. London: Routledge & Kegan Paul, pp. 3–27.

Feiner, A. H. (1979), Countertransference and the anxiety of influence. In: *Counter-transference*, ed. L. Epstein & A. H. Feiner. New York: Aronson, pp. 105–128.

Fink, G. (1967), Analysis of the Isakower phenomenon. *J. Amer. Psychoanal. Assn.*, 15:231–293.

Fisher, C., Byrne, J. V., Edwards, A. & Kahn, E. (1970), A psychophysiological study of nightmares. *J. Amer. Psychoanal. Assn.*, 18:747–782.

_____ , Kahn, E., Edwards, A. & Davis, D. (1974), A psychophysiological study of nightmares and night terrors. In: *Psychoanalysis and Contemporary Science, Vol. 3*, ed. L. Goldberger & V. Rosen. New York: International Universities Press, pp. 317–398.

Garma, A. (1955), Vicissitudes of the dream screen and the Isakower phenomenon. *Psychoanal. Quart.* 24:369–383.

Guntrip, H. J. S. (1969), *Schizoid Phenomena, Object Relations, and the Self*. New York: International Universities Press.

Heilbrunn, G. (1953), Fusion of the Isakower phenomenon with the dream screen. *Psychoanal. Quart.*, 22:200–204.

Isakower, O. (1938), A contribution to the patho-psychology of phenomena associated with falling asleep. *Internat. J. Psycho-Anal.*, 19:331–345.

Levenson, E. A. (1976), The aesthetics of termination. *Contemp. Psychoanal.*, 12:338–342.

Lewin, B. D. (1946), Sleep, the mouth, and the dream screen. *Psychoanal. Quart.*, 15:419–434.

———— (1948), Inferences from the dream screen. *Internat. J. Psycho-Anal.*, 29:224–231.

———— (1950), *The Psychoanalysis of Elation.* New York: Norton.

———— (1952), Phobic symptoms and dream interpretation. *Psychoanal. Quart.*, 21:295–322.

———— (1953), Reconsideration of the dream screen. *Psychoanal. Quart.*, 22:174–199.

Mahler, M. S. (1968), *On Human Symbiosis and the Vicissitudes of Individuation.* New York: International Universities Press.

Rycroft, C. (1951), A contribution to the study of the dream screen. *Internat. J. Psycho-Anal.*, 32:178–184.

Silberer, H. (1909), A method of producing and observing symbolic hallucinations. In: *Organization and Pathology of Thought,* ed. D. Rapaport. New York: Columbia University Press, 1951, pp. 195–207.

Sperling, O. E. (1957), A psychoanalytic study of hypnogogic hallucinations. *J. Amer. Psychoanal. Assn.*, 5:115–123.

———— (1961), Variety and analyzability of hypnogogic hallucinations and dreams. *Internat. J. Psycho-Anal.*, 42:216–223.

Stern, M. M. (1961), Blank hallucinations: Remarks about trauma and perceptual disturbances. *Internat. J. Psycho-Anal.*, 42:205–215.

Sullivan, H. S. (1953), *The Interpersonal Theory of Psychiatry.* New York: Norton.

———— (1973), *Clinical Studies in Psychiatry.* New York: Norton.

Tauber, E. S. & Green, M. R. (1959), *Prelogical Experience.* New York: Basic Books.

Winnicott, D. W. (1971), *Playing and Reality.* New York: Basic Books.

13

Eros Reclaimed
Recovering Freud's Relational Theory

STEVEN REISNER

Contemporary psychoanalytic theory has fallen into conflict over the question of the essentials of human motivation and the nature of desire. Is motivation irreducibly tied to a relational context, within which a self is constituted and differentiated? Or does desire arise from accessions of internal tensions, biological in origin, seeking relief? In recent overviews of the development of psychoanalytic theory (Greenberg and Mitchell, 1983; Eagle, 1984; Mitchell, 1988), these two perspectives have been described as predominant in contemporary psychoanalysis, the latter most often attributed to classical psychoanalytic theory, and the former to a variety of trends that have been grouped under the heading relational psychoanalysis (Mitchell, 1988).

The classical "drive/structure model" (Greenberg and Mitchell, 1983) has come to be associated with the legacy of Sigmund Freud. Freudians and anti-Freudians alike attribute to Freud a world view in which human interaction is described as secondary to drive tension, and psychic development is seen as motivated by the urge to reduce, defend against, or sublimate this endogenous drive energy. In a "Freudian" world, we are said to love those who reduce our discomfort and hate those who cause us tension.

In a recent article (Reisner, 1991), I argued that the metapsychology of drive tensions attributed to Freud is a narrowed and distorted view of his theories advanced by his followers, particularly A. Freud (1936), Fenichel (1945), Hartmann (1948), and Rapaport (1960a, 1960b), and that the rejection of Freud's ostensive metapsychology by

281

the group of theorists that emerged from the school of ego psychology (Gill, 1976; Holt, 1976; G. Klein, 1976; Schafer, 1976) can be
more correctly understood as the rejection of Freud's followers'
codification of that metapsychology. I argued further that those
aspects of Freud's theory which had been denuded by his followers
are precisely those which are most compatible with the seemingly
contradictory views offered by contemporary psychoanalytic theorists.

In this chapter, I make the case that throughout Freud's writings
there can be discerned a relational thread that is distinct from the
drive-discharge model traditionally attributed to him. Freud's theories have invariably benefited from an internal dialectic between the
influences of relational experience (and the subjective meaning derived from these influences) as well as those of bodily and genetic
tensions. However, the relational aspect of Freud's work has been
edited, reinterpreted, and often omitted altogether by the advocates
of classical psychoanalysis, in the interest of saving psychoanalysis
from Freud's "distracting" extra-analytical ideas (Rapaport, 1960b, p.
869). It is my aim to reclaim this relational side of Freud, and with it
a more richly textured foundation for contemporary psychoanalytic
theorizing.

Foremost among Freud's incontrovertibly relational concepts is that
of *Eros*, the "mischief-maker" (Freud, 1923, p. 59), the "instinct of
love" (Freud, 1933a, p. 209). This concept stands in marked contrast
with the presuppositions of the classical drive model: Eros represents
an urge *for* psychic tension and *for* the interrelationship of all living
things. In Eros, Freud (1920) posited love as one of the irreducible
primal human motivations that supersedes the pleasure principle. It
is not surprising, therefore, that this concept has not survived into
contemporary accounts of Freud's psychoanalytic theory;[1] it is antithetical to the received version of that theory.

It has been argued by classical psychoanalysts that Freud's final
dual-drive theory, of Eros and the death–drive, is an unnecessary
diversion from his essentially monistic, drive-discharge view of
motivation (Fenichel, 1945, p. 60). Those who reject the Freudian
view see this development similarly: "the essential assumption that
motivation is derived ultimately from endogenously arising, biologically determined drive is maintained" (Greenberg and Mitchell, 1983,
p. 64). In what follows, I will be arguing that, on the contrary, a full
appreciation of the development of the concept of Eros requires a

---

[1]References to Eros are not to be found in the basic textbooks of psychoanalysis, that
is, not in Fenichel (1945), Brenner (1973), or Zetzel and Meissner (1973).

complete rethinking of the "drive" theory that preceded it,[2] and furthermore, that through the understanding of Eros, we may recover the relational thread that stands alongside the traditional concept of drive and weaves through all of Freud's writings.

WHAT IS EROS?

Freud introduced the concept of Eros in *Beyond the Pleasure Principle* (1920), alongside that of the death instinct, or Thanatos. He described it as the drive to "establish greater unities among living things" (Freud, 1940). It has its manifestations in "sexual union with sexual intercourse as its aim . . . in self-love . . . love for parents and children, friendship and love for humanity" (Freud, 1921, p. 90). Its "purpose is to combine single human individuals, and after that families, then races, peoples and nations into one great unity, the unity of mankind" (Freud, 1930, p. 122). Where Thanatos represents the force in living substances that strives to "undo connections and so destroy things" (Freud, 1940, p. 148), human sexuality, according to Freud (1920), "coincides with the Eros of the poets and philosophers which holds living things together" (p. 50).

In this new dual-drive theory, particularly in highlighting the role of Eros, Freud made a number of apparent emendations to his view of the drives. Each of these represents a view of motivation distinct from the economic principles of traditional psychoanalytic metapsychology.

The traditional view of Freud's drive theory asserts that a drive is the psychic result of a build-up of endogenous tension, motivating the mind to action in the interest of reducing that tension. In the new theory, only one of the two drives could be seen to function in this

---

[2]It is essential to begin this rethinking with a challenge to the traditional understanding of what Freud meant by "drive." Freud referred to the drive concept as "our mythology" (1933b, p. 95) and the language of psychoanalysis as "figurative" (1920, p. 60). He referred to the languages of biology and physics as equally metaphorical, as in his letter to Einstein: "It may perhaps seem to you as though our theories are a kind of mythology. . . . But does not every science come in the end to a kind of mythology like this? Cannot the same be said to-day of your own Physics?" (Freud, 1933a, p. 211). Laplanche and Pontalis (1973) have been most clearly critical of those who would attribute a biological origin to Freud's concept of drive: "Far from postulating—as the instinct theorists so readily do—that behind each type of activity there lies a corresponding biological force, Freud places all instinctual manifestations under the head of a basic antagonism. What is more, this antagonism is derived from the mythical tradition: first, between Hunger and Love, and later between Love and Discord" (p. 216).

manner. Thanatos alone strove toward the "abolition of chemical tension, that is to say, to death." Eros, or libido, "*increases those tensions,* introducing what may be described as 'vital differences' " (Freud, 1920, p. 55, italics added). By 1923, Freud depicted the "process of life" as a balance between Thanatos, which seeks discharge and death, and Eros which "hold[s] up the falling level and introduce[s] fresh tensions" (p. 47). Freud's final dual–drive theory described motivation explicitly as the interaction of a striving for human relationship, with all its inherent vital tensions, and the longing to be relieved of such contact and to eliminate the tensions that stem from human interaction.

Furthermore, in his new theory, Freud changed the very defining characteristics of the drives, no longer presenting them as resulting from a buildup of tension, but rather as characteristics inherent in living substance. As Leowald (1971a) put it, "Instinct, or instinctual drive, as used in the terms life and death instinct, is no longer a stimulus impinging on the psychic apparatus, which latter seeks to extinguish the results of a stimulation coming from outside the apparatus" (p. 61). Rather, in his revised conceptualization, Freud depicted the drives as an interplay of forces, acting in consonance or in conflict, and aiming toward union and dissolution of living things. As Leowald has pointed out, this had consequences for the evolution of the structural model, which, as a result of these changes, had to be seen as responsive to "the interplay of forces and the conflicts within an organization and structuring this organization, in contrast to a theory of an apparatus designed to reduce or eliminate forces or stimuli impinging on it from the outside" (p. 62).

Finally, Freud transformed what he viewed as the prime, underlying psychic motivation from economics to *conservation.* He stated in *Beyond the Pleasure Principle* that "an instinct is an urge inherent in organic life to restore an earlier state of things" (Freud, 1920, p. 36). Freud asserted that Thanatos sought the restoration of an earlier inorganic state; whereas "Eros, by bringing about a more and more far-reaching combination of particles into which the living substance is dispersed, aims at complicating life and at the same time preserving it. Acting in this way, both the instincts would be conservative in the strictest sense of the word, since both would be endeavoring to reestablish a state of things that was disturbed by the emergence of life" (1923, p. 40). If the old pleasure principle survived at all in this reformulation, according to Freud (1920), it was not in response to a build-up of tension, but rather as part of the conservative nature of Thanatos: "The pleasure principle seems actually to serve the death instincts" (p. 63).

Freud (1920) presented his reformulation of drive theory tentatively at first: "I am not convinced myself and I do not seek to persuade others to believe in them" (p. 59). In *The Ego and the Id*, which Freud (1923) described as "a further development of some trains of thought which I opened up in *Beyond the Pleasure Principle*" (p. 12), he was not nearly so tentative: "I have lately developed a view of the instincts which I shall here hold to and take as the basis of my further discussions" (p. 40). By 1930, Freud was deeply committed to these new ideas, saying that "in the course of time they have taken such a hold on me that I can no longer think in any other way" (p. 170). In fact, he held firmly to these views of the drives for the last 19 years of his life, roughly half of his career as a psychoanalyst and theorist. Yet the theory of Eros and Thanatos is the only one in psychoanalysis that has been rejected out of hand by those who consider themselves most loyal to Freud and his theory. On what basis were these concepts, so central to Freud's thinking, repudiated by his followers?

Ostensibly, it was only the death drive that was being discarded; Rapaport (1957) put it most succinctly: "[Freud's] death instinct is as dead as a doornail" (p. 683). Hartmann (1948) based his rejection on the notion that the death drive is primarily a biological, rather than a psychological, concept: "These concepts are of a different order . . . [and] have to be proved or disproved biologically; . . . so far [they] have not added much to our understanding of the specific functions of drives (in the psychological sense)" (p. 72).

Brenner (1982) took the opposite point of view, arguing that the concept may make sense psychologically, but not biologically: "In men's minds, life and death are indeed polar opposites; not so biologically" (p. 17).

Each of these attacks can be understood to follow from Fenichel's early and most sustained critique of the concept. According to Fenichel (1945), a death instinct simply "would not be compatible with the approved biological concept of instinct" (p. 60). Fenichel attempted to use Freud against himself, paraphrasing Freud's own definition of drive from "Instincts and Their Vicissitudes":

> Instinctual need . . . begins in a somatic "instinctual source," which makes the psychological system excitable; . . . the instinctual action then results in changes at this source which are equivalent to a "discharge" of the excitation—that is, a relaxation of tension. A "death instinct" does not fit in with such a definition of instinct [Fenichel, 1935, p. 366].

It appears that, for Fenichel, it was the notion that the drive is motivational in and of itself, without a tension build-up, that was perceived to require rebuttal. It must be noted that in terms of the death drive this distinction is a minor one. Thanatos may not be the result of a tension build-up, but its aim of discharge of tension is not so far from the "approved" concept as to require so sustained and pronounced a critique. In fact, Fenichel admitted as much: "Indeed the concept of the 'Nirvana principle' as a point of departure does in fact permit a unitary view, not only of all psychological processes, but also of all life processes in general" (p. 366).[3]

If in fact the death drive is not incompatible with the "approved biological concept," on what basis did Fenichel and virtually all others of Freud's followers reject it? It was the notion that there might be a drive which *opposed* the Nirvana principle which Fenichel (1935) rejected:

> It cannot be that the "Nirvana principle" holds for one instinct, while the "craving for stimulus" holds for another; the craving for stimulus must be derived on genetic-dialectic lines from the Nirvana principle [p. 367].

In other words, although classical theorists have been most vociferous in their rejection of the death drive, it was really Freud's life drive, Eros, that was being rejected.

The rejection of Thanatos, I believe, is a theoretical smokescreen that has obscured the more profound threat to the classical view of psychoanalysis: the view that sexuality and libido are part of a drive for human interrelationship which seeks, innately, the creative tension of mutuality, and that these erotic forces are *opposed* by the striving for the reduction of tension. As Leowald (1988) has put it, "I cannot emphasize enough that it was the introduction of the idea of the life instinct (which encompassed different conceptions of pleasure and of the pleasure principle) that was a true and unsettling innovation in psychoanalytic theory" (p. 30). Laplanche (1989), too, states that the "innovation of 1915–1920 is not the death drive but the life drive" (p. 146).

If Eros and Thanatos have survived at all in classic psychoanalytic theory, they have survived denuded of their meaning in Freud's eyes. Eros was not criticized, it was co-opted. When Eros is discussed in the classical literature, it is as a synonym for libido in the original sense.

---

[3]Many have noted the compatibility of the concept of Thanatos with the classical view of the drives. As Laplanche (1989) has put it, "the death drive is not a fundamentally new innovation" (1989, p. 146). See also Leowald (1971b): "insofar as the death instinct can be equated with the constancy-inertia-unpleasure principle, the death instinct is nothing startlingly new in Freud's theory" (pp. 123–124).

Thanatos has been reduced to the "aggressive" drive. Each of these continue to be described as if *Beyond the Pleasure Principle* had never been written. They both are seen as derived from a build-up of somatic tension; the reduction of that tension is perceived as pleasurable (Brenner, 1973).[4]

It is my view that so much effort has gone into the rejection and redefinition of Freud's final drive theory because *if accepted as Freud intended, these views would require a radical rethinking, in relational terms, of the theory that preceded it.*

I believe that some variant of what was to become Eros was represented in Freud's psychoanalytic writings from the very beginning, and that Freud's endeavor was always to find a way to integrate a dualistic theory, combining endogenous motivation with others derived from the vicissitudes of human interrelationship.

Throughout Freud's writings, he presented a series of psychoanalytic axioms that he promptly undermined, often within the same paragraph, invariably within the same text. Casey (1990) termed this tendency in Freud's work "auto-deconstruction," citing it as the essential form of Freud's (1920) polemic in *Beyond the Pleasure Principle:* "When a text auto-deconstructs . . . it complicates or qualifies itself in such a way as to put into question a thesis already announced expressly in the same text" (p. 243). Essential psychoanalytic postulates which can be seen to autodeconstruct regularly in Freud's texts include the concepts conscious/unconscious; pleasure/unpleasure principle; and certainly the concept of the drive.

There is a consistency to this process that is worth noting. Each concept is presented initially as a postulate of the science of psychoanalysis, a science of psychic forces and energies that can be described economically, dynamically and topographically. From this point of view, consciousness is differentiated from unconsciousness on the basis of a quantity of psychic tensions that cannot be discharged due to conflict; the pleasure principle responds to the unpleasure experienced when psychic tension reaches a certain threshold and must be reduced; the drive is a continuously flowing endosomatic source of stimulation that aims at its own quiescence.

Freud's textual "autodeconstruction" consists of an undermining of

---

[4]In addition to revising the dual drive theory, Freud (1924) revised his conceptualization of the pleasure principle. Ultimately, what had been described as the pleasure principle became renamed as the Nirvana principle (the urge to reduce tension to zero). "Pleasure and unpleasure cannot be referred to an increase or decrease of quantity . . . but on some characteristic . . . which we can only describe as a qualitative one" (p. 160). This revision, connected as it is with the redefinition of the drive concept, has also been side-stepped by the classical psychoanalytic theorists (e.g., Brenner, 1973).

each of these concepts by examining them from a perspective that stands in opposition to the scientistic[5] one: he examines the effects of human relationship on psychic processes and presents the result as a corollary (at times contradictory) series of postulates. Thus, Freud adds to the concepts of consciousness and unconsciousness the notions of ego and repressed (Freud, 1900) and later the structural model of id, ego and superego (Freud, 1923). The former is constituted by the vicissitudes of desire, the latter by identification. Similarly, the pleasure principle is challenged by the concept of qualities of tension (Freud, 1905a, 1920), the yearning to reexperience the pleasurable tensions of relationship (Freud, 1905a, 1914a, 1920), and the pleasure derived from the pain of masochism (1920, 1924). Finally, the drive concept is repeatedly autodeconstructed in response to the subjective experience of longing for the absent object (Freud, 1900), by the concepts of "anaclisis" (Freud, 1905a; see Laplanche, 1976), narcissism (Freud, 1914a), and ultimately, Eros (Freud, 1920).

It was primarily these relational aspects of Freud's theory that were excised by his loyal followers in their attempt to present a consistent, "scientific" psychoanalysis. The concept of Eros was ignored by Freud's followers, not because it was inconsistent with Freud's theory, but because it restored to prominence precisely what the Freudians were trying to delete: the irreducible striving for human interrelationship side by side with the press of endogenous tensions seeking discharge.

In what follows, I make the case that the concept of Eros did not arise fully formed and independently from Freud's earlier work, but rather was the natural culmination of a relational self-critique evident throughout his writings. I focus on what orthodoxy has offered as the three turning points in classical drive theory: the so-called abandonment of the seduction hypothesis of 1897, the articulation of the infantile sexual drive of 1905, and the most often cited representation of classical drive theory, the metapsychology of 1915. I choose these moments in Freud's development precisely because they are most closely associated with the classical view of Freud's work. Yet under close scrutiny each turning point, I believe, has been interpreted narrowly in the literature. A full appreciation of Freud's subtle and complex texts reveals a constancy of reflexive reevaluation, placing the nature of human relationship, experience and longing alongside

---

[5] 'Scientism' means science's belief in itself: that is, the conviction that we can no longer understand science as *one* form of possible knowledge, but rather must identify knowledge with science" (Habermas, 1972, p. 4).

the more traditional presentation of endogenous tension seeking discharge.

THE SEDUCTION HYPOTHESIS

All psychoanalysts, whether they are classical or not, assert that the changes in his theory that Freud announced on September 21, 1897 irreversibly dictated the course of psychoanalytic thinking for years to come.

Classical theorists believe that psychoanalysis began when Freud realized that he was mistaken in his belief that parental seduction evoked sexuality in the infant; without this insight, he would not have been able to understand that sexuality was an innate force that produced wishes for sexual release. Arlow (1956), for example, stated that were it not for this reversal, "man's knowledge of the hidden depths of his mind might have been arrested at this point" (p. 31).

Coming from a very different perspective, Mitchell (1988) made the case that Freud's abandoning the seduction hypothesis mistakenly turned psychoanalysis away from the influence of relationship on the developing psyche: "The seduction hypothesis had placed the individual . . . in a social context. . . . With the abandonment of the theory of infantile seduction, other people, the cultural context, recede far into the background" (p. 43).

It is the received view that prior to September 21, 1897, Freud's emphasis was primarily environmental and that, rather suddenly, he came to believe that he had underestimated the importance of fantasies based on endogenous sexual tension. This paved the way, the argument goes, for the development of a psychoanalytic theory which "laid emphasis on infantile sexuality, on the centrality of the instincts as the agency of fantasy formation and as the source of the dynamic properties of the mental apparatus" (Zetzel and Meissner, 1973, pp. 75–76).

Yet a close reading of Freud's letters and papers during this early period reveals no such radical turnabout in Freud's thinking (See Garcia, 1987; Schimek, 1987; Gediman, 1991). It is certainly the case that Freud wrote to his friend Fliess (letter of September 21, 1897, in Masson, 1985), "I no longer believe in my neurotica" (p. 264), but it is not at all clear that from this we can determine that Freud had abandoned his belief in either the veridicality of seduction or the impact of the relational environment on the infant's developing psyche.

Many scholars, Masson (1984) foremost among them, take Freud's "neurotica" to mean his seduction theory; therefore disavowing the "neurotica" is seen as tantamount to disavowing the seduction hypothesis and all its ramifications. A turn to the text and its context may help elucidate to what Freud was referring as his "neurotica" and what impact this pronouncement had on his theoretical development.

In 1895, Breuer and Freud published the *Studies on Hysteria*, wherein the two argued that hysterical symptoms were the result of traumatic memories. In a section of the text written solely by Freud, he indicated his belief that "insofar as one may speak of the determining causes which lead to the *acquisition* of neuroses, their aetiology is to be looked for in *sexual* factors" (p. 257).[6]

His view at the time was that sexuality was associated with a physical "sexual substance" (Draft D, May 1894?, in Masson, 1985, p. 77), which became transformed or translated into a kind of psychical energy. "Actual neuroses" resulted from an overabundance of somatic sexuality, due to a failure in psychic transformation and motor discharge (leading to anxiety neuroses or neurasthenia). "Psychoneuroses" resulted primarily from traumatic exogenous stimulation, which, because of its noxious nature, was incapable of being psychically integrated or discharged (leading to the hysteria, obsessive-compulsive disorders, melancholia):

> the core and mainstay of the whole story remain, of course, the fact that as a result of particular sexual noxae even healthy people can acquire the various forms of neurosis. . . . Sexual affect is of course taken in its broadest sense, as an excitation having a definite quantity [letter to Fliess, May 21, 1985, in Masson, 1985, p. 75].

In the months following the publication of the *Studies*, Freud was confronted with patients' memories of sexual trauma which apparently predated puberty, prior to the period at which Freud believed sexuality began. As he wrote to Fliess on October 8, 1895: "I am on the scent of the following strict precondition for hysteria, namely, that a primary sexual experience (before puberty) . . . must have taken place" (in Masson, 1985, p. 141).

The prospect of prepubertal sexuality presented Freud with a dilemma. If sexuality causes neuroses as a result of psychic transformations in a somatic sexual substance, how could prepubertal sexual experience, that is, before there were such substances, be the cause of a neurosis?

---

[6]Breuer disassociated himself from this aspect of Freud's view, although later he became a supporter of Freud's theory.

Freud acknowledged the conceptual difficulty in "The Aetiology of Hysteria," one of a series of papers (Freud, 1896a,b,c) indicating his belief that sexual involvements in childhood were the cause of the psychoneuroses: "It is true we cannot help asking ourselves how it comes about that the memory of an experience that was innocuous at the time that it happened, should posthumously produce the abnormal effect of leading . . . to a pathological result" (Freud, 1896c, p. 213), but made no attempt to resolve it, stating that, "this is a purely psychological problem, whose solution may perhaps necessitate certain hypotheses about normal psychical processes . . ." (p. 213).

Freud's published work and posthumously published letters from this period indicate that he was attempting to resolve this dilemma in ways standing in stark contrast to the traditional view that his attention during this period was primarily on the influence of environmental events.

His first attempt at resolution was rather ingenious. He argued that sexual trauma preceding puberty may have pathogenic effects following puberty when the memory was revived by an association. This association, by a process of "deferred action," brought about "the release of sexual substances" (Draft I, October 1895?, in Masson, 1985, p. 144) postpuberty, beyond the capacity of the psyche to work over, resulting in a psychoneurosis: "Thanks to the change due to puberty, the memory will display a power that was completely lacking from the event itself" (Freud, 1896a, p. 154).[7]

Late in 1896 and early in 1897, Freud added a number of key concepts to his theory that lessened the impact of the transition of puberty and paved the way for his ultimate resolution of the dilemma: environmental trauma may have pathogenic effects in childhood because even in childhood there is already a potential for sexuality.

As early as May 30, 1896, Freud referred to the sexual experiences of childhood as producing a "surplus of sexuality" (letter to Fliess, December 6, 1896, in Masson, 1985, p. 187) even at age five. He elaborated this concept into a series of sexual "epochs" of childhood, wherein sexuality that is provoked prematurely takes on varied characteristics which may later lead to the different psychoneuroses. Soon afterward, he developed the concept of erotogenic zones of childhood (later to play such an important role): "During childhood sexual release would seem to be obtainable from a great many parts

---

[7]Alternatively, Freud (1894, 1896a) asserted in a series of articles published in the same period that an endogenous build-up of sexual substances postpuberty, with no avenue of discharge or psychic association, resulted in an "actual neurosis."

of the body" (letter to Fliess, December 6, 1896, in Masson, 1985, p. 212). He thus expanded the kind of sexual experiences that had infantile psychic effects. Actual sexual intercourse, or even genital stimulation, was no longer required to stimulate the release of sexuality (as it had been in his published papers).

By 1897, Freud had added the key notion of *hysterical fantasies,* "which regularly, as I see it, go back to things that children overhear at an early age and understand subsequently" (letter to Fliess, April 6, 1897, in Masson, 1985, p. 234). In May, Freud expanded his notion of sexual experience to include not only direct sexual contact, but *sexual scenes* that have been observed or overheard and understood subsequently, as well as sexual *impulses* derived from the primal scenes:

> Everything goes back to the reproduction of scenes. Some can be obtained directly, others by way of fantasies set up in front of them. The fantasies stem from things heard but understood subsequently, and all their material is of course genuine. . . . Their accidental origin is perhaps from masturbation fantasies . . . I realize now that all three [psycho-] neuroses exhibit the same elements (along with the same etiology) — namely, memory fragments, *impulses* (derived from memories) and *protective fictions* [letter to Fliess, May 2, 1897, in Masson, 1985, p. 239].

Thus, as early as May 1897, Freud had given up the notion that hysterics suffered from reminiscences; he replaced it with the view that neuroses were the result of repressed impulses derived from sexual scenes and the fantasies built upon them.

With these developments in mind, the ostensibly radical change heralded in the letter of September 21, 1897, turns out to be nothing of the sort. By this period, actual sexual seduction was no longer a requirement in Freud's theory of the neuroses. If not actual sexual seduction, then to what was Freud referring when he stated "I no longer believe in my neurotica"?[8]

---

[8]It is worth noting that a similar process of abandonment and revival can be detected during this period in Freud's communication to Fliess of his general psychological theory. For example, Freud abandoned his "Psychology for neurologists" (the "Project") in a letter to Fliess in November 29, 1895: "I no longer understand the state of mind in which I hatched the psychology . . . to me it appears to have been a kind of madness" (in Masson, 1985, p. 152). Nonetheless, Freud continued to expand upon these ideas in letters over the next two years and ultimately transformed it from neuropsychology to metapsychology, as the underpinnings of the general psychological theory of Chapter 7 of *The Interpretation of Dreams* (Freud, 1900).

It is best to take with a grain of salt the dramatic pronouncements that appear frequently in Freud's early correspondence. We find in the Fliess letters any number of

Although during this period Freud was enlarging his understanding of the types of experience that may be deemed sexual in
childhood, there was one particular aspect of his neurotica to which
he remained wedded. This was the notion that the source of sexual
overstimulation was invariably the *father*. This developed into his
theory of "paternal etiology" in which he speculated that there was an
intergenerational relationship between perversion and hysteria that
mimicked a genetic component to neurotic processes.

Freud wrote to Fliess on December 6, 1896:

> It seems to me more and more that the essential point of hysteria is that
> it results from *perversion* on the part of the seducer, and *more and more*
> that heredity is seduction by the father. Thus an alternation emerges
> between the generations: 1st generation—perversion; second genera-
> tion—hysteria [in Masson, 1985, p. 212].

Freud (1896b, c) published this concept as "pseudo-heredity" although in his published work he never implicated the father, whereas
in his letters of this period, it was the father alone who was blamed.[9]

I believe that this intergenerational aspect of his theory of the
neurosis was all that remained of the seduction hypothesis in its
original form. And it was this last vestige of what he had originally
referred to as a *"caput Nili* in neuropathology" (Freud, 1896c, p. 203)
which he was giving up in his letter of September 21, 1897: "in all
cases, the *father*, not excluding my own, had to be accused of being
perverse" (in Masson, 1985, p. 264).[10]

It is simply a misreading, albeit a widely held one, to construe this
letter as heralding the abandonment of the impact of environmental
influence on the developing psyche. I believe that the texts make
quite the opposite case: in minimizing the impact of parental seduction, Freud *expanded* the valence of all other interrelational experience.
In abandoning the requirement of a perverse father or parent, Freud

---

abandonments, breakthroughs, fears of being perceived foolishly, and anxiety about
the loss of his friend's love. It should not surprise us, therefore, that, although Freud
ostensibly rejected his "neurotica" during this period, a close reading of his work
reveals continued and repeated reference to the impact of seduction on the developing
psyche up until his death in 1939 (see Reisner, 1991).

[9]Freud did not assert that in each case the father had seduced his own child; it was
enough for the child to have seen or overheard the father in a perverse act with, for
example, a nursemaid (e.g., letter to Fliess, December 6, 1896, in Masson, 1985, p. 213)
for a neurosis to be the result.

[10]Even this abandoned concept was revived soon afterward, in a letter to Fliess dated
December 12, 1897: "My confidence in paternal etiology has risen greatly" (in Masson,
1985, p. 286).

was able to include a much wider variety of childhood experience as educing a sexual response with which the developing psyche must contend. As Freud would later put it: "the 'infantile sexual traumas' were in a sense supplanted by the 'infantilism' of the sexuality in these cases" (Freud, 1905b, p. 277).

The theoretical changes in the months following the ostensive abandonment of the seduction hypothesis, as well as the memories emerging from his self-analysis, show Freud widening still further the scope of environmental experiences coming under the purview of psychoanalysis. For example, of his self analysis, Freud wrote on October 3, 1897:

> [I]n my case the prime originator was an ugly, elderly, but clever woman [Freud is referring to his nursemaid] . . . later, my libido towards *matrem* was awakened . . . on the occasion of a journey . . . during which we must have spent the night together and there must have been an opportunity of seeing her *nudam* [letter to Fliess, October 3, 1897, in Masson, 1985, p. 268].

We see that Freud did not assert that the endogenous build-up of libido caused sexual fantasy, but rather that the wealth of environmental sexual and sensual stimulations evoked the libido. This was made even clearer in Freud's reformulation of the etiology of hysteria in his letter to Fliess of October 27, 1897:

> The infantile character develops during a period of "longing," after the child has been removed from the sexual experiences. Longing is the main character trait of hysteria. . . . During this same period of longing fantasies are formed and masturbation is practiced, which then yields to repression [in Masson, 1985, pp. 274–275].

We can see from this close reading of Freud's writings of 1897 that what is reputed to be his turning away from the relational origins of character and neurosis is something quite different. Freud actually expanded the role of social intercourse and the impact of the interrelational scenes of infancy and childhood. The child's sensuality was seen as easily evoked by his or her parents and caretakers. Not only what was experienced directly but what was heard and seen had its impact on the child's developing character. The child longed for the return of the earlier relationship and developed fantasies and models for future relationships based upon them. In short, where environmental influences had once to be sexually traumatic to have an impact on the developing psyche, now they simply had to be evocative of the child's fantasy and desire. The effect of relational experiences on normal psychology and psychopathology can be seen to have a broadened interaction with endogenous sexuality as a result of these changes.[11]

Even at this early stage certain relational antecedents to what would become the concept of Eros are present: experiences in relationship with others evoked a sensual longing for the repetition of those experiences. Sexuality at this stage was dualistic, derived from both an endogenous sexuality that arises in stages, beginning in infancy, and from the vicissitudes of relational experience, which provides a model for fantasy and longing.

THE THREE ESSAYS

It has been argued (Masson, 1984) that even where Freud continued to espouse the importance of relational experience on psychic development in the months following the abandonment of the seduction theory, this was simply a reflection of a temporary self-doubt. The full renunciation was to come soon thereafter, in Freud's (1905a) *Three Essays on the Theory of Sexuality*.

I am arguing quite the opposite: that the abandonment of the seduction hypothesis can be more accurately understood as Freud's progressive rebalancing of two essential aspects of human motivation, later to become the dual drive theory. On one side is the effect of the press of endogenous forces seeking discharge or transformation; alongside this pressure is invariably another motivation derived from the vicissitudes of relationship.[12]

In *The Interpretation of Dreams*, for example, Freud (1900) sustained and augmented this theory, indicating that, along with character,

---

[11]As Laplanche and Pontalis (1973) have put it: "Apparently, Freud could never resign himself to treating phantasy as the pure and simple outgrowth of the spontaneous sexual life of the child. He is forever searching behind the phantasy, for whatever has founded it in reality. . . . Indeed the first schema presented by Freud, with his theory of seduction, seems to us to epitomize this particular dimension of his thought" (pp. 406–407).

[12]In the text of the *Three Essays* (Freud, 1905a), what has been called Freud's rejection of the seduction theory reads more like a defense of the concept; his aim is clearly to place it in conjunction with an understanding of the influence of internal forces: "The reappearance of sexual activity is determined by internal causes and external contingencies. . . . I shall have to speak presently of the internal causes; great and lasting importance attaches at this period to the accidental external contingencies. In the foreground we find the effects of seduction . . ." (p. 190).

defenses, and symptoms, dreams, too, found their origins in the relational experiences of infancy:

> If we bear in mind how great a part is played in the dream-thoughts by infantile experiences or phantasies based upon them . . . a dream might be described as *a substitute for an infantile scene modified by being transferred onto a recent experience* [p. 585].

The *Three Essays* (Freud, 1905) has been described by Greenberg and Mitchell (1983) as "the height of the purest form of the drive/ structure model" (p. 35). This view is representative of the accepted interpretation of that work, not only among those who reject drive theory, but among those who consider themselves loyal to it. In the text, on the other hand, we find that although Freud presented his axiomatic definition of the drive in paragraph three, by paragraph four he had begun an autodeconstruction of the concept, departing significantly from the classical presentation. Freud (1905a) opened the text by "introduc[ing] two technical terms. Let us call the person from whom sexual attraction proceeds the *sexual object* and the act to which the instinct tends the *sexual aim*" (pp. 135–136). Immediately, he called the reader's attention to a quite different description of the sexual drive, indirectly associating it with the description of Eros found in Plato's Symposium, "the poetic fable which tells how the original human beings were cut up into two halves—man and woman—and how these are always striving to unite again in love" (p. 136).

In the preface to the fourth edition of the *Three Essays*, written in 1920, the association with Eros was made overt: "[Let us] remember how closely the enlarged sexuality of psychoanalysis coincides with the Eros of the divine Plato" (p. 134). Thus, right from the start, Freud overlaid his technical depiction of the drives with a mythological one, challenging the scientific concept of drive by redefining it according to the subjective longings derived from the separation of self and object.

The same autodeconstructive process can be seen at work in what Freud posited as the essential attributes of the drive: that sexual energy arises endogenously, that it stimulates the impulses of discharge in the interest of reducing tension, and that its aim is independent of its object. These attributes of drive reflected a turning, so the argument goes, away from the influence of the environment and relationship: "Once sexuality is posited as an internally arising force underlying human activity, seduction becomes theoretically vestigial, and the importance of childhood *events* correspondingly declines" (Greenberg and Mitchell, 1983, p. 32). Yet a turn to the text

uncovers an undermining of each of these attributes; this undermining can be derived once again from Freud's appreciation of the
impact of the relational scene on the development of the psyche and
its processes.

It is indeed the case that in the *Three Essays*, Freud (1905a) first
introduced into print the concept of an innate drive, stating that
"germs of sexual impulses are already present in the new-born child"
(p. 176). The concept itself was not at all new to Freud; its antecedents
can be found in the endogenous sexual energy of the Project (Freud,
1895), as well as in the endogenous sexual energy which as early as
1894 was implicated in the actual neuroses.[13] But what in fact was
Freud referring to as the germs of the sexual drive and how do they
"germinate" into the drive proper?

Freud began by attempting to model the sexual drive upon another
drive, that of *hunger*. However, this comparison rapidly turned out to
be inexpedient; sexuality was seen to differ from hunger both in
terms of its origin and its satisfaction.

According to Freud, the stimulation of the erotogenic zone of the
mouth through the taking of nourishment evoked a sexual sensation
in the infant. This sexual sensation was in itself pleasurable and, with
the satisfaction of the hunger and the withdrawal of the stimulation,
a drive for continued sexual stimulation came into play. The infant
resorted to self-stimulation or autoerotic activity to satisfy this newly
constituted sexual drive. Thus, "germs of sexual impulses" represented to Freud a kind of preparedness for the emergence and
localization of the sexual drive. The infant's preparedness was seen to
interact with a satisfying environmental stimulus by way of a specific
body part and process:

> The child's lips, in our view, behave like an erotogenic zone, and no
> doubt stimulation by the flow of warm milk is the cause of the
> pleasurable sensation. The satisfaction of the erotogenic zone is asso-
> ciated, in the first instance, with the satisfaction of the need for
> nourishment. . . . The need for repeating the sexual satisfaction now
> becomes detached from the need for taking nourishment—a separation
> which becomes inevitable when the teeth appear . . . [Freud, 1905a,
> pp. 181–182].

Laplanche (1976) has eloquently described the place of anaclisis (the
"propping" of the sexual drive upon a somatic function) in Freud's

---

[13]Here again, the traditional rendering of the abandonment of the seduction
hypothesis is contradicted. Not only did Freud sustain a respect for the impact of
environmental influences following September 21, 1897, but he had a concept of
endogenous sexuality prior to that date.

thinking during this period.[14] According to Laplanche, "propping is a leaning originally of infantile sexuality on the instincts. . . . Now the crucial point is that simultaneous with the feeding function's achievement of satisfaction in nourishment, a sexual process begins to appear" (pp. 16–17).

Whereas hunger arose endogenously, sexuality was evoked *as such* by the stimulation of an erotogenic zone:

> We can distinguish in the [sexual drives] . . . an instinct not in itself sexual which has its source in motor impulses, and a contribution from an organ capable of receiving stimuli (e.g., the skin, a mucous membrane or a sense organ). An organ of this kind will be described in this connection as an "erotogenic zone"—as being *the organ whose excitation lends the instinct a sexual character* [Freud, 1905a, p. 168n].

Thus, the notion of sexuality as an endogenously arising psychobiological force was undermined by the concept of anaclisis. From this perspective, sexuality was a psychic phenomenon derived from the linking of desire with an instinctual preparedness. It became a drive as a subjective longing for the restoration of a relational satisfaction now absent.

Similarly, Freud introduced and then contradicted the notion that the sexual drive was responsive to the pleasure principle, that is, that psychic tension is experienced as unpleasurable and that the drive is spurred to reduce such tension. Whereas the aim of the sexual drive was at first presented as "a release of the sexual tension and a temporary extinction of the sexual instinct—a satisfaction analogous to the sating of hunger" (Freud, 1905a, p. 149), this was rapidly transformed: "The sexual aim of the infantile instinct consists in obtaining satisfaction by means of an appropriate stimulation of the erotogenic zone which has been selected in one way or another. This satisfaction must have been previously experienced in order to have left behind a need for its repetition" (p. 184). Freud advanced a notion, derived from his Project (Freud, 1895), that, in addition to its quantity, stimulation had a quality and that "the quality of the stimulus has more to do with producing the pleasurable feeling than has the nature of the part of the body concerned" (Freud, 1905a, p. 183).

Freud (1905a) stated plainly, aware of the self-critique, that the sexual satisfactions of the relational matrix were *tension producing,*

---

[14]"What must unavoidably escape the reader of Freud in translation is the fact that the concept of *Anhenung* [anaclisis] is a cornerstone of the first Freudian instinct theory" (Laplanche and Pontalis, 1973, pp. 29–30).

rather than tension reducing. He asserted, in fact, that "In every case in which tension is produced by sexual processes it is accompanied by pleasure" (p. 209). He wrote, "This strikes us as strange only because in order to remove one stimulus it seems necessary to adduce a second one at the same spot" (p. 185). Freud's economic conceptualization was here, too, autodeconstructed with the postulation of a variation derived from interrelational experience.

Freud attempted to resolve the apparent contradiction by asserting a dialectical progression of pleasurable and unpleasurable tensions leading along a series of erotogenic zones and culminating in the search for a complete sexual object. But this resolution was only an apparent one, for the definition of the object itself was presented in two–fold fashion, the one undermining the other.

In the opening chapter of the *Three Essays*, Freud presented a view of the object that has since formed the basis of its classical representation; he asserted that the object of the drive and the aim of the drive were not intimately connected, giving the impression that the drive itself is paramount, the object of satisfaction secondary:

> We are thus warned to loosen the bonds that exist in our thoughts between instinct and object. It seems probable that the sexual instinct is in the first instance independent of its object; nor is its origin likely to be due to its object's attractions [p. 148].

Many theorists have inferred from this notion that the sexual drive arises endogenously and only later attaches itself to an object. Greenberg and Mitchell (1983), for example, cited Freud's statement that the drive "at its origin . . . has as yet no sexual object, and is thus autoerotic" (p. 182) in support of this traditional view. What Greenberg and Mitchell left out, however, was the clarification of this statement, which Freud added in 1915, rendering the complete quote as follows: "At its origin *it attaches itself to one of the vital functions;* it has as yet no sexual object, and is thus auto-erotic; *and its aim is dominated by an erotogenic zone*" (p. 182, italics added). This addition, coupled with Freud's description of the "finding of an object," turns the concept of the object in the *Three Essays* on its head.

Freud stated (and here I am drawing from Laplanche, 1976):[15]

---

[15]The citation is Mehlman's translation of the quote as found in Laplanche (1976, p. 19). Laplanche differentiates Freud's use of the word *instinkt* from the word *trieb* in order to highlight a transformation of the drive from the biological to the psychological realms. While it is propped upon the vital function, sexuality remains an *instinct*, as it becomes separate from the object and thereby spurs the formation of a conception of desire derived from the experience of the object, it is transformed into a sexual *drive*.

At a time when the first beginnings of sexual satisfaction are still linked
with the taking of nourishment [i.e., in the propping phase], the sexual
instinct has a sexual object outside the infant's own body in the shape
of his mother's breast. It is only later that he loses it, just at the time,
perhaps, when he is able to form a total idea of the person to whom the
organ that is giving him satisfaction belongs. As a rule the sexual drive
then becomes auto-erotic [*auto-erotism is thus not the initial stage*], and
not until puberty has been passed through is the original relation
restored. There are thus good reasons why a child sucking at its
mother's breast has become the prototype of every relation of love. The
finding of the object is in fact a refinding of it [p. 222].

Freud here asserted a quite different view of the evolution of the
sexual drive and its relationship to objects than the one with which he
opened his text. Sexuality in this passage is born of *longing;*[16] it comes
into existence in the absence of a relational satisfaction already
experienced.[17]

It is in this aspect that sexuality at its origin has no object, because
its creation is due to the withdrawal of the object: "On the one hand
there is from the beginning an object, but on the other hand *sexuality*
does not have, from the beginning, a real object" (Laplanche, 1976,
p. 19, emphasis added). In the transition from nameless instinct
to sexual drive infantile sexuality has taken the leap to infantile
love.[18]

Although the classical representation of the drive as endogenously
derived, independent of its object, and seeking the reduction of
tension can be found prominently in this seminal text, a close
examination reveals a countertheoretical view. Alongside the traditional point of view, simultaneously challenging and enriching it, is to
be found an alternative description of the sexual impulses. In this
alternative view, sexuality is brought into existence as such by an
absence of the previously experienced other and the longing for its
return; it is depicted as tension producing rather than solely tension

---

[16]Cf. letter to Fliess of October 27, 1897 (in Masson, 1985).

[17]Lear (1990) has recently highlighted the internal tension in this work between the
psychological and the scientific aspects of Freud's description of the drive: "Once one
defines a sexual object in terms of its psychological significance, the lesson of the Three
Essays seems to be the opposite of what Freud says it is. There is a sense in which the
sexual drive never abandons its object" (p. 131).

[18]As Bergmann (1987) put it, "Once Freud had recognized that the root of sexuality
goes back to infancy, it was only one further step to his recognition that love, too, has
its origins in the same years of infancy. . . . I regard Freud's statement that 'the finding
of the object is in fact a refinding of it' as Freud's most profound contribution to love"
(pp. 158–159).

reducing, and the perception of this tension is experienced as pleasure. The first of these can be seen as a continuation of the modification of the seduction hypothesis; the latter anticipates the transformations to come in the theory of Eros.

INSTINCTS AND THEIR VICISSITUDES

Whereas the *Three Essays* is cited as the true beginnings of classical drive theory, "Instincts and Their Vicissitudes" (Freud, 1915a) is generally viewed as its most complete elaboration. In the *Three Essays*, Freud defined the "object" and the "aim" of what has been depicted traditionally as an endogenous sexual drive; in "Instincts and Their Vicissitudes," he added the technical terms "impetus" and "source," and presented the definition of the drive that classical theorists and revisionists alike see as the most concise description of the drive-discharge model:[19]

> An 'instinct' appears to us as a borderland concept between the mental and the physical, being both the mental representative of the stimuli emanating from within the organism and penetrating to the mind, and at the same time a measure of the demand made upon the energy of the latter [the mind] in consequence of its connection with the body. [Freud, 1915a, p. 64].[20]

Yet, in this paper, no less than in the *Three Essays* and *Beyond the Pleasure Principle*, we see Freud "struggling against himself" (Bergmann, 1987, p. 173n). The process in each case is quite similar: Freud lays out, in technical terms, his axiomatic concepts, with all the earmarks of turn-of-the-century science; almost immediately he uses

---

[19]I am here making use of Joan Riviere's translations in the *Collected Papers*, rather than James Strachey's in the *Standard Edition*. I do this primarily to avoid Strachey's often cumbersome attempt to make a point about Freud while rendering Freud into English (Bettelheim, 1983). In addition, I am following Gay's (1988) lead that "the most vigorous translations into English, capturing Freud's virile and witty German speech better than any other, can be found in vols I-IV of Collected Papers, mainly tr. by the brilliant Joan Riviere" (pp. 741-742). Where Riviere's translation departs notably from the *Standard Edition*, I have placed Strachey's translation in a footnote.

[20]Cf. Strachey: "an 'instinct' appears to us as a concept on the frontier between the mental and the somatic, as the psychical representative of the stimuli originating from within the organism and reaching the mind, as a measure of the demand made upon the mind for work in consequence of its connection with the body" (Freud, 1915b, pp. 121-122). Strachey blurs the twofold nature of the origin of the drive, deemphasizing the additional formative impact of the environment's impact on the body.

his insight into the vicissitudes of human desire, love, and aggression to autodeconstruct these presumptions. This leads to a tension within his theorizing between a conceptualization of the press of internal forces, on one hand, and the striving for loving relationship, on the other.[21]

Bergmann has noted that "it was the reading and possibly misreading of this paper that was responsible for the widespread belief . . . that Freud confused love and sex" (p. 173). Fenichel (1935), it will be remembered, used the description of the biological processes of drive from "Instincts and Their Vicissitudes" to refute Freud's later theory of Eros and the death drive. And Mitchell (1988) cited it as evidence that "the center of gravity of the theory has shifted from interactions with others to the unfolding of inborn pressures. The entire field of interpersonal relations has been collapsed around spontaneously arising impulses with encoded a priori meanings" (p. 72).

Yet a close reading even of Freud's technical definitions of the aspects of the drive does not support the narrowed view of sexuality traditionally attributed to him. The drive, even in its most technical sense, remained a psychic transformation derived from two origins, resulting from what Freud (1905a) termed the "complemental series:"

> It is not easy to estimate the relative efficacy of the constitutional and accidental factors. In theory one is always inclined to overestimate the former; therapeutic practice emphasizes the importance of the latter. It should, however, on no account be forgotten that the relation between the two is a cooperative and not a mutually exclusive one. The constitutional factor must await experience before it can make itself felt; the accidental factor must have a constitutional basis in order to come into operation [p. 239].[22]

Freud did not say simply that the drive was the mental representation of endogenous stimulation, but rather that it combined the mental representative of endogenous stimuli with the demand arising from a sensual (erotogenic) experience. Hence, the *source* of the sexual drive, Freud (1915a) stated, was that "somatic process in an organ or

---

[21]Freud's attempts to resolve this tension led to his frequent recasting of the dual drive model, ultimately to the final version presented in *Beyond the Pleasure Principle* (Freud, 1920): "Our views have from the very first been *dualistic*, and today are even more definitely dualistic than before—now that we describe the opposition as being, not between the ego-instincts and the sexual instincts but between life instincts and death instincts" (p. 53).

[22]This passage was added to the *Three Essays* in 1915 about the time Freud was working on "Instincts and Their Vicissitudes."

part of the body from which there results a stimulus" (p. 65). Here, as in the *Three Essays*, Freud defined the drive as the psychological meeting point of the germ of a sexual impulse with the sensual stimulations of the human environment.

In other words, Freud sustained the notion that the drive is evoked *as such* by the vicissitudes of experience with an object, much as he had described it following the abandonment of the seduction hypothesis and in the *Three Essays*.[23]

In making the case against the later dual-drive theory, Fenichel first had to distort Freud's representation of this earlier definition of drive. Fenichel (1945) made no secret of his revision: "At first glance one finds many contradictory presentations of the essence of the instincts . . . in Freud's writings" (p. 54). He stated that where "Freud suggested that two kinds of excitations should be distinguished: one that is . . . external . . . and another that arises from . . . within. . . . Only the physical conditions that determine the urge, *the chemistry of the body*, and not the sensory stimuli can rightly be called the source of the instincts" (p. 54, italics added).

In Fenichel's version, the sexual drive was purely an endogenously derived force; since this was not the case in Freud's text, Fenichel amended it, thereby rendering Freud more appropriately "Freudian." It is this version of Freud's theory, distilled by Fenichel among others, which forms the basis of the classical view.[24]

Others in the classical tradition have compounded Fenichel's distortion; Rapaport (1960b), for example, would have us edit Freud's works in order to sustain this narrowed reading:

> Not until "Instincts and their vicissitudes" did Freud make an attempt to present the theory of instinctual drives more systematically. . . . In

---

[23]In fact, Freud's notion of the "complemental series" is among his oldest and most consistent, found in writings long before and long after the supposed abandonment of the seduction hypothesis. It is first alluded to in what is considered Freud's very first psychoanalytic writing, the draft of section 'III' of the "preliminary communication" sent to Breuer with the letter of June 29, 1892: "The hysterical disposition is therefore to be looked for where states of this kind either appear spontaneously (from internal causes) or are easily produced by external influences; and we may suppose a series of cases in which the two factors play a part of varying importance" (Freud, 1892, p. 149). In the "Aetiology of Hysteria," Freud (1896c) put it in different terms: "In the aetiology of the neuroses quantitative preconditions are as important as qualitative ones" (p. 210).

[24]This transformation of Freud's emphasis requires recasting Freud's history. It is only if one believes that Freud gave up his belief in the psychic impact of environmental interaction that the seduction hypothesis had to be "abandoned," and only if Freud is depicted as an advocate of a purely drive/discharge model of motivation does the theory of Eros appear to be a radical innovation.

the meanwhile, "On narcissism; an introduction" and later *Beyond the Pleasure Principle* and *The Ego and the Id* consistently distracted attention from the theory itself . . . [p. 869].

It was precisely in these "distracting" and "contradictory" texts, including the remainder of "Instincts and Their Vicissitudes" itself, that Freud presented a theory of the processes of love that undercut the technical, systematic one with which the paper opened. In its place, Freud advanced a view of love that stood independent from the vicissitudes of drive in the technical sense, a turning in his thinking that led naturally to the reconceptualization of the drive process in *Beyond the Pleasure Principle*.

Following Rapaport's lead (although in a manner opposite to that intended), it is helpful to trace the development of Freud's alternative theory of love as a driving force in its own right to "On Narcissism; an Introduction." In that paper, Freud (1914a), expanded upon the subtextual theory of sexual love first presented in the *Three Essays*.

Freud approached the study of narcissism "by observing the behavior of human beings in love" (p. 44).[25] He began with what appears to be a restatement of the origin of sexuality in the *Three Essays:* "The first auto-erotic sexual gratifications are experienced in connection with vital functions in the service of self-preservation." However, rather than defining sexuality as commencing upon the withdrawal of the object (as in the *Three Essays*), Freud here distinguished two aspects of sexuality. On one hand, "we have an indication of that original dependence in the fact that those persons who have to do with the feeding, care, and protection of the child become his earliest sexual objects . . . this type and source of object-choice . . . may be called the *anaclitic* type" (p. 44). Alongside the anaclitic type, and to an extent masked by it, was "a second type [of object choice], the existence of which we had not suspected" (pp. 44–45). To this aspect of sexuality, Freud gave the name narcissism, the love of the ego, or self-love.

Narcissistic desire was not evoked by the loss of the object, like the sexuality of the *Three Essays*, rather it was revealed in the object's absence. Freud (1914a) thus divided the earliest love relationship into two components: "We say that the human being has originally two sexual objects: himself [being loved] and the woman who tends him" (p. 45).

The division of sexuality into two types of love-relationship in the "Narcissism" paper brought to the surface what had up to that point

---

[25]Cf. Strachey: "by observing the erotic life of human beings" (Freud, 1914b, p. 87).

been a subtextual tension in the metapsychology of love. Where earlier Freud posited as paradoxical the simultaneous pleasure-in-sexual-tension and pleasure as the object-aided relief of tension, here Freud indicated that these were two types of object relationship: pleasurable tension was depicted as an idealized ontological state; side by side with this mode of experience was the anaclitic one, in which the object was experienced as aiding in self-preservation. Thus,

> a person may love, according to the narcissistic type: What he is himself (actually himself); what he once was; what he would like to be; someone who was once part of himself. According to the anaclitic type [a person may love]: The woman who tends; the man who protects; and those substitutes which succeed them one after the other [pp. 47–48].[26]

With the concept of narcissism, Freud presented a mode of love independent from the technical attributes of drive. Narcissistic love was not depicted as aiming toward satisfaction in terms of decreased tension, but rather sought the maintenance or restoration of the pleasurable tension experienced in the earliest relationship. Thus, Freud stated (1914a), "*to be loved* is the aim and the satisfaction in a narcissistic object-choice" (p. 55, italics added). Narcissism became noticeable as a motivational force only when the narcissistic state had been lost. Thus, like what would later be described as Eros, narcissism was depicted as the longing for the restoration of a state of unity with another: "The development of the ego consists in a departure from the primary narcissism and results in a vigorous attempt to recover that state" (p. 57).

In narcissism, we have the anticipation of the final transformation of the drive concept: rather than being an urge to reduce tension, the narcissistic desire, like Eros, is ultimately a conservative one, for the restoration of an earlier state of things.

In "Instincts and Their Vicissitudes," Freud (1915a) elaborated on the concept of narcissism; alongside it he added a qualitative dimension to the anaclitic drives. In so doing, he severed the ties that bound

---

[26]Erlich and Blatt (1985), in their review of this material, have designated the aims of these two object choices as "being" and "doing": In the narcissistic object choice, the object is experienced by the ego as in some state of *being*—in terms of what it "was," "is," "could be," or "would like to be." In the anaclitic object choice, on the other hand, the object is experienced as in some relation of *doing* to the ego: "tending" or "protecting" (p. 66).

sexuality and love to the technical characteristics of drive set out in the paper's opening pages.

Freud made it clear that "the primal narcissistic condition" was a subjective pleasure state made possible by the responsiveness of "fostering care." In this situation "the ego-subject coincides with what is pleasurable and the outside world with what is indifferent" thus, "the ego loves itself only" (p. 78). This narcissistic state was interfered with in two ways. There arose inner instinctual stimuli perceived by the ego as painful. As the anaclitic and self-preservative drives found objects in the external world, these, too, with their "afflux of stimuli" (p. 79) were perceived as painful.

The ego responded in a self-protective way to each of these interferences. First, via the mechanisms of introjection and projection, the ego was transformed into a purified pleasure ego that prized above all else the "quality of pleasure": "The objects presenting themselves, insofar as they are sources of pleasure, are absorbed into the ego itself . . . ; while, on the other hand, the ego thrusts forth upon the external world whatever within itself gives rise to pain" (p. 78). This process yielded two polarities, "ego-subject with pleasure, outside world with pain" (p. 79), and led to a second transformation, from subjective experience into affective motivation, from qualities of pleasure and pain to love and hate.

Thus Freud (1915a) stated that, "love . . . [which] is primarily narcissistic is then transferred to those objects which have been incorporated into the ego, *now very much extended,* and expresses the motor striving of the ego after these objects as sources of pleasure" (p. 81). On the other hand,

> when the object is the source of painful feelings, there is a tendency which endeavors to increase the distance between object and ego and to repeat in relation to the former the primordial attempt at flight from the external world with its flow of stimuli. We feel a "repulsion" from the object and hate it; this hate can then be intensified to the point of an aggressive tendency toward the object, with the intention of destroying it [p. 80].

Freud has here undercut the axiomatic principles with which he opened his text. Where he began with talk of pressures, quantities, and striving for discharge, he rapidly undermined these in his examination of the vicissitudes of love and hate. In the process, sexuality divided into aspects that perceive stimuli within and without as painful, and aspects that experience stimuli as loving. Freud has found himself again at the limits of his scientistic model;

once again, he transcends those limits by turning his attention to the vicissitudes of relationship, love, and aggression.

In fact, in "Instincts and Their Vicissitudes," Freud (1915a) intimated that the concepts of love and hate transcend the drives from which they are derived and require a reconceptualization of the motivating forces operating within the ego: "The attitudes of love and hate cannot be said to characterize the relations of instincts to their objects, but are reserved for the relations of the ego as a whole to objects" (p. 80). As Bergmann (1987) put it, "a new idea is in the process of being formulated. Love is not an instinct; it is the ego or the total ego that loves its objects. Libido and love are no longer synonymous. The sexual instinct as such cannot explain the nature of love" (p. 176). That "new idea" would find its full expression in *Beyond the Pleasure Principle* and in *The Ego and the Id*.

Here, then, in the very paper Fenichel used to critique the theory of Eros and Thanatos, are all the elements which make up that theory. Like Eros, the "love" of "Instincts and Their Vicissitudes" is derived from an original experience of undifferentiated connectedness, its subsequent loss, and the continual striving for its restoration. Where Eros "strives to make the ego and the loved object one, to abolish all spatial barriers between them" (Freud, 1926, p. 122), in the earlier paper it is love that "strives to bring the object near to and incorporate it into the ego" (Freud, 1915a, p. 79).

Hate, in "Instincts and Their Vicissitudes," is represented as the urge to project painful internal stimulation outside of the self; the projected excitation attaches to the stimulating objects of the external world, evoking the destructive impulse (Freud, 1915a, p. 80). This closely anticipates the vicissitudes of Thanatos in *Beyond the Pleasure Principle*: "Is it not plausible to suppose that this sadism is in fact a death instinct which, under the influence of the narcissistic libido, has been forced away from the ego and has consequently only emerged in relation to the object?" (Freud, 1920, p. 54).

Freud has thus prepared the way for the final transformations in his dual-drive theory. Where "Instincts and Their Vicissitudes" presents the autodeconstruction of the concept of instinctual drives, the work that followed can be understood as the result of that process.

In *Beyond the Pleasure Principle*, Freud severed love and hate altogether from the earlier concept of quantifiable drives, rendering these as irreducible motivations in their own right, and resolving the former narcissistic, anaclitic, self-preservative, and aggressive drive components into two primary motivations. Neither was seen any longer as arising as the result of accessions of internal tensions, nor the stimulations of the environment, rather each represented an a priori human urge toward loving relationships on the one hand, and quiescence on the other.

In *The Ego and the Id*, Freud (1923) transformed topography from one wherein the ego existed primarily to contend with the accessions of drive tension, to a structure evolving according to the interplay of essential human longings of Eros and the death drive (Leowald, 1971a).

CONCLUSION

In this chapter, I have argued that typical in Freud's work is a scientistic formulation of the precepts of psychoanalysis, couched in a language of tensions and forces, their facilitations and impediments, and that embedded within each text, typically, is a critique of those assumptions taken from the point of view of the subjectivity of human relationship and its impact on the developing self–concept. Furthermore, that the traditional reading of Freud's drive theory is a product of the codification and censorship of his work undertaken by his followers. Edited out in the process is the radical critique embedded in his own work.

I began with a reappraisal of the so-called abandonment of the seduction hypothesis in order to challenge the prevailing assumption that Freud's work can be understood as a progression from a purely environmental, relational theory to one based exclusively on a view of motivation as responsive to endogenously derived drives. A close reading of Freud's development during this period reveals the beginning of what was to be a lifelong process of balancing the psychical influences of relational experiences, endogenous tension states, subjective interpretations and longings, and objective memories and anticipations.

In the *Three Essays*, Freud (1905a) turned his attention from pathological symptoms to the universal unfolding of human sexuality. The traditional reading presents a sexuality of endogenous sexual tensions and infinitely substitutable objects. In the text, Freud critiqued and expanded upon these limitations by postulating a sexuality conceived in longing and transmuted by experience, the beginnings of a theory of love: "A mother would probably be horrified if she were made aware that all her marks of affection were rousing her child's sexual instinct. . . . [But] she is only fulfilling her task in teaching the child to love" (p. 223).

"Instincts and Their Vicissitudes" (Freud, 1915a) presented advances in both the technical description of the drives and the subjective experience of love that undermines it. Freud strove to perfect a series of axioms about the drives that might account, in the guise of science, for the influences of biology and sensual experience on psychosexual energy and motivation; simultaneously, he explored what emerge as the more primary human motivations of love and hate. These cannot be reduced to drives as presented in his opening pages, but call for a reevaluation of motivation in terms of "the relations of the ego as a whole to objects" (p. 80). Here the editing process of his followers has been more deceptive; not only has attention been focused away from aspects of the text that correct the opening postulates, but the technical descriptions themselves have been recast to fit an even more rigid Freudian paradigm than Freud's own.

What we find in evidence throughout Freud's work, in particular during what has been termed the height of his classical drive period (1905–1915), is a profound corrective to his own paradigm of drive and discharge. This corrective emerges, finally, in its own right as the theory of Eros, the love that binds. The remnants of the drive discharge model can be discerned, transformed, in the death drive.

Ironically, in the final dual-drive theory, the drives are indeed seen as irreducible, endogenous forces; but only one of the two, the death drive, seeks the reduction of tension. Eros is depicted as the unyielding motivation for relationship. As such, it is irreducibly object-seeking, rather than pleasure-seeking: "In no other case does Eros so clearly betray the core of his being, his purpose of making one out of more than one" (Freud, 1930, p. 108).

A close reading of even those texts most commonly associated with the classical psychoanalytic tradition reveals how consistently Freud departed from that tradition. Where Freud has been portrayed as emphasizing economic motivations over relational ones, we find the progressive autodeconstruction of the pleasure principle. Where the traditional representation of Freud's history posits an historical development from an environmental emphasis to one of endogenous tensions seeking discharge, we find a continuous complemental series of pressures for discharge and longing for the (re-)finding of relationship.

Alongside the development of the theory of the drives as endogenous forces, with their sources, pressures, aims, and objects, we can trace an alternative relational development in Freud's thought. It is found in the widening of the seduction concept (the sexual scene) of the late 1890s, in the wish model of the *The Interpretation of Dreams* and in the concept of anaclisis in the *Three Essays*. It reemerges as a function of narcissism, and soon thereafter in the loving aspect of the ego. Relational longing is, ultimately, elevated to the stature of a drive in its own right and given mythic proportions and cosmological implications in *Beyond the Pleasure Principle*, a stance from which Freud does not retreat.

In ignoring Eros, psychoanalysts have ignored not just the core concept of Freud's last 20 years, but a major portion of the canon that preceded it. In editing out his relational contribution, classical theorists have deprived Freudian psychoanalysis of the creative internal tension that inspired Freud to some of his most profound theoretical insights. In accepting this distortion of Freud's theory, present-day relational and self-psychologists have deprived him of his rightful place as originator of many of the key concepts in contemporary psychoanalysis.

REFERENCES

Arlow, J. (1956), *The Legacy of Freud*. New York: International Universities Press.

Bergmann, M. (1987), *The Anatomy of Loving*. New York: Columbia University Press.

Bettelheim, B. (1983), *Freud and Man's Soul*. New York: Knopf.

Brenner, C. (1973), *An Elementary Textbook of Psychoanalysis* (rev. ed.). New York: International Universities Press.

_____ (1982), *The Mind in Conflict*. New York: International Universities Press.

Breuer, J. & Freud, S. (1895), *Studies on Hysteria, Standard Edition*, 2. London: Hogarth Press, 1955.

Casey, E. S. (1990), The subdominance of the pleasure principle. In: *Pleasure Beyond the Pleasure Principle*, ed. R. A. Glick & S. Bone. New Haven, CT: Yale University Press, pp. 239–258.

Eagle, M. (1984), *Recent Developments in Psychoanalysis*. Cambridge, MA: Harvard University Press.

Erlich, H. S. & Blatt, S. J. (1985), Narcissism and object love: The metapsychology of experience. *The Psychoanalytic Study of the Child*, 40:57–80. New Haven, CT: Yale University Press.

Fenichel, O. (1935), A critique of the death instinct. In: *The Collected Papers of Otto Fenichel*. New York: Norton, 1953, pp. 363–372.

_____ (1945), *The Psychoanalytic Theory of the Neurosis*. New York: Norton.

Freud, A. (1936), *The Ego and the Mechanisms of Defense*. New York: International Universities Press.

Freud, S. (1892), Sketches for the 'preliminary communication' of 1893. *Standard Edition*, 1:147–154. London: Hogarth Press, 1966.

_____ (1894), On the grounds for detaching a particular syndrome from neurasthenia under the description 'anxiety neurosis.' *Standard Edition*, 3:90–115. London: Hogarth Press, 1962.

_____ (1895), Project for a scientific psychology. *Standard Edition*, 1:283–387. London: Hogarth Press, 1966.

_____ (1896a), Heredity and the aetiology of the neurosis. *Standard Edition*, 3:143–156. London: Hogarth Press, 1962.

_____ (1896b), Further remarks on the neuro-psychosis of defense. *Standard Edition*, 3:163–185. London: Hogarth Press, 1962.

_____ (1896c), The aetiology of hysteria. *Standard Edition*, 3:191–221. London: Hogarth Press, 1962.

_____ (1900), *The Interpretation of Dreams. Standard Edition*, 4–5. London: Hogarth Press, 1953.

_____ (1905a), *Three Essays on the Theory of Sexuality. Standard Edition*, 7:125–248. London: Hogarth Press, 1953.

_____ (1905b), My views on the part played by sexuality in the aetiology of the neurosis. *Collected Papers*, 1:272–286. London: Hogarth Press, 1950.

_____ (1914a), On narcissism. *Collected Papers*, 4:30–59. London: Hogarth Press, 1950.

_____ (1914b), On narcissism. *Standard Edition*, 14:67–102. London: Hogarth Press, 1957.

_____ (1915a), Instincts and their vicissitudes. *Collected Papers*, 4:60–83. London: Hogarth Press, 1950.

_____ (1915b), Instincts and their vicissitudes. *Standard Edition*, 14:117–140. London: Hogarth Press, 1957.

_____ (1920), *Beyond the Pleasure Principle. Standard Edition*, 18:1–144. London: Hogarth Press, 1955.

_____ (1921), *Group Psychology and the Analysis of the Ego. Standard Edition*, 18:65–143. London: Hogarth Press, 1955.

_____ (1923), *The Ego and the Id. Standard Edition*, 19:13–59. London: Hogarth Press, 1961.

_____ (1924), The economic problem of masochism. *Standard Edition*, 19:159–170. London: Hogarth Press, 1961.

_____ (1926), *Inhibitions, Symptoms and Anxiety. Standard Edition*, 20:77–178. London: Hogarth Press, 1959.

_____ (1930), *Civilization and Its Discontents. Standard Edition*, 21:57–157. London: Hogarth Press, 1961.

_____ (1933a), Why war? *Standard Edition*, 22:203–215. London: Hogarth Press, 1964.

_____ (1933b), New introductory lectures on psycho-analysis. *Standard Edition*, 22:1–182. London: Hogarth Press, 1964.

_____ (1940), *An Outline of Psycho-Analysis. Standard Edition*, 23:139–207. London: Hogarth Press, 1964.

Garcia, E. E. (1987), Freud's seduction theory. *The Psychoanalytic Study of the Child*, 42:443–468. New Haven, CT: Yale University Press.

Gay, P. (1988), *Freud: A Life for Our Time*. New York: Norton.

Gediman, H. K. (1991), Seduction trauma: Complemental intrapsychic and interpersonal perspectives on fantasy and reality. *Psychoanalytic Psychology*, 8(4):381–401.

Gill, M. M. (1976), Metapsychology is not psychology. In: *Psychology vs. Metapsychology, Psychological Issues*, Monogr. 36. New York: Basic Books, pp. 71–105.

Greenberg, J. R. & Mitchell, S. A. (1983), *Object Relations in Psychoanalytic Theory*. Cambridge, MA: Harvard University Press.

Habermas, J. (1972), *Knowledge and Human Interests*. Boston, MA: Beacon Press.

Hartmann, H. (1948), Comments on the psychoanalytic theory of instinctual drives. In: *Essays on Ego Psychology*. New York: International Universities Press, 1964, pp. 69–89.

Holt, R. R. (1976), Drive or wish? A reconsideration of the psycho-analytic theory of motivation. In: *Psychology vs. Metapsychology, Psychological Issues*, Monogr. 36. New York: Basic Books, pp. 158–197.

Klein, G. (1976), *Psychoanalytic theory*. New York: International Universities Press.

LaPlanche, J. (1976), *Life and Death in Psychoanalysis*. Baltimore, MD: Johns Hopkins University Press.

_____ (1989), *New Foundations for Psychoanalysis*. Cambridge: Basil Blackwell.

_____ & Pontalis, J.-B. (1973), *The Language of Psychoanalysis.* New York: Norton.

Lear, J. (1990), *Love and Its Place in Nature.* New York: Farrar, Straus & Giroux.

Leowald, H. (1971a), Discussion of *The Id and the Regulatory Principles of Mental Functioning* by M. Schur. In: *Papers on Psychoanalysis.* New Haven, CT: Yale University Press, 1980, pp. 58–68.

_____ (1971b), On motivation and instinct theory. In: *Papers on Psychoanalysis.* New Haven, CT: Yale University Press, 1980, pp. 102–137.

_____ (1988), *Sublimation.* New Haven, CT: Yale University Press.

Masson, J. M. (1984), *The Assault on Truth.* New York: Farrar, Straus & Giroux.

_____ ed. & trans. (1985), *The Complete Letters of Sigmund Freud to Wilhelm Fliess, 1887–1904.* Cambridge, MA: Harvard University Press.

Mitchell, S. (1988), *Relational Concepts in Psychoanalysis.* Cambridge, MA: Harvard University Press.

Rapaport, D. (1957), Letter: Response to Robert W. White's review of Heinz L. & Rowena R. Anspacher's *The Individual Psychology of Alfred Adler.* In: *The Collected Papers of David Rapaport,* ed. M. M. Gill. New York: Basic Books, 1967, pp. 682–684.

_____ (1960a), *The Structure of Psychoanalytic Theory. Psychological Issues,* Monogr. 6. New York: International Universities Press.

_____ (1960b), On the psychoanalytic theory of motivation. In: *The Collected Papers of David Rapaport,* ed. M. M. Gill. New York: Basic Books, 1967, pp. 853–915.

Reisner, S. (1991), Reclaiming the metapsychology: Classical revisionism, seduction and the self in Freudian psychoanalysis. *Psychoanal. Psychol.,* 8:439–462.

Schafer, R. (1976), *A New Language for Psychoanalysis.* New Haven, CT: Yale University Press.

Schimek, J. K. (1987), Fact and fantasy in the seduction theory: A historical review. *J. Amer. Psychoanal. Assn.,* 35:937–965.

Zetzel, E. R. & Meissner, W. W. (1973), *Basic Concepts of Psychoanalytic Psychiatry.* New York: Basic Books.

14

Some Historical Aspects of Contemporary Pluralistic Psychoanalysis

BENJAMIN WOLSTEIN

In this paper, I distinguish within the structure of psychoanalytic inquiry a variety of perspectives on the human psyche—Freud's instinct, Adler's power struggle, Jung's collective unconscious, Rank's absolute will, current ego, object, and interpersonal relations, and the psychic center of the self. They are all interpretive and speculative metapsychologies of psychoanalysis, radically distinct from its empirical and systematic psychology. Psychoanalysis does not stand or fall, it is now clear, with the changing visions and revisions of such metapsychologies. Its structure of therapeutic inquiry is designed, rather, to study the relation of conscious and unconscious processes and patterns arising directly within a unique and shareable field of experience that evolves in and through the self-supporting psychic connectedness of a particular psychoanalyst and patient.

A close review of some neglected aspects of the development of psychotherapeutic inquiry from hypnosis to early psychoanalysis, from the vantage point of contemporary pluralism, throws new light on the distinction between empirical and systematic psychology on

This chapter, in substance, comprises a report originally entitled "Aspects of the Distinction between Psychology and Metapsychology in Hypnosis and Psychoanalysis," and prepared for Symposium 37, The Contribution of Psychoanalysis to Psychology, 21st International Congress of Psychology, Paris, July, 1976. In the concluding section, its central theme is brought to bear on the New York University Postdoctoral Program. For a detailed discussion of the structure of psychoanalysis on which this theme is based, see *Theory of Psychoanalytic Therapy* (Wolstein, 1967).

one hand, and the many different interpretive metapsychologies on the other, thereby also strengthening the current foundations and clarifying the possible future directions of the relation between theory and practice.

There is little question about the original therapeutic aims of both hypnosis and early psychoanalysis. The major aims of those two procedures were, in fact, the same—namely, from a dynamic transformational point of view, to overcome the resistances caused by the unconscious repressions; and from a descriptive observational point of view, to recover the lost memories found to cause the pathological symptoms. Those two procedures of psychotherapy were carried out, however, under two radically different sets of psychic conditions: that of hypnosis constructed under directive inquiry during the trance experience; and that of early psychoanalysis, by way of contrast, constructed during free–associative inquiry into waking experience.

In his major, yet hardly complete, 1915–1917 synthesis, Freud summarized the change in therapeutic inquiry from the one procedure to the other. He based his consideration of the sources of free-associative inquiry, among other things, on Breuer's report, in the early 1880s, of Anna O.'s remarkable talking cure through cathartic abreaction during autohypnotic experience, and on Bernheim's somewhat later experiments with hypnotic subjects who, under concentrated inquiry after emerging from their trance state, could actually recall the posthypnotic suggestions they took while undergoing that state.

GREEK MYTH AND LIBIDO METAPHOR

Psychoanalytic inquiry, from the late 1890s onward, developed into a new and independent clinical procedure of direct psychological inquiry. The development of that early procedure was, as it emerged, sui generis, and so was its open inquiry into the new and indefinitely extended field of unconscious psychology. Rooted in strong precursors, without peer among weaker contemporaries, it proved capable of generating great exploratory power in depth. That early procedure now stands, by common agreement, solidly beyond question as the original precursor of the present structure of psychoanalytic inquiry within which it is possible to coordinate both its empirical and systematic, and its interpretive constituents with a reasonable degree of confidence.

The therapeutic procedure of early psychoanalysis, as is now well known, was also built up around something far more imaginative and

far-reaching than its exploratory psychology. It was very closely—
indeed inextricably, some id and ego psychoanalysts still assert—
entwined with a uniquely created chain of carefully selected, presumably universal myths and metaphors stretching back to ancient Greek
culture. And that, in the psychotherapies of the 1890s, was unprecedented. A clue to the introduction of classical Greek myths and
metaphors as the critical interpretive and speculative symbols, aside
from their hold on Freud's psyche, may be traced to the abreactive
results brought about by suggestion in hypnosis and cathartic therapy
and, soon after that, by the autohypnotic procedure of the talking
cure. Greek myths and metaphors were used to represent and give
meaning to the various stages and dramatis personae of the regressive process of early psychoanalytic inquiry.

Freud's appeal to the psychodramatic metaphors of ancient Greek
mythology no doubt marked an absolutely new departure from the
working context of psychotherapeutic inquiry previously established
by such outstanding, late 19th-century hypnotists and cathartic
therapists as Bernheim, Breuer, Charcot, and Janet. Freud, in fact,
departed from all the established interpretive contexts of psychotherapeutic inquiry then in use. Even now, however, nearly 100 years
later, it has yet to be demonstrated that the aims and procedures of
early psychoanalytic inquiry could be inextricably tied into that
speculative and highly symbolized chain of ancient myths and
metaphors in which the first generation of psychoanalysts thought it
necessary, following Freud's lead, to couch the empirical and systematic psychology of their new therapeutic inquiry.

Since the turn of the century, moreover, other psychoanalysts have
found it equally valuable—and, in some instances, even more compelling—to provide their psychotherapeutic inquiries with the interpretive support of still other cultural myths and metaphors. They did
this without undergoing any reduction of their therapeutic striving,
on the contrary being energized to make their best effort instead.
Witness, for example, such rather widely known perspectives on
metapsychology as evolve from the terms of power, race, and will;
adaptation, satisfaction, and security; self-fulfillment, self-realization,
and mystical self-love.

Those early instinctual psychoanalysts of the libido, it is now clear,
arbitrarily affirmed the particular chain of myths and metaphors that
they arbitrarily applied to their work in the concrete individual case as
a matter of abstract generalized commitment. I refer to it below, and
elsewhere (Wolstein, 1971), as the biological model. Even into the
1940s, the later id and the new ego psychoanalysts continued to
embrace and to embellish this biological model without rethinking

and fundamentally reworking its interpretive metapsychology. They followed this path on the basis of strong personal preference—unexamined and, in the nature of the case, perhaps ultimately unexaminable. Yet that interpretive metapsychology was not of their own making in fact; it took root in someone else's personal needs instead. The biological model was first envisioned by Freud in the 1890s, and he laid such strong stress on the trope of that particular interpretive metapsychology as a matter of firm personal belief.

Meanwhile, a broad and varied range of post-Freudian psychoanalysts has been able to march to many different drummers in interpretive metapsychology without, however, losing track of their fundamental focus on the empirical and systematic activities of their daily therapeutic inquiry. They have continued, instead, to employ and extend the early procedures of psychoanalytic inquiry, to modify and enlarge the two aims of those early procedures beyond hypnosis, and to restate and refine the controlling theory of unconscious psychic experience, the better to coordinate and cover the structure of psychoanalytic inquiry with the umbrella of post-Freudian pluralism. The post-Freudians changed both the aims and the procedures of direct therapeutic inquiry, and they reformulated the diverse constituents of the overall structure of psychoanalysis. Yet they did not, however, find it necessary or possible merely to re-echo Freud's strong insistence on expressing as their generalized metapsychology his personal preference for the instinctual context of the libido metaphor to interpret the experience of others.

The use of labels ordinarily tends to be constricting, rather than productive, of deeper understanding. It's worth noting here that by post-Freudian I mean literally to include all who have worked in this field since the early Breuer-Freud transformation of hypnosis into psychoanalysis. This opens the radius of pluralism to a very wide number of psychoanalytic interpreters—among others, from the early defenders of the biological model, such as Abraham (1927), Ferenczi (1950), and Jones (1953-1957), to its early critics, such as Adler (1917), Jung (1927), and Rank (1945); from its later reconstructionists in the biological wing of the sociological model, such as Reich (1945), Anna Freud (1946), and Hartmann (1958), to those in the cultural wings of that model, such as Sullivan (1940), Thompson (1950), and Fairbairn (1954); to those, more recently, who are taking a fresh look at various dimensions of the experience of the self around which to envision a psychological model, such as Arieti (1967), Wolstein (1971), and Kohut (1971).

All the above, among numerous others, are post-Freudians. They were free to discover their own uniquely individual slants by which to interpret themselves and their patients during their psychoanalytic inquiries precisely because they were all aware—if, in some cases, only implicitly—of the enduring and ineluctable distinction that obtains between psychology and metapsychology. As a direct consequence of that distinction, they were able to extend their psychoanalytic inquiries—if, again, only implicitly—around a pluralism of perspectives on interpretive metapsychology.

These, then, are the major innovative turnings in the development of psychoanalysis over the years being considered here: first, the change from hypnosis and the talking cure to early psychoanalytic inquiry; second, the change from open to closed perspectives on the interpretation of actual clinical experience; and, finally, the probable changes that arise in the structure of psychoanalysis from including the many uniquely individual perspectives on metapsychology held by practicing psychoanalysts, and, it should also be noted, by their diverse patients.

THE BIOLOGICAL AND SOCIAL MODELS OF PSYCHOANALYSIS

From its earliest beginnings in the 1890s, psychoanalysis has taken the field of experience created and shared by any two particular coparticipants to be the active context of therapeutic inquiry. A careful reading of the overall structure of psychoanalytic inquiry would soon reveal, moreover, that this shared field of cocreated experience, and not the various general metapsychologies set forth to interpret it, generates the empirical and systematic boundaries, as well as the special sources, limits, and possibilities, of clinical therapeutic inquiry. As a matter of direct clinical experience, this special character of psychoanalytic psychology was, most likely, clearer from the late 1890s to the middle 1920s than it is today. During those first three decades, most clinical psychoanalysts, in their personal work history, had already been engaged in the practice of various forms of hypnosis and cathartic therapy, some having done that long before they had even begun to experiment with the new psychoanalytic approach to therapeutic inquiry.

As a consequence, the roots of their approach to this new psychotherapy already were deeply implanted in a two-way field of experience. So the roots of early psychoanalysis in the hypnotic, hypnocathartic, and autohypnotic therapies remained very prominent—without revisioning, without reshaping—both in the aims and in the procedures of the descendent clinical context of the biological model of psychoanalysis. Hence, those special origins of psychoanalytic psychology were far more explicitly understood by the first generation of psychoanalysts during that early period of id therapy, from the late 1890s to the middle 1920s, than by the next generation of psychoanalysts during the later period of ego, object, and interpersonal therapy, from the middle 1920s to the early 1950s, that marked out the interpretive and speculative basis for the sociological model.

The second generation moved psychoanalysis forward on two levels: it changed the aims and procedures for many different versions of that second model in the terms of ego, object, and interpersonal relations; and proposed new interpretations of psyche, self, and persona to point up the average and expectable conditions of a homogeneous environment. In a number of innovative yet parallel terminologies—for example, character armor, ego defense mechanism, and interpersonal security operation—they moved the focus of clinical psychoanalytic inquiry over to the adaptive and internalizing aspects of the total personality. However, with this later development of the theory and practice of ego, object, and interpersonal therapy— designed essentially to correct for the social and cultural oversights and inadequacies of the original model of id therapy—the psychic connections generated and directly undergone by the two coparticipants in the psychoanalytic field of inquiry had, in major respects, disappeared into those armored, defensive, and security-operating presuppositions of the sociological model.

The dominant themes of the second model of psychoanalysis were, instead, mapped and pursued in a variety of environmental perspectives set forth in other-oriented terminologies—for example, Hartmann's ego psychology adapting the ego's mechanisms of defense to their environing conditions; Fairbairn's object relations as the internalized patterns of the social self; or Sullivan's interpersonal relations as the consensual validation of operational dynamisms for satisfaction and security.

From a historical point of view, the psychic connections both first-hand and distant, both first-personal and ego-object-interpersonal, of the particular psychoanalyst and patient who cocreate and share the therapeutic experience of psychoanalytic inquiry were never at issue to such major 19th-century hypnotists as Bernheim, Breuer, Charcot, and Janet, who were among Freud's most important precursors and mentors in his studies of hypnosis and the cathartic procedures. The existence of those psychic connections were, in fact, beyond question.

From our current vantage point, it is, moreover, quite clear that all those strong and innovative hypnotists were themselves very actively and deeply involved in the conduct of the trance experience with the particular patient undergoing it, and that, in the course of it, they had to work most closely with that individual's unconscious processes and patterns—and most intimately as well, if they were indeed going to work hypnotically with the patient at all—from the original, uniquely individual, unconscious resources of their own psyches. This inevitably made for a high psychic drama with wide-ranging practical effect in the direct connectedness of hypnotist and patient— as Charcot, for example, so amply demonstrated during his grand rounds in a seemingly scripted performance with his patients dovetailing their shared experience through hypnotic traction.

It may also be observed, in brief amplification of this historical point, that while Breuer and Anna O. were originating the psychotherapeutic context of the talking cure together, he could develop so clear and profound a grasp of the special psychic meaning of her autohypnotic processes and patterns precisely because they had become directly available to him in unmediated experience with her during that genuinely new therapeutic procedure. Breuer, as is well known, with great originality—yet, interestingly enough, without further striving in interpretive metapsychology—proceeded to subsume Anna O.'s autohypnotic experience under the unprecedented theory of the hypnoid state. Freud, in turn, first followed Breuer in the intensive study of those newly theorized hypnoid states, and, after renaming and reconstructing them as unconscious terms, later followed both Breuer and Bernheim in his continued effort to work with those states, by instructing the patient under ordinary waking conditions to report, without any feeling or thought or act of suppression, whatever comes to mind in sequence.

However, on the basis of that most ingenious plan of procedure unparalleled in the history of psychotherapeutic inquiry, Freud could only move the fundamentals of his lifelong approach into two distinct and irreducible—and, for him, ultimately inseparable—domains of psychoanalytic inquiry. He first proposed the general terms of transference and resistance under which to define the observable psychology of suggestibility and dependency, and sought to transform their unconscious roots into conscious awareness; and second, as the special self-ascribed mark of his therapeutic originality, he claimed to understand their metapsychology as the highly symbolized derivatives of what he named the instinct and libido theories, which they were not, instead of the instinct myth and the libido metaphor, which they were.

THE PSYCHIC CONNECTION IN HYPNOSIS

As background for the present point of view, recall a relatively neglected aspect of the Breuer–Freud (1895) *Studies on Hysteria*. For that landmark collaboration on the hypnocathartic and autohypnotic therapies, Breuer and Freud implicitly agreed on depicting the new talking context of psychotherapeutic inquiry as emergent and explorable within the shared field of experience that each particular coparticipant would, could co-create with the other in his or her own uniquely individual way.

However, in making this gradual but thoroughgoing change from the hypnoid model in use through the 1880s to the middle 1890s, to the biological model in use from the late 1890s to the middle 1920s, Freud articulated still another yet closely related aspect of his ongoing therapeutic inquiry, which, as already mentioned, gave rise to an unanticipated gap or split between this psychoanalyst and his patient: the authoritarian overload of the foreground of the psychoanalytic inquiry with the burden of his absolutism in interpretive metapsychology. And a very special perspective on metapsychology it was: tightly bound to the intellectual ideals of 19th-century philosophy and natural science; neither yielding nor modifiable in the one-dimensional movement of its biological myth and metaphor; yet supreme in uniform application, without welcome to other alternatives of interpretive metapsychology.

I am referring here, in rough sketch, to the instinctual reduction of the striving, affective, and cognitive processes and patterns—that is, the psychic connectives of psychoanalyst and patient in the therapeutic inquiry—to their, so to speak, subpsychic origins that are conjectured, first, to extend beyond behavior and experience, and then speculated to derive from biological instincts and libido.

This special authoritarian aspect of the biological model arose quite unawares, I think, in the ongoing psychoanalytic inquiry. The gap or split it introduced between the two coparticipants was an arbitrary personal limit that Freud built into this model of the therapeutic experience. Most relevant to the present discussion, however, was his speculative decision to reduce such processes and patterns as could be explored under the conditions of direct therapeutic relatedness. In that way, they became the putative instinctual derivatives of the id, in further support of the stipulated subpsychic perspective of the biological model.

It is as though, under its own conditions, the psyche lacked the substance and structure and function to supply the boundaries of a self-sufficient field of scientific knowledge; as though, in its own terms, the analysis of the psyche were not capable of generating the elements of a coordinated empirical and systematic inquiry within those boundaries; and as though, on its own grounds, the manifold experience of the ongoing coparticipant connectedness that makes the actual therapeutic inquiry coherent were a psychic wasteland, in itself beyond visioning, reconstruction, and healing.

THE DISPLACEMENT OF PSYCHIC CONNECTEDNESS

Largely influenced by the strong evolutionary approaches to 19th-century biology, the first generation of psychoanalysts found the myths and metaphors of interpretive biological metapsychology they chose to impart to their patients. By so doing, however, they actually created a sense of intellectualized distance from their patients during the shared therapeutic experience. That generation of psychoanalysts, in my view, went too far in that interpretive direction. In other words, they undervalued the empirics and systematics of psychoanalytic inquiry in favor of the interpretable contents, or, in more recent terminology, sought the finished product of therapy at the expense of the exploratory process of inquiry.

But that clinical pragmatism proved short-sighted, for it covered up how the formal aspects of the process were unavoidably embedded in the therapeutic meanings of the content produced. The distinction between psychology and metapsychology played a crucial role in maintaining in this model a distance between psychoanalysts and patients, and between patients and their therapeutic problems. The first generation of psychoanalysts accomplished this distance in the following way. They first separated the process from the product in terms of psychology and metapsychology, and then treated the unique experience of psychic connectedness directly generated by the individual psychoanalyst and patient as representative of some antecedently elaborated biological myth and metaphor, and, by that means, actually let go of the diverse characteristics of every shared experience of psychic reality. They preferred, strangely enough, to work with a highly interpreted, intellectualized, and, in that measure, even distortive facsimile of the original.

This strong appeal to interpretive metapsychology was intrinsically distancing from the direct interpersonal experience. Those early psychoanalysts, after invoking the principle of determinism in further support of the reduction of integrally psychic experience to its speculated instinctual-libidinal underpinnings, also succeeded, in effect, to transform the experiential field of therapy they shared with patients into a metatheoretical field of epiphenomena—one that the particular psychoanalyst and patient could, as a matter of the psychoanalyst's choice of metapsychology, once again recover through the interpretive medium of that myth and metaphor. In this model of therapeutic inquiry, the point of invoking metapsychology was literally the re-covering of disturbed psychology, the reason for which becomes clearer in the retrospect of history. When the biological model was in its prime, the anxiety underlying disturbed psychology (counteranxiety, then still beyond conceiving) was not yet systematically treated as being armored, defended, or security-operated, nor yet empirically defined in direct clinical inquiry for observation by experience.

Instinctual-libidinal interpretation, first reinforced by the principle of psychic determinism and then linked to a historiogenetic bias in the ostensibly free-associative inquiry, led to a peculiar imbalance in the development of the overall structure of psychoanalytic inquiry. The actual field of the unique and shareable experience of therapy no longer appeared capable of holding the center of inquiry on the psychic connections of psychoanalyst and patient, but centered it on the metapsychics of those connections instead.

Implicit in this therapeutic approach, the unfolding experiential field of therapy was not considered capable of providing the psychic resources for psychoanalysis that could stand on their own grounds: that is, a psychological therapy that could be self-corrective within its own processes and patterns, or self-supporting under its own conditions, or self-consistent for its own facts and hypotheses, or, in summary, intelligible in its own terms. In the biological model, the experience of therapy provided but another situation, occasion, or opportunity for unloading a particular burden of interpretive metapsychology.

As a result, the therapeutic inquiry of psychoanalysis, emerging in antithetical correction to the hypnocathartic and autohypnotic therapies, did not attain its full sense and adequacy, nor, finally, its full psychic outcome in the direct study of the psychic connectedness of psychoanalyst and patient, that is, through the empirical relativity of transference, resistance, anxiety, and countertransference, counter-resistance, and counteranxiety moving back and forth in the unique psychic medium they cocreate. Nor, of course, did its substantive outcome remain a matter of direct psychic experience. Early psychoanalytic inquiry did not, for the purposes of a therapeutic experience, include among its psychic resources for the inquiry any notion of the original, spontaneous, generative sense of the first-personal self that emerges from its own ground, by its own movement of itself, in relation to the ego, object, or interpersonal relation with some particular or generalized other.

However, as a clinical side effect of the heavy interpretive bias of the biological model, psychoanalysis grew apart from hypnosis in an unexpected way. The strong psychic connection that holds between the hypnotist and the patient gradually disappeared from the affective foreground and into the preconscious shadows of clinical psychoanalytic interest. In other words, the biological model, being primarily interpretive, could do without a firm empirical and systematic analysis of those processes and patterns of the human psyche. The method of interpretation, because of its abstract and highly symbolized nature, bypassed the experience of psychic connectedness made directly available to a particular psychoanalyst and patient during their clinical inquiry. Attention to this psychoanalytic experience was not paid, I think, because it is directly given and ultimately unmediated. This is the connective experience often termed, in ordinary language, as a particular psychoanalyst and patient clicking, resonating, hitting it off, getting it, or, more formally, as establishing a good working relationship with one another.

Psychoanalysis as a structure of clinical inquiry – to interpret it in its own dynamic transformational terms – repressed its early roots in the hypnotic, hypnocathartic, and autohypnotic therapies, and, by the application of a highly speculative biological perspective on metapsychology, turned its therapeutic approach into yet another abstract intellectualized defense against the emergence of the concrete experiential psychology of the two unique coparticipants that involved them with one another. It became a complex and convoluted reductionism whose major outlines extend far beyond the psychic experience directly had in the first person – psychic experience that is both original and relational, both active and passive – and branch out into a more distant transcendental metapsychology about the vicissitudes of the instinctual libido. It developed, in short, as a magnificent displacement.

PSYCHICS AND METAPSYCHICS

In response to this state of affairs in the history of psychoanalysis, the full character and significance of the distinction between psychology and metapsychology may now once again be considered in the coordination of psychoanalytic knowledge, this time, however, from a pluralistic point of view.

The many differences between these two distinct sides of psychoanalytic knowledge may be traced back to the earliest origins of the Western scientific traditions. Most importantly, to the ancient Greek philosophers who first clearly saw the point of marking out the differences between a particular science and its metascience. That distinction is, at present, very familiar in its widely established usage for setting off the empirical and systematic terms of physics on one hand, from the interpretive and speculative notions of metaphysics on the other.

To speak of psychics and metapsychics as a parallel rendering of the distinction in contemporary psychoanalysis, psychiatry, and psychology may not seem congenial to the ways psychoanalysts ordinarily think about these matters. Yet, however they choose to articulate the differences between psychology and metapsychology, the distinction is, nonetheless, applicable and fruitful in all psychotherapeutic inquiries. It is the difference between what they observe, define, and infer about unconscious psychic experience, and why they proceed to project speculative interpretations of that acquired empirical knowledge.

The substance of this distinction has come down, of course, as a strong philosophical inheritance. In spite of its studied neglect in early psychoanalytic inquiry, it remains, without question, unexpendable in the study of the human psyche in depth. When clinical psychoanalysts, psychiatrists, or psychologists formulate a philosophy, a system of beliefs and values, a metaphysics, or a model of human nature, they are, in my view, referring, perhaps without acknowledgment, yet unerringly to the metapsychology of therapeutic inquiry, and not to its psychology.

The difference between the two may be summed up as: psychoanalytic psychology is both empirical and systematic, being based on the specific clinical orders of observations, definition, transformation, and explanation; psychoanalytic metapsychology is both interpretive and speculative, being based on a number of general and highly conjectural perspectives built around a variety of myths and metaphors. Psychology, it is clear, is no more a metapsychology than a body of scientific knowledge is a critical philosophy of life.

The point, then, is not that metapsychology has no place or significance in psychoanalysis. It does, and obviously so. It is an inevitable part of the field of experience and inquiry that any particular psychoanalyst cocreates and shares with any particular patient—essentially because each uniquely individual coparticipant owns the rudiments of a system of beliefs, values, and ideals considered, in some sense, ultimate, yet derived, in the main, from adaptation to the society and from individuation within the culture into which a person is born and lives out a given psychic endowment.

The point is, rather, that early psychoanalytic inquiry represents a special case of the relation between psychology and metapsychology in the history of psychotherapy. It represents that special case in which all the effective terms and conditions of its empirical and systematic inquiry were made to fit into the absolutism of instinctual-libidinal or drive metapsychology, while the empirical and systematic features, it turns out, were all treated within the unacknowledged narrowing of that interpretive focus—and, indeed, the unnoticed constriction of the actual clinical range of the overall structure of psychoanalysis.

Early psychoanalytic inquiry was fatefully aligned with the perspective of a single interpretive metapsychology. It was a reductionist perspective at that, based largely on a varied series of instinctual dualisms. It excluded, and continues to exclude, a large number of such other perspectives as, for example, struggle for power, archetypes of the collective unconscious, absolute will, adjustment and adaptation, satisfactions and securities, as well as the wide varieties of existentialism and mysticism, Eastern and Western, and the various naturalist, pragmatist, and humanist—in addition to the dialectical, countercultural, and even theological—metapsychologies of the present. About these exclusions from the traditional biological model the major points of controversy continue to reverberate.[1]

In view of this ever-increasing abundance of philosophical and highly speculative efforts in psychoanalytic metapsychology, it becomes appropriate for the heirs of this profusion of voices to undertake a thorough review, revision, and revaluation of the basic constituents of the structure of psychoanalytic inquiry. In the current historical situation, the recipients of this babel-like inheritance are required to understand how it is possible that so many serious and equally responsible psychoanalysts, compelled by the uniquely indi-

---

[1]A current question, for example, whether psychoanalysis is a one-person or a two-person psychology puts the focus of discussion back into the framework of that singular interpretive metapsychology of the biological model. The question has a certain merit in its own historical terms, but what psychoanalysts now face is a different sort of question, which is whether the experiential field of psychoanalytic therapy is a one-metapsychology or a two-metapsychology field of therapy—the psychoanalyst's, the patient's, or both. In other words, whether clinical psychoanalysis can hold more than one metapsychology within its overall structure of inquiry without prejudice to its therapeutic goals. On the workings of contemporary pluralistic psychoanalysis, see Addendum to this chapter.

vidual views, visions, and values of so many personally fulfilling metapsychologies, actually manage to work with a coherent structure of inquiry running through their psychoanalytic therapies, and still make room for the diverse metapsychologies of their patients as well.

It becomes necessary, in addition, to reconsider with a fresh eye still another aspect of all psychoanalytic inquiry, perhaps of all psychotherapeutic inquiry: namely, whether it is the direction of the special perspective on metapsychology, or the freedom of the special exploration of the psychic connectedness of the two coparticipants involved with one another in the experiential field of therapy, or whether it is some other now untouched, still unknown, even unimagined factor that spells out the difference between success and failure in the many varieties of psychological therapy, as well as in the three dominant models of psychoanalytic therapy: the biological, the social, and the psychological.

UNCONSCIOUS PSYCHIC EXPERIENCE AND
PSYCHOANALYTIC INQUIRY

When disentangled from total dependence on any single perspective on interpretive metapsychology, psychoanalysis moves into empirical and systematic focus as a psychology of unconscious psychic experience considered the theory and practice of a special mode of therapeutic inquiry. To point up its distinctiveness requires a reconsideration of the body of clinical psychoanalytic knowledge from the standpoint of its structure of inquiry, so as to coordinate that structure around the central theory of unconscious psychic experience, and base the inquiry on such empirical conditions and systematic terms that govern the transformation of unconscious into conscious psychic experience.

Psychoanalysis is, moreover, the one variety of therapeutic inquiry with the self-assigned task of exploring the psychic connections of a particular psychoanalyst and his patient, as far as any two coparticipants, individually, can take it. They may define their connections as observed in transference, resistance, and anxiety, and in countertransference, counterresistance, and counteranxiety; then transform the originally defined observations by the postulates of genesis and function, structure and dynamism, immediacy and reflection, as warranted; and then, of course, explain those defined observations, now transformed, in accordance with the theory of unconscious psychic experience.

Psychoanalysis, its structure so demarcated, is not a philosophy of human life and experience—biological and social—nor primarily a metapsychology whether of Freud's instinctual libido, or Adler's struggle for power, or Jung's collective unconscious, or Rank's absolute will, or anyone else's particular preference in myth and metaphor that neither originates nor derives from the empirical and systematic results of clinical psychoanalytic inquiry. Perspectives on the interpretation of those results belong, instead, at the order of plural metapsychologies, as matters of personal preference. All clinical psychoanalytic psychology may be organized around them. Yet such clinical knowledge is self-corrective—it concerns matters of fact—while plural metapsychologies are not: they concern matters of belief. This knowledge has foundations in a structure of psychoanalytic inquiry capable of persisting without absolute dependence on any single preferred perspective on interpretive metapsychology.

Following this distinction between fact and belief, psychoanalysis is that special branch of the study of the human psyche developed especially to explore the relations of conscious and unconscious psychic experience arising directly within the experiential field of therapy that is cocreated and shared through the unique and shareable, yet self-supporting, psychic connectedness of a particular psychoanalyst and patient. The therapeutic experience of psychoanalytic inquiry does not, finally, come down to a philosophy of human nature, nor, therefore, does it stand or fall with the changing visions and revisions of the meaning of human life and human psyche, in which the structure of that therapeutic inquiry may be placed for interpretive finish and speculative embellishment.

ADDENDUM

What psychoanalysts explore differs from why they interpret it. Empirically, they observe, define, and make inferences about the conscious-unconscious dimensions of transference and countertransference, resistance and counterresistance, anxiety and counteranxiety, and the self: which makes their therapeutic inquiry psychoanalysis. Interpretively, they appeal to diverse myths and metaphors of contemporary pluralism about the conjectured and reconstructable meanings of those observations and inferences: which makes for their varieties of perspective in psychoanalysis.

Observations of the empirical facts of transference and countertransference, and so on, and their systematic transformation in accordance with the unconscious psychic experience psychoanalysts share with patients in the field of therapeutic inquiry, are the core of clinical psychoanalytic psychology. Interpretations of those defined and transformed observations in that shared field of inquiry and experience, in accordance with a particular perspective such as ego, object, or interpersonal relations, are the core of clinical psychoanalytic metapsychology. While psychology and metapsychology coalesce in the particular personalities of a unique psychoanalyst working with a unique patient, they remain, nonetheless, conceptually distinct orders of a coordinated structure of psychoanalytic inquiry.

This distinction is central to the ordering of psychoanalytic knowledge from a pluralistic point of view. It provides for the large variety of disparate orientations among psychoanalysts as well as for their common field of therapeutic inquiry. The two best publicized models, the biological and the social, took shape through the addition of new proposals and conjectures at the order of metapsychology. Yet the instincts, drives, or needs of the first model, and the ego, object, or interpersonal relations of the second, are not now, nor have they ever been, mutually exclusive concerns. The biological was always viewed as reaching into the social domain; the social was always viewed as retaining a biological point of reference. There is, I think, clinical psychoanalytic space for still a third model built around the psychology of the self, from which both the drives and the relations, among all the other things in the psychic domain, derive their meanings and functions in individual psychic experience. First, of course, came the instinctual–libidinal model, which moved into the relational area guided by the metapsychology of adaptation and consensus in the ego, object, or interpersonal model, which moved into the selfic area guided by the metapsychology of individuation and uniqueness, hence the psychic model.

The drawing of this line in psychoanalytic knowledge between psychology and metapsychology, or more generally, between fact and value, is not recent. It was done rather early in the history of psychoanalysis, nearly 100 years ago, in clear language, in the Preface to the first edition of the landmark *Studies on Hysteria*. The line is ineradicable. Breuer and Freud explicitly noted their full agreement on the observational data, alongside their failure to agree on the interpretive and conjectural approach to those data. "If at some points divergent and indeed contradictory opinions are expressed, this is not to be regarded as evidence for any fluctuation in our views," they wrote in 1895. "It arises from the natural and justifiable differences between the opinions of two observers who are agreed upon the facts and their basic reading of them, but who are not invariably at one in their interpretations and conjectures" (pages xxix–xxx).

This stated position of the first generation of psychoanalysts greatly surprises. Lost though it later was in the polemical shuffle, it may now be considered a major early source of contemporary pluralistic psychoanalysis. It shows, among other things, that Breuer and Freud unambiguously saw the central point of pluralism in psychoanalysis. From our current point of vantage, it supports the growing shift in therapeutic procedure away from the onesided emphasis on interpretation—since, a fact they did not mention, pluralism applies to patients as well—and it directs attention over to exploratory inquiry (where agreement is possible) and away from interpretation singly or jointly arrived at (where agreement is not necessary).

Moving to the immediate present, the New York University Postdoctoral Program exemplifies the contemporary emergence of pluralistic psychoanalysis. Its four tracks or orientations are each strong in their own right, yet cohesive in the postdoctoral community at large. They all depend on the value and validity of distinguishing psychology from metapsychology, or observation from interpretation, or fact from belief. One thing, moreover, it makes very clear: that while psychoanalysts may differ among themselves—and, worth noting here, with their patients as well—in matters of interpretive metapsychology, their clinical psychoanalytic inquiries converge in matters of empirical and systematic psychology. That is why they are capable of organizing a psychoanalytic four-track program in common, in spite of the deep personal and axiological differences among them.

Thus, for example, they now deal with the clinical manifestations of transference and countertransference, and so on, in the perspective of metapsychologies other than those in which the major empirical areas of psychoanalytic inquiry were first discovered and defined. It is possible, they find, to accept the myths and metaphors of a preferred orientation—(1) Freudian ego, (2) object–relational, (3) interpersonal-humanistic, or (4) independent—without, on that account, prejudging the therapeutic inquiry of any particular psychoanalyst and patient. Unless, of course, that prejudgment were part of the orientation; in which case it would defeat the psychoanalytic pluralism around which the NYU Program is now organized.

No necessary connection has been demonstrated to exist between metapsychology and psychology, or between orientation and practice. That is an ineluctable fact of psychoanalytic life. Nothing in psychoanalytic knowledge restricts the practice of psychoanalysis to any single orienting perspective and to the exclusion of all others. That is why the training program may offer an overall catalogue of training with four orientations, and remain open to the probable addition of still others in the foreseeable future. On the other hand, however, the NYU Program actually holds a number of logical and practical convictions about the existence of a common field of empirical and systematic psychoanalytic inquiry.

Absent any established connection between psychology and metapsychology in psychoanalytic knowledge, a perspective on metapsychology may be formulated apart from any involvement with clinical psychoanalytic inquiry. One may, for example, believe the classical Freudian, Adlerian, Jungian, or Rankian orientation without ever practicing psychoanalytic therapy, or practice psychoanalytic therapy without, of course, being a classical Freudian, Adlerian, Jungian, or Rankian metapsychologist.

The distinction between psychology and metapsychology applies to all the psychoanalytic orientations at this or any other psychoanalytic institute. That is to say, proposing new models of interpretation or reformulating old ones neither diminishes nor augments the psychological focus of psychoanalytic inquiry from the standpoint of the theory of unconscious psychic experience. A new model may indicate some changes in the shape of some myth or other, or it may suggest some revised views of the surrounding context in which clinical psychoanalytic inquiry is done. Any claim to innovative modeling recommends itself to its developer on its own terms, as a matter of personal interpretive preference. Which does not, of course, signify new empirical and systematic discovery with the exploratory power of transference and countertransference, resistance and counterresistance, anxiety and counteranxiety, or the self, and with the *explanatory power of unconscious psychic experience*. And in the development of the four orientations at New York University, this is clear all around.

REFERENCES

Abraham, K. (1927), *Selected Papers on Psychoanalysis*. London: Hogarth Press.
Adler, A. (1917), *The Neurotic Constitution*. New York: Moffat, Yard.
Arieti, S. (1967), *The Intrapsychic Self*. New York: Basic Books.
Breuer, J. & Freud, S. (1895), Studies on Hysteria. *Standard Edition*, 2. London: Hogarth Press, 1955.
Fairbairn, W. R. D. (1954), *The Object-Relations Theory of Personality*. New York: Basic Books.
Ferenczi, S. (1950), *Sex in Psychoanalysis*. New York: Basic Books.
Freud, A. (1946), *The Ego and the Mechanisms of Defense*. New York: International Universities Press.
Freud, S. (1916–1917), Introductory lectures in psycho-analysis. *Standard Edition*, 15 & 16. London: Hogarth Press, 1963.
Hartmann, H. (1958), *The Ego and the Problem of Adaptation*. New York: International Universities Press.

Jones, E. (1953–1957), *The Life and Work of Sigmund Freud*, Vols. 1, 2, & 3. New York: Basic Books.

Jung, C. (1927), *Psychology of the Unconscious*. New York: Moffat, Yard.

Kohut, H. (1971), *The Analysis of the Self*. New York: International Universities Press.

Rank, O. (1945), *Will Therapy, and Truth and Reality*. New York: Knopf.

Reich, W. (1945), *Character Analysis*. New York: Orgone Press.

Sullivan, H. (1940), *Conceptions of Modern Psychiatry*. Washington, DC: W. A. White Psychiatric Foundation.

Thompson, C. (1950), *Psychoanalysis*. New York: Hermitage.

Wolstein, B. (1967), *Theory of Psychoanalytic Therapy*. New York: Grune & Stratton.

_____ (1971), *Human Psyche in Psychoanalysis*. Springfield, IL: Thomas.

Index

333